HEALTHY LIVING IN
LATE RENAISSANCE ITALY

Healthy Living in Late Renaissance Italy

SANDRA CAVALLO
and
TESSA STOREY

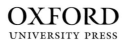
OXFORD

UNIVERSITY PRESS

OXFORD
UNIVERSITY PRESS

Great Clarendon Street, Oxford, OX2 6DP,
United Kingdom

Oxford University Press is a department of the University of Oxford.
It furthers the University's objective of excellence in research, scholarship,
and education by publishing worldwide. Oxford is a registered trade mark of
Oxford University Press in the UK and in certain other countries

© Sandra Cavallo and Tessa Storey 2013

The moral rights of the authors have been asserted

First Edition published in 2013

Impression: 1

Published in the United States of America by Oxford University Press
198 Madison Avenue, New York, NY 10016, United States of America

British Library Cataloguing in Publication Data
Data available
Library of Congress Control Number: 2013942159

ISBN 978–0–19–967813–6

As printed and bound by
CPI Group (UK) Ltd, Croydon, CR0 4YY

Acknowledgements

First of all we would like to thank the Wellcome Trust whose generous funding in the form of a History of Medicine Project Grant (087266/Z/08/Z January 2009–September 2012) meant that we have been able to research and write this book. We are also grateful to the Isobel Thornley Fund for a grant that has helped with the expenses related to the publication of the images in this book and to the Archive of the Vicariato in Rome for permission to photograph documents.

In the course of such a long project many people have contributed in various ways and firstly we would like to acknowledge our debt to Marta Ajmar who has acted as our adviser on various aspects of the project. She not only shared her ideas and expertise on material culture, but identified several of the objects we discuss in the book. Furthermore, she has written some of the text relating to objects in the chapter on 'Air' as well as several of the extended captions for the illustrations. We acknowledge these latter contributions with her initials on the captions.

We are particularly grateful to those who read early drafts of chapters and gave us their valuable comments: Carol Rawcliffe and Marlyn Nicoud read Chapter 1; Silvia de Renzi Chapter 3; and Francois Quiviger Chapter 6—as did Maria Pia Donato who also gave us extensive advice on the passions. We have also benefited from the expertise of Hugo Blake on objects of everyday use and archeological findings; Elaine Leong, Silvia de Renzi, Christelle Rabier, and Giulia Calvi for helpful references, discussions, and suggestions; and Hugo Crespo, for providing information about the Fonseca family.

Others have helped us in other very important ways. Viviana Tagliaferri has offered valuable assistance in tracking down images and getting permissions, at times a very trying business indeed. Alessandra Chessa has done so too, as well as giving us useful insights into some of the objects and images. Roberto Benedetti was meticulous in his efforts to help us ferret out, photograph, and organize many of our documents. We would also like to thank Maria Conforti for her help at the Biblioteca di Medicina in Rome. Finally, a huge thank you to Suzy Knight who has sat up many a late night conscientiously copy-editing our chapters with great care and patience.

We have also greatly appreciated the opportunity to give our ideas a first airing at numerous conferences and seminars and we thank the participants for their comments and questions: SCSC Geneva (2009); RSA Venice (2010); 'From Space to Place: the Spatial Turn in History', German Historical Institute, London (2010); Anglo-American Conference of Historians: Environment in History, London (2010); Sheffield University History seminar series (2010); 'Indoors: Spaces, Families and Communities (16th–18th Centuries)', Instituto de Ciencias Sociais, Lisbon (2011); Southampton University History seminar series (2011), IHR Late Medieval and Renaissance Italy Seminar (2011); Anglo-American Conference of Historians: Health in History, London (2011); 'Sport in Early Modern Culture',

German Historical Institute, London (2011); 'Clothing and the Culture of Appearance in Early Modern Europe', Fundacion Camberes, Madrid (2012); 'History of Medicine in the Household', University of Warwick (2012); SSHM conference 'Emotions, Health and Wellbeing', Queen Mary, University of London (2012); and 'Objects as Historical Evidence', European University Institute Seminar, Florence (2012).

    Finally, Tessa would like to thank her family, but particularly James, Emily, and Edward for their endless support and patience throughout and Sandra thanks Clare Coope and Laurence Lumley for their insightful comments about the images used in this study.

S.C. and T.S.

Contents

List of Plates

List of Figures

List of Abbreviations

ASG	Archivio di Stato di Genova
ASR	Archivio di Stato di Roma
ASVR	Archivio del Vicariato di Roma
FSV	Fondo Spada Veralli
MCI	Monastero delle Convertite, Inventari
Misc.Fam.	Miscellanea Famiglie
Notai AC	Notai Archivio Capitolino
Notai UG	Notai dell'Ufficio del Governatore
TCG	Notai del Tribunale criminale del Governatore
TNC	Trenta Notai Capitolini
Uff.	Ufficio

Introduction

In 2011 a report was published announcing the findings of a UK government-sponsored research project which included an assessment of the health benefits to be derived from the natural environment. Amongst other things, they estimated that the value of 'living with a view of green spaces' was £300 per annum per individual. Moreover, they concluded that 'green exercise', i.e. exercise which took place outside in a natural environment, especially in the presence of open water, 'produces a significantly larger degree of improvements in mental well-being particularly amongst those with mental health problems'.[1]

The fact that such a study was undertaken at all is symptomatic of the increasing awareness in Western European societies that in order to preserve our health and prolong our lives, rather than simply depending on the timely intervention of powerful drugs and surgery, we must focus on prevention in our daily lives; by taking regular exercise, living in a clean or 'pollutant'-free environment, and eating a 'good' diet.

Yet we would be profoundly mistaken if we considered this concern with prevention and the desire for longevity to be a purely modern phenomenon. For example, although the idea that one can assign a monetary value to the impact of nature on one's health is novel, there is certainly nothing new in the observation that taking walks in green spaces and contemplating pleasant landscapes and water are beneficial to health. On the contrary, this knowledge lay at the core of the humoral tradition which underpinned medical thinking until as late as the eighteenth century, and its teaching on the management of both physical well-being and what we term 'emotions'. Although the physiological premises which formed the framework of this tradition were gradually dismantled and replaced by new understandings of the working of the body, many key notions are still with us, embedded in European languages, proverbs, and cautionary advice. In Italy one is often warned never to leave the house with damp hair or to drink milk after a meal; in England we still might speak of 'being in good spirits', or note that 'a breath of fresh air will do you good'. Although these expressions still convey meaning, they have been 'hollowed out' and their full import lost, along with the medical understandings which underlay them. Yet the fact that certain elements of preventive humoral medicine still litter our speech is surely a testament to how profoundly it penetrated European understandings of the body and health.

---

[1] The report runs to over 1,400 pages; Pretty et al., 'Health Values', 1154.

This book explores the efforts made by our predecessors to maintain their health in the course of their daily lives and in their home environment. Homes have been convincingly portrayed as the principal locus of health care in the early modern period and recent historians have documented the extent of the medical practices taking place there.[2] Considerable attention has been given to the sources of domestic medical knowledge: from the rising tide of medical books in the vernacular directed to a lay audience to the circulation of medical advice that took place through oral and written exchanges between neighbours, relatives, and friends.[3] Moreover, there has been an extraordinary surge of interest in printed and manuscript recipe collections, which allowed for the experimentation of domestically produced medicinal remedies.[4] The focus of these studies however has been the provision of medical treatment in the household; in other words they have mostly been concerned with the domestic care of the sick body. We still know very little about the precautions taken within the home to preserve the health of its members, and whether health considerations affected the ways in which people addressed routine activities such as sleeping, exercising, drinking, and attending to personal hygiene. Diet constitutes perhaps the exception to this trend, as scholars have long been aware of the medicinal significance that contemporaries attached to different foodstuffs.[5]

However, to judge from the advice contained in the dozens of vernacular guides to healthy living that were published in Italy during the Renaissance and the early modern period, health concerns prompted a much wider range of domestic activities than historians have so far recognized.[6] Besides cooking and producing medicines, the emphasis on prevention implicit in contemporary ideas about health had a profound influence both on the way in which the body was managed and on how the house was chosen, built, and furnished. Whilst historians of medicine have devoted considerable attention to the measures taken by civic institutions to improve public health and the quality of air and water, particularly in the urban environment and in times of plague, they have disregarded the fact that the quality of domestic surroundings, and the lifestyle adopted by private citizens in their homes were also matters of concern. Scholars of private life, on the other hand, have often underestimated health concerns and the extent to which these affected internal domestic arrangements.[7] As research on the materiality of domestic life is burgeoning, this is the ideal time to turn to households.

[2] For an overview, Fissell, 'Introduction'.
[3] Slack, 'Mirrors'; Fissell, 'Readers'; Fissell, 'The Marketplace'; Harkness, 'A View'; and Cabré, 'Women'.
[4] See the wide bibliographies in Leong and Rankin, 'Introduction' and in Storey, 'Face'.
[5] O'Hara May, 'Food'; and Albala, *Eating Right*.
[6] Studies on this genre have so far largely focused on Britain and America: Slack, 'Mirrors'; Horrocks, 'Rules'; Wear, *Knowledge*, ch. 4; Rawcliffe, 'The Concept'; Fissell, 'Popular Medical Writing'; and Richards, 'Useful Books'.
[7] See e.g. Chartier (ed.), *A History*; Roche, *A History*; and Thomas, *The Ends*.

A STATIC BODY OF KNOWLEDGE?

Medical thought and practice in the early modern period were still informed by the classical medical tradition that assigned equal importance to prevention and treatment. Avicenna's *Canon*—the most popular medical textbook in the Renaissance—held that medicine and what the ancients called 'hygiene', that is the art of taking care of one's health, were two complementary practices.[8] In Hippocratic treatises, as well as in Galen's works, medicine was not just conceptualized as a healing art but as the art of well-being and of conserving health. While Hippocratic medicine emphasized the importance of the balance between nourishment and exercise, Galen significantly expanded the number of factors to be attended to in order to stay in good health. In his view, moreover, the physician's task was not confined to treating disease, but he played a key role in popularizing 'dietetic' methods (where 'diet' stands for a healthy lifestyle)—that is, in educating patients in the precautions necessary to pursue a long and healthy life.[9] These ideas were then systemized in the Middle Ages. The dietetic doctrine that first became available to Europeans in translations from the Arabic in the eleventh and twelfth centuries was structured around the 'Six Non-Natural things' on which health was seen to depend (air, sleep, movement and rest, food and drink, repletion and evacuation, and emotional life). It was further consolidated in the regimens of health compiled in Europe in the thirteenth and fourteenth centuries by figures such as Petrus Hispanus, Taddeo Alderotti, Aldobrandino da Siena, Arnau de Villanova, and Maino de Maineri.[10] Some authors, such as Aldobrandino da Siena, went so far as to suggest that the art of healthy living was the main constituent of the science of physics.[11] At the onset of the Renaissance prevention was therefore seen as a branch of medicine, and the idea was further theorized by sixteenth-century academic thought.[12]

Though the preventive paradigm appears to have been firmly established in medical theory at the beginning of the early modern era this has had little impact on the medical histories of the period: the study of healthy living has been addressed almost exclusively from the perspective of the history of medical ideas. Social historians of medicine have concentrated on the demand and offer of cures and medicinal remedies rather than on the measures actively designed to preserve health. The emphasis on the medical marketplace that has informed these studies in the last decades might perhaps be held responsible for distracting attention away from preventive practices and for directing it onto cures.[13] This appears to be particularly true in relation to the highly commercialized and consumer-oriented economy of Renaissance Italy.[14] Recent commentators have, in fact, extended the rise of medical

---

[8] Gil-Sotres, 'The Regimens of Health', 298; Palmer, 'Health', 75–6.

[9] On Galen: Bergdoldt, *Wellbeing*; Mikkeli, *Hygiene*; and Galen, *De sanitate tuenda*, ch. 1.

[10] On this process Gil-Sotres, 'The Regimens of Health' and especially Nicoud, *Les Régimes*.

[11] Nicoud, *Les Régimes*, 117.

[12] Mikkeli, *Hygiene*, 45–56.

[13] On the historiography on the medical marketplace and its limitations see Jenner and Wallis, 'Introduction'.

[14] On the Italian consumer economy in the Renaissance see Goldthwaite, *Wealth*; Jardine, *Worldly Goods*.

consumerism—initially associated with the eighteenth century—back to the Renaissance. It is argued that the Italian medical economy boomed as early as the sixteenth century, accelerating the demise of traditional regimens, which stressed the importance of a healthy lifestyle for maintaining and restoring one's health. In the Italian peninsula this paradigm supposedly gave way to a new attitude to health, whereby cures available on the market and the possibility of eliminating disease through treatment became more important than the need to regulate one's lifestyle and maintain the body well 'tempered'.[15] Various factors contributed to this shift: the arrival of hitherto unknown exotic substances from the East and, later, from the New World that were commercialized on the market as repositories of wondrous medicinal properties; the influence of Paracelsus' theories that defined disease as an entity rather than the result of a humoral imbalance; and the proliferation and appeal of charlatans and empirics who sold ready-made remedies designed to treat an impersonal disease rather than the individual body and who often used the rhetoric of secrecy to promote their nostrums.[16] Taken together, these elements are seen to lead to a new confidence in the possibility of targeting specific illnesses, which replaced and invalidated the idea that health depended on diet, hygiene, and the maintenance of a good humoral balance. For why give so much value to a healthy lifestyle if disease could be treated? It would seem that we are already in a modern ontological framework, in which the sick body rather than the healthy (or imperfectly healthy) body is the main object of medicine.

Very little attention has been given therefore to the role that concerns about health maintenance occupied in everyday life: whether doctors were consulted on issues of prevention, whether laypeople were familiar with medical principles of healthy living, and whether these were adhered to or disregarded. Harold Cook has cogently documented the important role that doctors were expected to play as health counsellors in this period and how central their pastoral tasks were to their professional image, but his suggestions have not been followed up.[17] Early modern medical historians have only recently begun to explore the relationships between individual patients and their medical advisers over the management of lifestyle, and mainly with reference to the court environment.[18] With very few exceptions the scholarship on prevention has been confined to intellectual studies of the philosophical and medical ideas regarding the preservation of health. The broad chronological scope and the pan-European perspective adopted by these overviews inevitably present a rather uniform picture of attitudes to prevention, which fails to differentiate between texts published in different countries and belonging to different cultural contexts, and between learned medical treatises and tracts for a larger readership.[19]

---

[15] This view is summarized in Eamon, 'Markets' and 'The Scientific Renaissance', 412–14. See also Eamon, *Science*, 412 and 414; and Siraisi, *The Clock*, 73.

[16] On the expansion of pharmacists and on the influence of Paracelsus in Italy see Palmer, 'Pharmacy'. On charlatans see Gentilcore, *Medical Charlatanism*.

[17] Cook, 'Good Advice'.

[18] Palmer, 'Medicine'; and Andretta, 'Les Régimes'.

[19] Cook, 'Physical Methods'; Wear, 'The History'; Mikkeli, *Hygiene*; and Bergtold, *Wellbeing*. See also n. 25.

In this book we intend to shift attention away from academic writing on prevention and verify the penetration of healthy living precepts into actual life. We will do this by mobilizing a range of textual visual and material evidence. Our core source is represented by an important but neglected textual genre: the guides to healthy living in the vernacular (regimens of health), largely authored by doctors, which were published in great numbers in Italy between 1500 and the last third of the seventeenth century, often in cheap, portable format. They provide detailed recommendations on how health could be promoted in everyday life. The close and diachronic analysis of these texts will enable us to clarify what doctors presented to patients as healthy lifestyles and whether their views changed over time.

Health regimens have been studied extensively as far as the medieval period is concerned, largely thanks to Marilyn Nicoud's comprehensive reconstruction of their development as a separate literary genre, independent from academic medical treatises, between the thirteenth and the late fifteenth centuries.[20] However, no systematic study of this source has been carried out for the later period. Long assumed to be a static genre, just repeating advice found in classical sources, the early modern regimen has attracted very little interest, even more so if one compares it with the attention sparked by another contemporary health-related genre: the printed recipe book. Andrew Wear's judgement that, despite some changes in emphasis, the advice found in regimens remained largely unaltered throughout the centuries, providing an example of *histoire immobile*, seems to be widely shared.[21] The only significant change signalled is the shift towards 'cold regimes', which encouraged a more Spartan approach to ventilation, clothing, bathing, eating, and drinking; a fashion which started to take hold in England at the end of the seventeenth century—that is, outside the time frame and geographical scope of our study.[22] But as far as the sixteenth and seventeenth centuries are concerned, the genre is deemed to be uneventful and therefore unworthy of detailed analysis. Even the in-depth studies of medieval regimens, on the other hand, have paid little attention to their contents: the focus in Nicoud's monumental work on medieval preventive literature has been on the development of the genre rather than the advice this contains.

But are the recommendations found in these books really so static and repetitive? Only a diachronic analysis of their contents can ascertain this. Hence we will compare the precautions recommended in regimens over a period of nearly two centuries to identify changes and continuity in the advice. We will structure our discussion around the six areas of well-being these books tend to consider, the Non-Naturals—that is, the air one breathes, sleep, food and drink, evacuations, movement, and emotions—and their management.

The individual Non-Naturals have also suffered from comparative neglect as historians have focused on the development of the concept in medical thought

[20] Nicoud, *Les Régimes*. See also Gil-Sotres, 'The Regimens of Health'; Rawcliffe, 'The Concept'; Hardingham, 'The *Regimen*'; and Bonfield, 'The *Regimen sanitatis*'.
[21] Wear, *Knowledge*, 155 and 'The History', 1288.
[22] Wear, 'The History', 1295; and Smith, *Clean*, 217–23.

rather than on which practices were regarded as healthy and unhealthy in these various spheres of life.[23] The only exception in recent years has been the boom in research on recommendations concerning food and diet while the other Non-Naturals have been the object of a few general surveys.[24] Yet a focus on each of these activities and how they should ideally be performed in order to maintain the body's good health can provide much insight not only into changing ideas about preventive measures but into how these aspects of everyday life were seen to impact on the working of the body. In other words, by paying attention to the explanations given in regimens as to why disregarding certain healthy living rules could generate pathogenic processes, we hope to widen our understanding of how early modern humoral physiology was conceptualized.

Our awareness of how the early modern body was supposed to work is indeed rather limited. For radically new insights into early modern perceptions of the body see Stolberg, *Experiencing Illness*, part II. Many of its suggestions are confirmed by our findings. We regret that as the work came out in English when this book was already advanced, its contents could not be considered in this study. References to humoralism abound in historical works, so that it has assumed an explanatory value far beyond the boundaries of the history of medicine. However, these accounts are normally rather sketchy and just reiterate the basic ideas regarding the four humours, their characteristics, and the need to balance them. Barbara Duden's work has been very influential in proposing an idea of the humoral understanding of the body as made of fluids in continuous motion, and hence in promoting a view of the early modern body as unstable and unpredictable as a result of this constant flux.[25] This picture—which is based on evidence from eighteenth-century Germany—has been reproposed again and again without further investigations into the working of early modern humoral physiology. Little attention has been given, for example, to the fact that in the two previous centuries, the medical literature also refers extensively to 'vapours' and 'fumes' or 'fumosities', 'spirits', 'exhalations', and 'excretions'—and these tended to refer to the evacuation not so much of fluids but of solid particles and invisible, volatile matter. Moreover it is questionable that Duden's findings can automatically be generalized and applied without nuance to earlier periods.

These generalizations reflect the common assumption that humoral theory remained a largely adaptable and unchanging body of knowledge in spite of the challenges posed by anatomical discoveries and the appearance of mechanistic ideas of the body that encouraged a view of disease as an entity, curable through specific remedies rather than by restoring humoral balance. Indeed historians of medicine have generally stressed the plasticity of the system, and its ability to integrate new elements in its medical practice (especially the increased emphasis on medicines and chemical therapies) without substantially altering its theoretical framework, diagnostic principles, and narratives of disease.[26] But is this emphasis

[23] Intellectual histories on the Non-Naturals include Rather, 'The "Six Things Non-Natural"' and García Ballester, 'On the Origins'.

[24] For studies on food see Ch. 7. On sleep, hygiene, and exercise see Dannenfeldt, 'Sleep'; Smith, *Clean*; and Arcangeli, 'Del moto'.

[25] Duden, *The Woman*, esp. ch. 4.

[26] e.g., on the absorption of Paracelsian ideas in Italian medical practice, Clericuzio, 'Chemical Medicine'.

on the endurance and elasticity of humoral theory perhaps too static? Should we talk more accurately of progressively shifting views of the functioning of the body rather than of the persistence of an adapted but still basically unchanged paradigm? Our research on preventive ideas and measures may bring a different dimension to this debate on the long life of humoralism: what sort of picture do we get if we focus on how the healthy body was seen to work rather than on how the sick body was understood and treated? Do we find similar continuities if we address questions such as whether the importance attributed to individual spheres of health maintenance (or Non-Naturals) changes over time, and whether definitions of what is regarded as dangerous and beneficial to health modifies over the period. And is the idea of the body and its vulnerabilities which underpins these views subject to any transformations? Or do substantial changes emerge during the early modern period within this corpus of physiological and preventive knowledge?

In this study therefore, we would like to explore the possibility that humoral theory might have been subject to a more significant internal evolution than is often assumed. We are aware that early modern accounts of the working of the body can be very detailed and complex and appear at times hard to decipher for the modern reader, even in a source directed to a lay readership like the regimens. Our aim in analysing these sources has been therefore to grasp the thrust of the major transformations in advice and in the logic underpinning changing rules of health taking place over the period and convey them in an accessible language to the non-specialist.

A NEW CULTURE OF PREVENTION?

The first aim of this study is to demonstrate that a sophisticated and pervasive culture of prevention developed in Italy in the sixteenth century and increasingly informed domestic practices. Inevitably, due to the highly urban character of the peninsula, our focus is on cities and urban culture, though, as we will see, the dissemination of preventive advice through various printed genres also involved small rural towns. An in-depth and diachronic analysis of the vernacular regimens published in Italy since 1500 and a comparison between these texts and some of their medieval and ancient precedents conducted in Chapters 3–8 will represent a first step towards probing the expansion of preventive discourse in the early modern period and its innovative features. But why were concerns for healthy living growing? The classic explanation for the first surge of interest in preventive measures at the end of the Middle Ages has been that it was a response to epidemics and, in particular, the plague. In the sixteenth and part of the seventeenth centuries however, bouts of plague were a recurrent presence in the Italian peninsula, which suggests that other elements need to be taken into account in our explanations for the increasing emphasis on prevention. A more promising line of explanation points to the rising presence of doctors who present themselves as advisers in matters of health maintenance at the Italian princely courts and the new demands of the growing urban classes for this type of advice.[27]

---

[27] Nicoud, *Les Régimes*, esp. 339–41; and Crisciani, 'Histories', 309.

Certainly, much was going on in the Italian medical world in this period: Renaissance Italian states were unrivalled for their very high number of doctors and medical faculties, and the early development of medical services ranging from hospitals to municipal health boards. The Italian medical experience was often seen as an influential model inspiring new health policies and provision introduced in other European countries. One can expect therefore that Italian society was more attuned to health concerns than its European counterparts. Italy in this period was also the cradle of humanism and saw an early development of courts and courtly models, as well as of levels of material and cultural consumerism unknown in other parts of Europe. Moreover, after the Council of Trent, it was the site of a religious reform that profoundly affected everyday behaviour. These and other social and cultural processes deserve to be taken into account when we try to understand the appeal that preventive concerns seem to have exercised on Italian citizens.

Rather than confining our analysis to medical sources therefore, texts by physicians will be considered as part of a broader canvas of contemporary textual genres which might have contributed to shifts in emphasis in the discourse on health. Humanism for example was responsible not only for the growing availability of medical works from antiquity that had discussed healthy lifestyles but also for the recovery and dissemination of texts representing other scholarly traditions, such as architecture and natural history, that also promoted well-being and salubrious houses. Worth noting also is the influence that new intellectual trends, such as the growing interest in geography and local climates brought about by overseas exploration, might have had on late Renaissance notions of prevention.

Alongside the intellectual environment, broader cultural trends also deserve attention. Processes such as the early demilitarization of Italian society and the early development of courtly life in the peninsula had a particularly influential role in the emergence of new models of manners and deportment appropriate to the elite, prompting a new emphasis on physical appearance and a concomitant increase in the attention devoted to caring for the body. Starting from the late sixteenth century, new routines of household and corporeal management developed in the courts and then spread into the palaces of the nobility and the better-off. This process was given impetus by the rise of an urban, aristocratic culture that extended well beyond the boundaries of the court. The emergence of new models of genteel life, of a quest to increase social distance, and of an ethos of comfort also led to the emergence of new practices, such as a culture of *villeggiatura* and *otium* (leisure time spent withdrawing from public affairs in the country villa, inspired by classical precedents) which were profoundly linked to ideals of healthy living.[28]

The need to formulate and transmit the ideals and rules developed at the princely court to wider domestic arenas was also responsible for the development of a broad range of conduct literature that provided detailed guidelines about the perfect management of the household and of physical appearance and well-being. We therefore

---

[28] Burke, 'The Invention'; and Arcangeli, *Recreation*.

extend our attention to this flourishing literature. Its success testifies to the growing importance that the culture of the time ascribed to homes and bodies and contributes to an explanation of the new emphasis on personal health and the salubriousness of domestic spaces that pervades late Renaissance regimens.

Other key developments also had a bearing on attitudes to the body in the Italian context. By the late sixteenth century the Counter-Reformation Church was vocal in its attempts to discipline bodies and promote physical decorum and emotional restraint. Articulated not just through the pulpits but through various strands of pedagogical literature, these ideals were disseminated to a broad stratum of society, also affecting ideas of health and well-being. Whether addressing a courtly environment, an aristocratic household, or the disciplined home of the modest devout Christian family, what all these texts had in common was a focus on the management of the body within a well-regulated domestic arena.

This surge of interest in domestic preventive measures occurred during a period in which the Italian states were profoundly affected by a remarkably dynamic consumer culture. In particular the increased production and circulation of a wealth of material goods radically transformed the domestic surroundings of rich and poor alike. This phenomenon has been researched from multiple perspectives over the past two decades: whether focusing on material magnificence and display, or the relationships between consumers, producers, and retail practices;[29] whether through analyses of the evolution of domestic furnishings or more locally based studies of the economic anthropology implicit in the hierarchies and circulation of goods.[30] Of particular relevance for our project, however, has been the recent wave of studies on the material culture of the domestic interior, which also signals the increased importance that the home and domestic life acquire, in the course of the sixteenth century, in the experience of Italian urban dwellers.[31]

This broad contextualization of medical discourse will enable us to explore the relationship between shifting medical views about prevention and wider social and cultural trends. Indeed a central question that runs through the chapters concerns the extent to which changing medical recommendations about healthy living were stimulated by these new lay and religiously inspired models of conduct and lifestyles. Were doctors simply adapting their advice to the transformations taking place around them and to the changing habits of their patients, or did they have a role in these changes? Putting it another way, how was medical authority maintained in the face of radical transformations in lifestyles and changing fashions? Influential but crude accounts of the power relationship between patient and practitioner have presented the latter as subordinate to the demands and views of the former in terms of choices of treatment and the formulation of diagnoses.[32] Though this simplistic view has subsequently been rejected, the nature

---

[29] Goldthwaite, *Wealth*; and Welch, *Shopping*.

[30] Thornton, *The Italian*; Ago, *Il gusto;* Fantoni, Matthew, and Matthews Grieco (eds.), *The Art Market*; and O'Malley and Welch, *The Material Renaissance*.

[31] Ajmar-Wollheim and Dennis (eds.), *At Home*; Ajmar-Wollheim, Dennis, and Matchette (eds.), 'Approaching'; and Hohti, 'Conspicuous'.

[32] Jewson, 'Medical Knowledge'.

of the relationship between patient and practitioner remains elusive and we hope that looking at it from the perspective of prevention may contribute to throw new light on this issue.

A context that deserves special attention is the growing exposure of the reading public to preventive advice following the introduction of print (Chapter 1). How was the professional image of physicians affected by the spread of a print culture of prevention? It may appear paradoxical that medical authors engaged enthusiastically in a textual genre that by disseminating the principles of healthy living would make their patients more independent from their services as health advisers. And was the philosophy of medical preventive advice transformed by engagement with this wider form of communication, in which doctors were expected to cater for universal needs? In particular, was the emphasis on the unique 'complexion' (individual humoral balance) of each patient undermined, as some authors have suggested, or simply differently articulated?[33]

The study also intends to shed light on the thorny issue of the relationship between medical advice and lay practice. To what extent were medical recommendations heeded and put into practice? Were they ignored or appropriated, transformed or adapted by lay culture? Using Rome as a case study we draw on household inventories from across the social spectrum and sets of family correspondence as evidence for exploring lay conceptions and practices of healthy living and how they compared with the recommendations found in the prescriptive literature.

The choice of focusing on Rome for this study of both elite and lower-class households has been motivated not only by its importance as a centre for intellectual, medical, and cultural development but by the existence of an unrivalled background of scholarship on both the material culture of the city and its medical setting in the early modern period.[34]

This evidence will also be used in combination with visual sources and museum artefacts to explore the impact that principles of healthy living had on the transformation of the material culture of the home and its design. Health concerns have only been marginal to any explanation of how the domestic material environment changed over time. Work on health and the home has concentrated mainly on the modern period and on the actual impact that the design of domestic space, the presence of filth and sanitation had on health.[35] Little attention has been paid to the perspective of their inhabitants and to their perception of certain features of the house and of domestic objects as significant in promoting health. However, one striking characteristic of the early modern regimen is the attention given to the material culture of the home and its role in health maintenance. Hence guides to healthy living are concerned with furnishings and the arrangement of furniture, and

[33] e.g. Cook, 'Physical Methods', 949.
[34] On material culture Ago, *Il gusto*; Storey, *Carnal Commerce*. On Roman medical culture Palmer, 'Medicine'; Donato and Kraye (eds.), *Conflicting Duties*; De Renzi, 'Medical Competence'; De Renzi, 'A Career'; De Renzi, 'Tales'; Andretta, *Roma medica*; and Siraisi, '*Historiae*'.
[35] e.g. Jackson (ed.), *Health*.

references to the health value of specific household objects (from bed canopies to wall hangings, from fireplaces to combs) abound. We hope therefore that the focus on surviving artefacts and on those mentioned in texts, letters, and inventories will contribute to assess the role that the new culture of prevention had in the appearance of specific household objects in the domestic environment, their social dissemination, and finally their demise, enabling a better understanding of the still unexplored relationships between health concerns and the construction of the physical domestic environment.

More broadly, this study will explore the possibility that the process of medicalization, which according to medievalists was ongoing in the states of northern and central Italy from the thirteenth century, was broadening in the sixteenth century to include other, more intimate spheres of individual life, such as domestic space and culture. 'Medicalization' is understood in these medieval studies as the extension of medical expertise to new domains, not previously affected by medical concerns.[36] They argue that, over the previous two centuries and a half, qualified medical treatment had progressively become available to many and access to medical knowledge had expanded through the production of texts for the non-specialist; medical expertise had extended to the legal sphere and to judicial practices and had acquired a public role, as governments came to see doctors as arbiters in the healthiness of the population. Building on these works, our study adopts an even broader notion of medicalization and explores the extension of ideas of healthy and unhealthy to everyday routines and the home surroundings, paying attention to the role of both medical and sociocultural perspectives in this shift. Did the sixteenth century mark a step forward in the expansion of medical discourse to new aspects and moments in a person's life, and if so why? Moving away from a notion of medicalization as simple 'colonization' of new territories by the medical profession we hope to identify the role that patients, changing patterns of behaviour, and ways of thinking about the body and the home had in promoting this process.[37]

Clearly the use of a broad range of written, visual, and material sources at the basis of this study poses many methodological challenges and we devote the first chapters of the book to an in-depth discussion of our material. Chapters 1 and 2 introduce the broad historical framework, as well as the sources and their characteristics, and highlight the ways in which they can help in addressing the questions at the core of the study. Then the book adopts a thematic structure, reproducing the organization of the regimens themselves and hence the way in which early modern people thought about their well-being. Chapters 3–8 each focus on one of the activities involved in the management of the six separate areas of everyday life which affected health—the Non-Naturals. Whenever possible the guidelines

---

[36] Nicoud, 'Formes et enjeux'. For a similar perspective on Spain, McVaugh, *Medicine Before the Plague*, ch. 7. These authors' definition of medicalization differs from the way in which the concept was used in earlier studies, that is, as effectively encapsulated by Brockliss and Jones's critical comment (*Medical World*, 32), as an 'overarching modernization process invariably figured as being engineered by the state'.

[37] For a critique of the 'colonization' approach see Conrad, *The Medicalization of Society*, especially the 'Introduction'.

associated with each of these spheres of life are compared with actual practices, paying special attention to the material culture deployed in fulfilling these recommendations and to the ways in which changing health concerns also contributed to assign a new significance to particular areas of the house, such as the garden, the kitchen, and the bedroom. We hope that this detailed analysis of how health was managed within households will provide a better understanding of the holistic culture of well-being that pervaded the period, contributing in the meantime to various areas of historical debate related to the influence of medicine on everyday practices.

1

Print and a Culture of Prevention

The key evidence for the increasing importance of the preventive paradigm in the Italian peninsula is provided by the growing number of vernacular guides to healthy living, known as regimens. These enjoyed considerable publishing success between the beginning of the sixteenth and the third quarter of the seventeenth century. It may come as a surprise that these handbooks, which instructed readers on how to preserve their own health, were largely authored by physicians despite the threat the genre potentially posed to the medical profession. As well as examining the authorship of this literature, and its rise and decline, in what follows we will explore the reasons why doctors became increasingly involved in this form of communication, how they dealt with the expansion of preventive concerns, and what their engagement with the vernacular and printed health advice tells us about their strategies for professional self-fashioning. By placing the best-selling vernacular regimens in the context of the authors' overall print production we also hope to contribute to the reflection upon the role of print in Renaissance medical writing and in particular in the highly commercialized Italian medical economy.

In recent years historians have started to consider books not just as scripts but as artefacts displaying significant material features (ranging from size to paper quality, from the page layout to the presence of paratext) and marks of use (signatures, marginalia).[1] Treating regimens as both texts and objects, this chapter will therefore analyse their styles and physical characteristics as a way of understanding their target readerships. Evidence of ownership, circulation, and usage of these books will also enable us to compare intended and actual readers and to identify examples of reading practices.

But regimens were not the only means for disseminating the principles of healthy living. A variety of other medical and non-medical genres that developed in the sixteenth and early seventeenth centuries also contributed to this process: 'recipe books' provided readers with practical instructions for making their own preventive remedies, whilst various strands of prescriptive literature and conduct books by secular and religious authors engaged with the preventive health paradigm. As we will see, the appearance of this extensive advice literature is closely intertwined with wider social and cultural transformations in Italy at this time: the early development of courts in northern and central Italy, where codes of behaviour were elaborated that would soon extend beyond the boundaries of the court; the related

---

[1] On materiality Daniels, *Boccaccio*; on readers' interventions, Sherman, *Used Books*.

emergence of new ideals of social distance; changing notions of what constitutes nobility; and the subsequent rise of a genteel urban society, where life centred on learned conversation, polite social intercourse, and recreational activities, and in which maintaining one's health became a key value. In the final section of this chapter we will therefore explore the wider contexts in which the emergence of these genres took place and the reasons why health concerns were enhanced by these developments.

Overall, this chapter aims to explore the role of print in the establishment of this vast and composite preventive culture. Arguably, in a period in which books became much more numerous and affordable, and a familiar element in people's lives, even amongst women and members of the popular classes, print did not simply satisfy the existing demand for health advice but was in itself a factor that contributed to fuel it.

A FLOURISHING BOOK CULTURE

By the first decades of the sixteenth century the steady progress of the print industry in Italy had ensured that the availability of health regimens had increased significantly by comparison with the earlier period of typography considered by Marilyn Nicoud in her study of the genre in the late Middle Ages. Not only had the number of titles available on the market increased dramatically but these were also printed in far greater quantities. In Venice a print run of 400 copies was required in order for a book to be granted *privilegio* (the exclusive right to print a work within the state) but by the mid-sixteenth century runs of 1,500 copies were already common and at the close of the century the number had increased to 3,000 for certain titles to meet demand.[2] From the beginning of the century the diffusion of pocket-size editions encouraged new approaches to the book. Reading casually and for pleasure rather than for study, in a variety of environments and at different times also became much more common.[3] The price of books was largely determined by the cost of paper (books were normally sold unbound, and the binding was then added by the buyer according to his taste and means), and this significantly dropped as result of the increased productivity of the paper industry. Thanks also to the increased number of titles in the vernacular, a phenomenon that in Italy manifests itself from an early date, the printing press was reaching out to a greater and more socially diverse number of readers. People were more likely to encounter books as retail outlets multiplied. The number of bookshops doubled in a few decades, in Verona alone going from five in 1544 to twelve in the 1580s (see Plate 1). Printed books were also on sale at the more humble *cartolaio* shops which provided a more inviting environment for customers not used to mixing with the academic clientele of bookshops, where readers congregated to discuss their interests and

---

[2] Nuovo, *Il commercio librario*, 40–3.
[3] On the relationship between size and function of the book, Petrucci, 'Alle origini'. On the increase in pocket editions, Richardson, *Printing*, 190–6.

compare their readings.[4] Books were also part of the varied merchandise of the itinerant pedlars who distributed them in smaller centres. They specialized in particular in 'popular' publications which not only presented content in a simplified version but were characterized by specific physical features such as rough paper, a limited number of pages, the use of old-style typefaces, and printing arranged on two columns to save space, that targeted an uneducated and unrefined audience.[5] These cheap publications, written to be easily grasped by readers of limited means and abilities, experienced a boom in the second half of the sixteenth century. All these developments reflected and at the same time promoted the rise of literacy. Already significant in fifteenth-century Italian cities by comparison with other European regions, the ability to read increased even further starting from the last decades of the sixteenth century, thanks to the efforts of evangelization promoted by the Counter-Reformation.[6] Church educational policy led in fact to the creation of a capillary network of catechism schools for girls as well as boys that had a dramatic impact on levels of popular literacy.[7]

In Italy the diffusion of books and the expansion of reading also owed much to the sophisticated distribution networks of the print industry.[8] Books were sold well beyond their place of production. Italian printers and publishers (the two roles did not necessarily overlap) were often members of mercantile families who also traded spices, silk, paper, and other goods, taking advantage of established trade routes and merchants and agents. Already in the first half of the sixteenth century they were capable of selling books all over Italy as well as abroad. In 1514, Soardi, a publishing house based in Ferrara, sent its books to Lyons, Salamanca, Pavia, Naples, Ancona, Rimini, Bologna, Rome, and Lisbon. They also had two bookshops in Venice and deposits in Lanciano and Recanati in central Italy, which were sites of important fairs, and this ensured a diffusion of the printed word in smaller centres.[9] The same can be said of Valgrisi, Giolito, and other large publishers. It was particularly the development of these complex distribution networks, rather than significant advances in printing techniques, which was responsible for the proliferation of titles and subject areas available in print, as can be seen from the booksellers' catalogues. One should also consider that in this period books were highly mobile goods: they were frequently donated, lent, or resold by owners, feeding in this way a flourishing market for second-hand books. Most copies of a book therefore had multiple readers.

It is in the context of this rising interest in books and increased reading opportunities that the first vernacular texts entirely devoted to preventing rather than curing disease (regimens) made their appearance in print.

---

[4] Carpané, 'Libri', 210.   [5] Grendler, 'Form'.
[6] On levels of literacy, Grendler, *Schooling*, 42–7.
[7] Toscani, 'Catechesi'; Roggero, 'L'Alphabétisation'. Some scholars hold a much more negative view of the impact of the Counter-Reformation upon reading. Focusing exclusively on the introduction of censorship, they have suggested that Church policy had the effect of lowering levels of literacy and even discouraged the development of a solid middle-class readership. For a summary of these views, which remain isolated, Harris, 'The History of the Book', 262–3.
[8] What follows is largely based on Nuovo, *Il commercio librario*; and Richardson, *Printing*.
[9] Nuovo and Sandal, *Il libro*, 166.

DOCTORS AND PRINTED VERNACULAR REGIMENS

As mentioned earlier, a regimen is a compendium of guidelines on how to preserve one's health. In more or less depth it provides advice about the 'Six Non-Natural Things' upon which health was traditionally seen to depend: the air we breathe; the control of emotions; how, when, and for how long one should sleep and exercise; what and when one should eat and drink; and how to cleanse the body. Its practical content and the fact that it is addressing a non-specialist public distinguish it from academic medical treatises. As in the medieval period, various organizational models coexist in regimens—at times even within the same text. The advice might be arranged according to the stages of life, with some regimens focusing largely or entirely on how to keep healthy in old age. Others focus on the organs and limbs prescribing rules for the maintenance of body parts from head to toe. Others are organized according to the season or months of the year.[10] Sometimes a regimen might concentrate largely or entirely on one Non-Natural, for example on air, sleep, or food. But usually in the early modern period regimens addressed all six Non-Naturals, with separate sections devoted to advice on each one. Over the period we can also observe changes in the space devoted to each Non-Natural, so while attention to food is prominent in the first vernacular regimens, written in the late fifteenth century, in texts written in the following century the different Non-Naturals receive a more even treatment.[11] We witness, in other words, the emergence of a more balanced approach to the preservation of health which is no longer centred mainly on diet.

This holistic attitude is perhaps a factor in the lukewarm reception that contemporaries gave to the theories advanced by Luigi Cornaro in his treatise on the sober life, where he saw diet alone as holding the secret of health and longevity. In spite of the attention that this work has received from recent scholars of prevention, it is interesting to observe that the text, first published in 1558, only reached the height of its popularity in the eighteenth and nineteenth centuries, when it was reprinted several times.[12] By contrast attempts to get it published were initially thwarted in sixteenth-century Italy and even once published, Cornaro's views sparked considerable criticism. Even in the next century the treatise received a much warmer reception in northern than in southern Europe, perhaps because of the explicit links the author established between sin and illness, uncommon elsewhere in the genre.[13] His venturing onto a territory, that of preventive advice, seen as the domain of doctors, certainly played a part in the hostility towards Cornaro's theories, but these appear extravagant even in relation to the dietetic principles commonly held

---

[10] Nicoud, *Les Régimes*, 16 and 151.

[11] However, there are exceptions as the regimens authored by Durante, Petronio, and Paschetti devote far more attention to food than to the other Non-Naturals. See Ch. 8.

[12] Wear, 'The History', 1292–4; and Smith, *Clean*, 201–2.

[13] See the documents in Milani (ed.), *Scritti*. Milani also publishes a list of the book's editions. Her analysis shows that with the exception of the 1591 posthumous edition, organized by Cornaro's nephew, the 16th-century reprints of the work were all promoted by the author and included responses to the criticisms the work had received. On the success of the text in England, Milani, 'La fortuna'.

at the time. The fact that between 1630 and 1712 the text was published five times as an annex to the popular regimen *Scuola salernitana*, and hence directed to a poorly educated readership, is revealing in this context.

Let us turn now to the development of the printed vernacular regimen and its changing features. Most of the works considered in our study have been identified by searching for texts that included the words *sano, sani, sanità* (healthy, health) in their extended titles and this method has allowed us to single out approximately fifty texts that can be considered regimens of health according to the definition outlined earlier. We have also included some re-editions of extant titles. As will become clear, in this period a new edition of an existing regimen often constituted a work in its own right, as it frequently contained numerous editorial changes such as additions, cuts, and reorganization of the text that in many cases may have significantly altered its content. The distinction in terms of role and status between author and editor was not nearly as strong during the early days of print as it is today. Obviously the texts we have identified do not encompass all the regimens published in the period considered. Those works whose titles do not include our chosen keywords are left out and so are the many early printed books published in just one edition which, as historians of the book have repeatedly suggested, have simply not survived.[14]

The first vernacular works entirely devoted to healthy living appeared in the first decade of the sixteenth century. The year 1508 saw the publication of two regimens authored by distinguished fifteenth-century doctors. The first, the *Tractato circa la conservatione de la sanitade* was attributed to Ugo Benzi (d. 1439), personal physician of the Duke d'Este and university professor of philosophy and then of medicine at Siena, Bologna, Parma, and Pavia, but was in reality the translation of a Latin regimen by Benedetto Reguardati (1398–1469), doctor to the Sforza dukes. The second, the *Libreto . . . de tutte le cose che se manzano*, was written in the vernacular around 1450 by Benzi's successor at the Este court and professor of medicine at Ferrara, Doctor Michele Savonarola (d. 1469).[15] Both these works focus in large part on food and diet, a topic that according to Chiara Crisciani came to dominate the genre, prompted by the simultaneous development of courts and their banqueting culture in the Italian principalities of northern Italy.[16]

The publication of these two regimens was followed, in 1549, by the adaptation into Italian of one classical and one medieval work: *Di Galeno*, an apparently faithful translation of Galen's *De tuenda sanitatis* by the historian, Latinist, and Greek specialist Giovanni Tarcagnota;[17] and the *Opera utilissima di Arnaldo da Villanova*

---

[14] e.g. Sinclair in his *The Code*, vol. ii, entries 304 and 961, signals two regimens, authored in 1662 and 1690 respectively by doctors Bruno Cibaldi and Fabrizio Paravicino, but we could not find them in any library.

[15] On Benzi, Lockwood, *Ugo Benzi*. On the attribution of this text to Reguardati see Hill Cotton, 'Benedetto Reguardati'; and Nicoud, *Les Régimes*, 429–35. There was already an incunabular printing of this work, dated 1481; the translator is unknown. The 1508 edition was in 4°, three editions in 8° format followed in 1514, 1515, and 1554.

[16] Crisciani, 'Histories', 309.

[17] The comparison has been made with Montraville Green's *A Translation of Galen's Hygiene*.

di conservare la sanità, which, despite the reference to Arnau, is actually a translation of a regimen written in the fourteenth century by Doctor Maino de Maineri (d. 1341).[18] Both these works were printed in 8° by Michele Tramezzino, a publisher with presses in both Venice and Rome who specialized in the popularization of pocket editions of classical texts.

Prior to this however, rules for healthy living had appeared in more composite texts alongside a variety of other topics. These included the translation into the vernacular of the pseudo-Aristotelian text known as *Secretum secretorum* by the Greek specialist Giovanni Manenti in 1538 and the numerous reprints and re-editions of the *Libro de homine/Il perché* which first appeared in 1474, authored by Gerolamo Manfredi, a highly esteemed doctor and astrologer from Bologna.[19] The *Secretum secretorum* includes a regimen amongst a compendium of pronouncements on political and ethical matters which, arranged in epistolary form, claims to be the advice given by Aristotle to Alexander the Great during his campaign in Persia.[20] Manfredi's text takes the form of a popular encyclopaedia organized in question-and-answer format and aims to satisfy the curiosity of the common man about a number of more or less bizarre issues, in the tradition of the pseudo-Aristotelian *Problemata*.[21] Book I consists of straightforward prescriptions for the management of the six Non-Naturals, while book II is a treatise on physiognomy. Thanks to its simplified but very broad contents and its accessible language, Manfredi's text had great popular appeal and became an astonishing publishing success: by 1678, twenty-seven editions had been printed under three different titles (*Liber de homine*; *Opera nova intitulata Il perché*; *Libro intitulato Il perché*).[22] Over its long life, however, the text, like other best-sellers, changed significantly. As a result of editorial alterations 110 of the 568 original questions were removed from the late sixteenth-century editions, partly because they touched on matters that could incur the censorship of the post-Tridentine Church (about twenty were queries about sexual life) and partly to adapt contents to the new times.[23]

As the publishing history of the texts discussed so far suggests, the dissemination of preventive principles through print in the first decades of the sixteenth century was not achieved by members of the medical profession. Rather, it was due entirely to professional writers who translated, edited, and published works written by or attributed to distinguished medieval or ancient physicians and philosophers. They also adapted texts which had already been published as incunabular texts in the previous century. It is well known that such 'polygraphs', as recent scholars have defined these professional writers, were at the heart of the publishing industry in

[18] This has been ascertained by Soler, *Arnau de Villanova*, 18 and 163 n. 9. On the enduring popularity of Arnau see Paniagua, 'El regimen'.

[19] Manente, *Col nome de Dio*. On Manfredi, Duranti, *Mai sotto Saturno*.

[20] The *Secretum secretorum* reached Europe through Hispano-Arabic translations in the 13th century and circulated in manuscript form until the 16th century. On its fortunes, Eamon, *Science*, 45–53; and Milani, 'La tradizione'.

[21] Carré and Cifuentes, 'Girolamo Manfredi's *Il perché*: I'.

[22] Carré and Cifuentes, 'Girolamo Manfredi's *Il perché*: II', 44–6.

[23] Carré and Cifuentes, 'Girolamo Manfredi's *Il perché*: II', 46–7.

this period. Little attention however has been paid to their involvement in popular medical publications.[24] These learned men, often from relatively modest social backgrounds, earned their livings partly through court service, as secretaries of powerful patrons, and partly by the proceeds from engagement in the printing industry, an activity that was becoming lucrative at the time, especially if one could secure a share of the profits on sales.[25] It is interesting to note, therefore, how preventive themes were regarded by publishers and polygraphs alike as a profitable field in which to focus their initiatives.

It was one such man, the professional writer and classical scholar named Lucio Fauno, who was responsible for the Italian translation and posthumous publication of Marsilio Ficino's *De le tre vite*. A philosopher also trained as a physician, Ficino had composed this regimen specifically for scholars and it was circulating in Latin editions by 1489. The Italian version was published in a pocket-sized edition in 1548 by Tramezzino, a publisher who once again appears to have been particularly active in the promotion of medical knowledge. The aim underpinning the translation of works of this type was that of reaching out to a wider public and this is made explicit in the preface and dedication signed by the publisher and the translator. Tramezzino argues that Ficino's text should be in everyone's hands, since, 'Who is the man who does not wish to live a healthy life, and a long one?' Meanwhile he notes that Ficino's reputation as the principal philosopher of the time goes before him and that will persuade the reader not just to read his recommendations, 'But surely also to carry out what he teaches, so as to live a long and healthy life.'[26] Then the book's reader is described by the translator as someone not yet acquainted with the principles of healthy living and the medical terminology used to present them. Hence he includes a kind of disclaimer in which he justifies his choice not to remove difficult medical terms (*voci di medicina*) from the text (terms such as phlegm, pituity, bile or choler, and the 'other bile' or *melancholia*), but to accompany them with an explanatory note that clarifies the nature of each of these humours and the effects they have on one's health, physiognomy, and temperament.

The same didactic aim characterizes the publication in Italian, in 1560, of a regimen by the German doctor Pictorius, which had originally been issued in Latin (Basel, 1530). For the first time in the history of printed vernacular regimens we find that a doctor (Pamfilo Fiorimbene), rather than a professional writer, was responsible for the translation.[27] In the introduction he makes explicit that by translating the work he intended to empower readers to look after their own health. Pictorius himself had also underlined the educational intent of his book in his address to his *candido lettore* (open-hearted reader). He assumes that his public is

---

[24] See, however, Maclean, 'The Diffusion', 67–70.

[25] On the social background and economic strategies of this category, Bareggi di Filippo, *Il mestiere*.

[26] 'Chi é colui che non desideri di vivere sano, e di vivere molto?'; 'Ma sicuramente anco essequire quello che egli ci insegna, per potere vivere sano, e gran tempo . . .'; Ficino, *De le tre vite*, iiii.

[27] Pictorius, *Dialogi*.

completely ignorant on matters of prevention and tries to draw the reader in with witty exchanges and by adopting a dialogue form that enables him to introduce the subject each time in a simple way rather than talking down to the reader. Moreover, the publisher evidently hoped to reach an even wider readership by including a very brief work on how to keep young and postpone ageing (once again falsely attributed to Arnau de Villanova) which offered, through a series of short pieces of practical advice arranged in no evident logical order, an even more accessible version of preventive recommendations.[28]

A similar strategy can be seen in another work published by Tramezzino in 1560 in 8° format. Only seventeen pages long, this regimen was attributed to another distinguished foreign physician, Robert Grospré, and provided basic and eminently practical instructions for a healthy lifestyle, largely centred around diet and exercise.[29] It was annexed to a non-medical text, Domenico Romoli's *La singolare dottrina*, one of many treatises on the ways of choosing, storing, preparing, and serving foods and drinks known as *libri dello scalco*. These texts were compiled by stewards in noble households who were in charge of all matters pertaining to dining and they sometimes also touched briefly on topics related to preventive health. Within the *libri dello scalco* genre (to which we will shortly return) Romoli's work was particularly successful (it was re-edited five times between 1587 and 1637). The inclusion of the healthy living guide by Grospré might have contributed to its success.[30]

The fact that publishers chose to append highly simplified regimens to the more complex and learned treatises by Pictorius and Romoli seems to suggest that by 1560 a preventive culture had been established and was now being extended to a less educated and sophisticated public. A differentiation had started to develop between the health advice literature directed to a relatively intellectual readership—one that appreciated the occasional reference to classical authors and explanations of the physiological rationale behind specific recommendations—and purely prescriptive regimens that simply offered practical advice, often in easy-to-memorize forms, aimed at the less well-educated reader.

Whilst a stream of translations had initially satisfied the thirst for preventive knowledge, from the 1560s onwards Italian physicians, by now aware that a market existed for tracts of this kind, started to publish their own compilations of rules for healthy living in Italian and in smaller, portable formats than the traditional 4°, still reserved for academic medical treatises.[31] In some cases these were in reality vernacular translations of works previously published in Latin. This trend was

---

[28] On which see Paniagua, 'El regimen sanitatis', 356–9.

[29] It was an abridged version of the *Regimen sanitatis* that Grospré had published in Latin in Ghent in 1539.

[30] Only 23 of the 30 chapters in the Ghent edition had been included in the Italian version; the plague tract was also removed.

[31] On 4° as the dominant format for academic monographs in Italy see Maclean, 'The Diffusion', 74. There were already Italian editions of regimens in Latin that had concentrated in particular on one Non-Natural: food. e.g. Accoramboni, *Tractatus de lacte*; Laguna, *De victus*; and Corti, 'De prandii ac caenae modo libellus', published posthumously by his son in 1562. On these and their relationship with the re-edition of Hippocrates' treatise *De diaeta*, see Andretta, *Roma medica*, 294–7.

probably started by the doctor and astrologer Tommaso Giannotti Rangoni (*c*.1493–*c*.1577). His regimen was first published in 4° format and in Latin, and three editions were issued between 1551 and 1560, but from 1556 onwards several vernacular editions of the text came out in pocket format (some of them published posthumously), four of which were shortened versions of the original, which had been reduced from eighty to only sixteen sheets. Each of these pamphlets had a different dedicatee, another expedient aimed to boost the circulation of the work, not only through the appeal of a prestigious name but also in the hope that the patron would become an active sponsor of it.[32] Similarly the regimen by the distinguished doctor Alessandro Petronio first appeared in Latin in 1581 and was rendered into the vernacular by another doctor, Basilio Paravicino, and published posthumously as *Del viver dei Romani*, in 1592.

Provincial doctors, too, now began composing vernacular regimens, inspired by the ideal of educating their public. For example, Traffichetti, a physician active in the small town of Rimini, published *L'arte di conservar la salute tutta intiera* in 1565 with the declared intention of presenting preventive advice by the best authors on the subject in concise and accessible language ('in ordine essentiale e assai facile') for those who did not know about medicine.

It has been suggested that Latin long remained the language of choice for learned medical treatises and that only at the end of the sixteenth and the beginning of the seventeenth century did some doctors break with this cultural tradition and begin adopting local vernaculars—though they still felt obliged to justify their choice of language in prefaces.[33] As far as preventive medicine is concerned, however, the vernacularization of medical knowledge pre-dates these developments. It is true that a certain reluctance to publish in the vernacular still characterized the medical world in the last quarter of the sixteenth century. Indeed, there was even a degree of contempt for those who resorted to the printed word! For example much ink was spilt in a dispute between Traffichetti (mentioned earlier) and Matteo Bruno, another doctor also active in the small town of Rimini. In 1569 Bruno published a rebuke of the errors allegedly present in Traffichetti's regimen, which was followed by a response from the latter in 1572.[34] In his introduction, Bruno blames Traffichetti precisely for not writing in Latin, and furthermore for writing in 'low' Italian, unadorned and unpolished, revealing how new it was for doctors to engage with the vernacular language. Bruno also indicates how unusual it was for provincial doctors to get their works printed, as he claims that there are many physicians in Rimini no less worthy and learned than Traffichetti, who, however, 'don't tire themselves every moment of the day trying to get into print'.[35]

But prejudice against the printed word and vernacular publishing in the medical world was dying out. In the next two decades the number of regimens written by

---

[32] Rangoni, *Thomaso philologo*. This was followed by the much shorter editions of 1557, 1565, 1570, and 1577.
[33] Carlino, 'Introduction', 18–19, and 22.
[34] Bruno, *Discorsi*; Traffichetti, *Idea*.
[35] 'che Rimini, oltra voi, e fors'a voi non inferiori, ha altri medici suoi, li quali se ben non s'affaticano ogni hor per entrar nelle stampe'. Bruno, *Discorsi*, 9–11.

Italian doctors directly in the vernacular increased steadily. These were both re-editions of published texts, like the expanded version of Savonarola's regimen by Boldo, a physician from Brescia, in 1575, and regimens that were entirely new. Two among these are particularly noteworthy: Castore Durante's *Tesoro di sanità* (1586), which would become the best-seller within the genre, counting as many as thirty-three editions up to 1679 (see Fig. 1.1); and the highly successful *Trattato della natura de' cibi et del bere* (1583) by Baldassarre Pisanelli, entirely devoted to healthy food and drink.[36] Initially printed in folio and dedicated to the Duke of Mantua, the work was reprinted at least twenty-seven times, in various formats, between 1584 and 1676 (and once again in the late eighteenth century). Moreover, a considerably revised edition of the text by Gallina, a physician in the little Piedmontese town of Carmagnola, came out in 1589.[37]

Whether as authors, editors, or translators, physicians were now responsible for the increase in printed health regimens which had until then been published by the *poligrafi* described earlier, and the trend continued into the seventeenth century. At this point, however, signs of a certain saturation of the market become evident. In this period we start to see a tendency towards specialization, with preventive literature tending to concentrate on specific aspects of health, and authors trying to carve a niche for themselves within the genre. So, for example, in 1610 Camaffi wrote a regimen that focused specifically on how to keep healthy in hot weather and several regimens published between the 1590s and the 1620s centre on the benefits and drawbacks of drinking hot or cold liquids.[38] In the mid-seventeenth century, Doctor Panaroli wrote a regimen entirely devoted to one Non-Natural, air.[39] And even when they maintained a holistic approach, authors now sought to clearly differentiate the new regimen from the existing ones at least at a stylistic level. They were at pains to underline the traits that distinguished their work from that of other authors. In 1626, for example, Viviani declared his intention to write a text as concisely as possible on the ways of keeping healthy, avoiding references to sources and disputes among medical authors that would appear 'useless, highly tedious and obscure' ('inutile, piena di tedio, e d'oscurità') to those who do not practise the art of medicine.[40] Panaroli justified including poetry in his text on the grounds that it 'recreates the spirit and the noble intellects, tired by long studies or similar strains'. Frediano, in 1656, explained that his aim in compiling a regimen was to illustrate the particular benefits of dressing for warmth ('vestire caldo') given that none of his distinguished predecessors had dwelt on this subject in their regimens.[41]

After the 1650s, however, the genre came to a standstill. No new regimens were written, no revised editions of existing ones appeared, and even reprints of the

---

[36] For a full list of Durante's editions see Rhodes, *La vita*, 63–7.

[37] Gallina's re-edition extends and rearranges the original text. It was reprinted twice, in 1589 and 1612, and in 1620 was annexed to the re-edition of Benzi's regimen by the Turin doctor Bertaldi.

[38] Camaffi, *Reggimento*. For treatises on drinking hot and cold liquids see Ch. 8.

[39] Panaroli, *Aerologia*.

[40] Viviani, *Trattato*, dedication and introd., 9.

[41] 'ma per ricrearne l'animo e gli ingegni nobili ancora che stanchi da lunghi studij, o fatighe simili'; Panaroli, *Aerologia*, 3; Frediano, *Arca novella*.

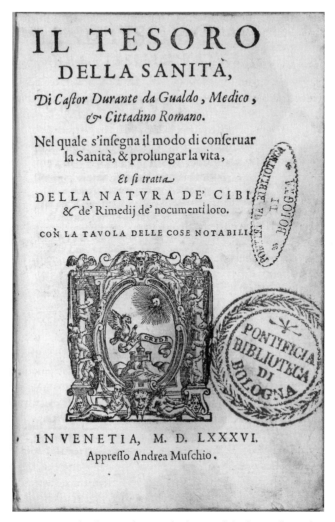

Fig. 1.1. Frontispiece to the first pocket-sized edition of the best-selling *Il tesoro di sanità* by Castore Durante (1586).

best-sellers stopped, as we have seen, in the 1670s. In the last decade of the century only one new regimen was published, Barnaba Ciccolini's (1697), while Rangoni's text was reissued under the new title *Svegliarino ai signori veneziani.* By and large the production of preventive literature had now shifted towards treatises which examined the advantages and disadvantages for health of new substances such as tobacco, chocolate, or coffee.[42] The holistic approach that saw the correct management of

---

[42] e.g. Gufferi, *Il biasimo dello tabacco*; and Stella, *Il tabacco medico.* On treatises on coffee and hot chocolate see Ch. 8.

bodily routines as being the key to a long and healthy life seems to have been abandoned, along with the mission to instruct readers on how to carry out the different aspects of this management properly.

Nonetheless, for about a century, many members of the medical profession had been eager to associate their names with printed preventive advice addressed to non-specialists. Prevention had gradually acquired a distinguished status and writing or editing a regimen, or translating a regimen into the vernacular, came to be viewed by physicians of different backgrounds as a means of promoting their professional image. Medical authors fashioned themselves as champions of preventive medicine arguing that, contrary to the Hippocratic dictum, this had been neglected by modern authors. In the prefaces to their regimens, Durante, Paschetti, and Viviani use almost identical phrasing to reiterate that there are two parts to medicine, one aimed at preserving health, the other at restoring it, but that the former has been almost entirely abandoned.[43] By giving new impetus to classical understandings of the doctor as a figure devoted to educating their patients to take good care of their health, early modern doctors were paradoxically raising their professional credibility.

REGIMENS' PHYSICAL AND FORMAL FEATURES

The didactic intent of late Renaissance regimens is evident both in the choice of the vernacular and in their format. In the great majority of cases these books were issued at some point in a more 'portable' edition, known as 8° (approximately 15 centimetres on the long side) or even in 12° (13 centimetres) or in the even smaller pocket-sized 16°. However, the reasons why many healthy-living books had only one edition while others had more than twenty in just a few decades do not simply depend on size. Other formal elements such as the length of the book, the style in which information was presented, the layout of the page, and the presence of divisions within the text acting as signposts are also important factors. Despite the didactic intentions declared in the preface, a regimen like Traffichetti's was not very 'user-friendly' and stood little chance of becoming a publishing success, both because of the very dense prose and, visually, because of the print style, which adopted a small font size (9 or 10 pt) and ran on continuously, with very few cross-headings or breaks.[44] Such stylistic and formal aspects played a key role, creating major differentiations within the genre that also marked out different readerships.

Indeed, the health-advice literature we have examined is rather diverse in terms of its target audiences. Some regimens were clearly oriented towards a learned public of experts. This group of texts includes, for example, the translations of Petronio's regimen which was a thick book in 4° format of more than 400 pages, written in a dense, erudite style, which provides very complicated advice, and Pietragrassa's regimen which was nearly 500 pages long and only published in folio format.[45] The

---

[43] See Paschetti, *Del conservar*, dedication to Giacomo Doria.
[44] Traffichetti, *L'arte*.   [45] Petronio, *Del viver*; Pietragrassa, *Politica medica*.

800-page re-edition of Benzi's regimen by Doctor Bertaldi also looks like a compendium for the learned, despite its small format. Each topic considered has Benzi's advice followed by Bertaldi's comments and updatings which are put in italics. A third layer of comments is then added to the food section, which also includes text from Pisanelli's regimen, thus creating a kind of general reference tool.[46]

At the other end of the spectrum we find a group of texts that were not written by university-trained physicians as were most regimens, but by members of other categories of the medical profession: astrologers and charlatans like Rosaccio, and herbalists and surgeons like Tartaglini and Latino de Grassi.[47] These are often very short tracts, sometimes made of just a few folded and unbound sheets with the script running on from start to end without any division into paragraphs or sections; at other times the paper is thick and the print rough and dark. They frequently present a mixture of advice and recipes, thus overlapping with the 'book of secrets' genre, which only included recipes of various kinds. They provide no rationale for their instructions on healthy living, which are schematic and reductionist, written in simple, popular language and often presented in no detectable order. These types of texts clearly aimed to reach a wide, uneducated audience of limited means—'all those who can read, including women'—as is declared in the preface to the vernacular edition of the puzzling *Regimen sanitatis salernitanum* (1581). This presents randomly-organized brief prescriptions for healthy living in short rhymes and proverbs that could be easily memorized.[48] In reality, in spite of their 'popular' appearance and style, it is likely that these texts also held an appeal for more sophisticated readers, who from time to time liked to rely on their direct, uncomplicated message.[49]

The great majority of the texts published in this period, however, were most likely aimed at a well-read public of non-specialists and non-professionals, who nonetheless could be intellectually curious and critical readers. These are regimens of medium length (most commonly 150 to 250 pages long, but sometimes shorter), normally issued in small format, printed on fine paper, and written by doctors. Importantly, it seems that physical and formal characteristics, more than the originality of their contents, made some texts particularly appealing. Considerable effort was being expended to make these books readable. They are characterized for example by the adoption of medium to large print, a clear layout, the inclusion of an alphabetical index, headings in italics, and summaries of key ideas in the margins. The text is divided up into sections and short chapters and the language is not too technical. It includes a few references and quotes to prove the credentials of the author but without rehearsing all the arguments, unlike more erudite ones. The

---

[46] Bertaldi, *Regole della sanità*.

[47] Rosaccio, *Avvertimenti*; Tartaglini, *Opera nuoua*; Grassi, *Opera nuova*.

[48] *Scuola salernitana*. The translator was Father Serafino Razzi, from the religious order of the Predicatori. The involvement of an ecclesiastic in the publication of regimens of health is exceptional in the Italian context, while it seems to have been much more common in England; Rawcliffe, 'Concept of Health', 333. Several versions of this text, erroneously attributed to the Salernitan School, exist both in the manuscript and edited traditions, to the extent that, according to Nicoud, one should talk of *regimina sanitatis salernitanum*, in the plural; Nicoud, *Les Régimes*, 368 and 'Il *Regimen*'.

[49] On the broad appeal of the popular press see Grendler, 'Form', 453.

instructions are straightforward and succinct but simple explanations highlighting their rationale are normally provided (see Figs. 1.2, 1.3, and 1.4 for comparison). Some regimens, like those authored by Rangoni, Durante, Fonseca, and Frediano, are interspersed with contemporary observations and local colour and frequently mention objects of current use and everyday practices. Though the combination of these features varies from text to text, such ingredients are crucial in determining the commercial success of a book; indeed a clear link seems to exist between the systematic use of these editorial and typographical strategies and the number of published editions of the different titles.

As regards content, innovation in the genre only emerged gradually and cannot be identified with any one title in particular. Novelties there certainly were, however, and Chapters 3–8 will identify a number of new ways of thinking about preventive health, but such changes were introduced almost imperceptibly from one text to the other. Similarly, slightly newer recommendations can coexist with traditional advice, and we rarely find an openly critical stance towards the wisdom of the author's predecessors. Hence the reasons why one text rather than another becomes a success are to be found more in the way in which information is communicated stylistically and visually than in any particular novelty in its contents.

Sixteenth- and seventeenth-century regimens are patchworks incorporating substantial elements from contemporary and earlier works. The practice of reworking existing texts was routine, yet most re-editions were presented as new works. These certainly included variations and additions to the original script, but it was also the way in which the material was presented that made a text new. For example, Boldo reworked Savonarola's *Libreto* in 1575, 'set out in better order, expanded and amended and almost made anew', as stated in the title.[50] Indeed Boldo's regimen included new entries, was far more detailed, and introduced a better subdivision of the text. For example while Savonarola had twenty-six chapters, Boldo had twenty-five treatises further divided into chapters. But the work also displayed a far more effective page layout. Whereas the 1515 edition of Savonarola was still printed in two columns without any spacing between the chapters, the treatises and chapters were now visually separated and there were headings on each page, and Boldo also included an alphabetical list of contents.

Translators, too, were not averse to making their own additions to the text or to changing the organization and layout of contents. In the preface to his translation of the *Scuola salernitana*, Serafino Razzi proudly alerted the reader to the new order he had imposed on the work by collating information on the same topic, organizing the entries in alphabetical order, trimming it of unnecessary detail, and finally adding some words and sentences commonly approved by the 'common people' (*volgo*) and by 'specialists in the arts and professions'.[51] Even the translation of a centuries-old text could therefore constitute a relatively new work.

---

[50] Boldo, *Libro della natura*: 'poi di nuovo con miglior ordine ordinato, accresciuto e emendato e quasi fatto un altro per Bartolomeo Boldo medico bressano'.
[51] *Scuola salernitana*, 'Prefazione'.

By the closing decades of the sixteenth century, doctors had also acquired better knowledge of the presentational techniques that could make a book particularly popular and certainly in retrospect, stylistic and formal aspects seemed to count more than the author's fame in ensuring the marketable value of the book. The authors of the two best-selling regimens, Durante and Pisanelli, were far from being celebrities when they published their books. Pisanelli was a physician at the hospital of Santo Spirito in Rome. Durante had been a town physician in the small centre of Gualdo in the Marche region (central Italy), and was now practising in Viterbo—an unremarkable career. The success of Durante's regimen was the springboard for his professional advancement, and not vice versa. It would seem, in fact, that Durante obtained the chair of botany at the Roman Archiginnasio and the title of personal physician to the Pope in his mid-fifties after the publication of both his regimen (1586) and the *Herbario nuovo*, a year earlier, which was another great publishing success.[52]

Durante's regimen arranged information in a simple, straightforward way, devoting one chapter to each Non-Natural and adopting a range of graphic devices to make the text easily searchable. In Pisanelli's regimen, too, the structure was clearly evident. His text was organized with a grid like a reference book, adopting a style of presentation of data from nature that was increasingly used by scientists at the time. For each item considered the author provided a number of standardized entries, each filling one or two pages, specifying its qualities, impact on health, medicinal uses, and humoral characteristics. Within each entry there would be succinct descriptions of the season, age group, and complexion for which it was recommended, each only taking up between two and four lines (see Fig. 1.3). These are followed by a longer and unstructured section titled 'Historie naturali' (natural histories), tracing the origin of the item's name, describing how it was cooked in the past, and looking at curious facts or tales surrounding it. Though the way in which the items follow one another appears chaotic to the modern reader (they are not systematically listed in alphabetical order, nor consistently arranged by category, nor is a list of contents included to guide the reader), for those interested in finding out about the beneficial or harmful nature of particular foods this work was much more accessible than the other guides to healthy food printed around the same time. Boldo's re-edition of Savonarola, which had appeared ten years earlier, had a treatise for each category of food (grains, herbs, citrus fruits, etc.) divided internally into chapters devoted to the individual grain, herb, or fruit, but the information supplied for each item was several pages long and unstructured, without any internal subdivisions or thematic order.[53] In Pisanelli's regimen readers would find the detail they were interested in much more easily once they had identified the relevant item. As for Bertaldi's, published in 1618, this was a learned book that presented a tedious compendium of what had been said about individual foods, first by Benzi, then by Gallina in his re-edition of Benzi, and then by Pisanelli in his regimen, to which were added Bertaldi's own views.[54] Clearly Pisanelli's work had been structured and paginated with a different reader and type

---

[52] Rhodes, *La vita*, 25–33.   [53] Boldo, *Libro della natura*.
[54] Bertaldi, *Regole della sanità*.

of reading in mind, to facilitate quick consultation even by readers who were not particularly well educated.

This applies even more strongly to the way in which Durante organized his section on food, basically merging the two structures found in Boldo's and Pisanelli's regimens and imposing a more precise order. Like Boldo he grouped the various items by category, starting with grains and then dealing with the various grains individually, arranged in alphabetical order, then moving on to herbs and treating them in the same way, and so on. However, as in Pisanelli's regimen, the information about each food stuck to the essentials and followed a fixed template, although the longer and diverse section, 'Historie naturali', was dropped, making the text even more direct and accessible (see Figs. 1.2, 1.3, 1.4).

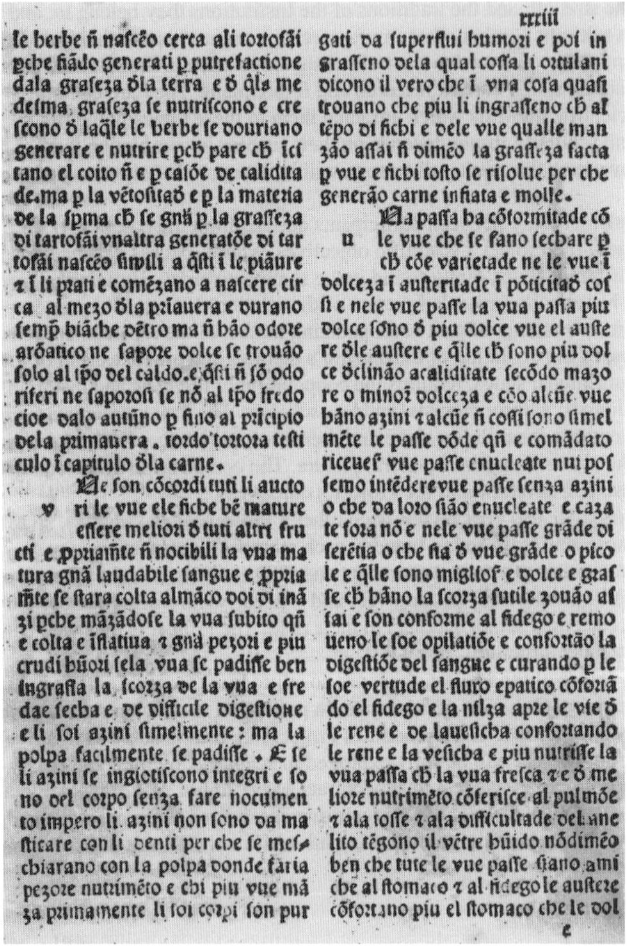

xxxiii

le herbe ñ nascẽo cerca ali tortofãi
pche fiãdo generati p putrefactione
dala graseza dla terra e d qls me
desma graseza se nutriscono e cre
scono d laq̃le le herbe se douriano
generare e nutrire pch pare ch ici
tano el coito ñ e p casõe de calidita
de ma p la vẽtositad e p la materia
de la spma ch se gnã p la grasseza
di tartofãi vnaltra generatõe di tar
tofãi nascẽo simili a q̃sti i le piãure
e i li prati e comẽzano a nascere cir
ca al mezo dla priauera e durano
semp̃ biãche dẽtro ma ñ hão odore
arõatico ne sapore dolce se trouão
solo al tpo del caldo. e q̃sti ñ sõ odo
riferi ne saporosi se nõ al tpo fredo
cioe dalo autũno p fino al pricipio
dela primauera. tordo tortora testi
culo i capitulo dla carne.

Ve son cõcordi tuti li aucto
ri le vue ele fiche bẽ mature
essere meliori d tuti altri fru
cti e ppriamẽte ñ nocibili la vua ma
tura gnã laudabile sangue e ppria
mẽte se stara colta almãco doi di inã
zi pche mãzãdose la vua subito qñ
e colta e iflatiua e gnã pezori e piu
crudi hũori sela vua se padisse ben
ingrassa la scorza de la vua e fre
dae secha e de difficile digestione
e li soi azini simelmente: ma la
polpa facilmente se padisse. E se
li azini se ingiotiscono integri e so
no del corpo senza fare nocumen
to impero li azini non sono da ma
sticare con li denti per che se mes
chiarano con la polpa donde faria
pezore nutrimẽto e chi piu vue mã
za primamente li soi corpi son pur
gati da superflui humori e poi in
grassano dela qual cossa li ortulani
dicono il vero che i vna cosa quasi
trouano che piu li ingrasseno ch al
tẽpo di fichi e dele vue qualle man
zão assai ñ dimẽo la grasseza facta
p vue e fichi tosto se risolue per che
generão carne infiata e molle.

Va passa ha cõformitade cõ
le vue che se fano sechare p
ch cõe varietade ne le vue i
dolceza i austeritade i põticitad cos
si e nele vue passe la vua passa piu
dolce sono d piu dolce vue el auste
re dle austere e q̃lle ch sono piu dol
ce dclinão acalidita te secõdo mazo
re o minor dolceza e cõo alcũe vue
hãno azini e alcũe ñ cossi sono simel
mẽte le passe dõde qñ e comãdato
riceuer vue passe enucleate nui pos
semo intẽdere vue passe senza azini
o che da loro sião enucleate e caza
te fora nõ e nele vue passe grãde di
ferẽtia o che sia d vue grãde o pico
le e q̃lle sono miglior e dolce e gras
se ch hãno la scorza sutile zouão as
sai e son conforme al fidego e remo
ueno le soe opilatiõe e confortão la
digestiõe del sangue e curando p le
soe vertude el fluxo epatico cõfortã
do el fidego e la milza apre le vie d
le rene e de la uesicha confortando
le rene e la vesicha e piu nutrisse la
vua passa ch la vua fresca e e d me
liore nutrimẽto cõferisce al pulmõe
e ala tosse e ala difficultade del ane
lito tẽgono il vẽtre humido nõdimẽo
ben che tute le vue passe siano ami
che al stomaco e al fidego le austere
cõfortano piu el stomaco che le dol

e

Figs. 1.2–1.4. Comparison between layouts adopted for the sections on food in Benzi, *Tractato* (1508) (Fig. 2.1); Pisanelli, *Trattato della natura de' cibi* (1587, 1st edn. 1584) (Fig. 1.3); and Durante, *Il tesoro* (1616, 1st edn. 1586), showing advice on grapes (Fig. 1.4).

2 DELLA NATVRA

FICHI.

Elettione. PRima i bianchi, ſecondariamente i roſſi, & vltimamente i negri: perche quei che hanno la ſcorza ſottile, ſono piu digeſtibili; ma tutti ſenza ſcorza, mondi, netti, & maturi.

Giouamẽti Nutriſcono ottimamente, purgano le reni dalla renella, preſeruano dal veleno, e nutriſcono piu de gli altri frutti, cauano la ſete, e nettano il petto.

Nocumẽti Generano ventoſità quando ſe ne mangiano molti: e però offendono lo ſtomaco a quei che patiſcono dolori colici, e che ſono pieni di crudità.

Rimedio. Mangiandoſi appreſſo granati, ò aranci acetoſi, ouero altri cibi che ſiano conditi con l'aceto.

Gradi. Sono caldi nel primo grado, & humidi nel ſecondo.

Tempi, Etadi, Cõpleſſioni Sono buoni in tutti i tempi, maſſime nell'Autunno. A tutte l'etadi, eccetto che a' vecchi, & a tutte le compleſſioni, ma che ſiano ben maturi.

VVA.

Elettione MAtura, bianca, dolce, e che ſia di ſcorza ſottile: perche paſſa piu preſto, e genera manco ventoſità.

Giouamẽti Nutriſce ottimamente, fa ingraſſare preſto, rinfreſca il fegato infiammato, & prouoca l'orina, & accreſce il coito.

Nocumẽti Apporta ſete, fa ventoſità, conturba il ventre, & genera dolori colici, quando ſe ne mangia aſſai: & fa gonfiare, & dolere la milza.

Rimedio. Mangiandoſi appreſſo alcuna coſa ſalata, e granati, ò aranci, ò altri cibi acetoſi, ouero che ſiano con l'aceto conditi.

Gradi. E calda nel primo grado, & humida nel ſecondo: ma temperatamente, e ſenza eceſſo.

Tempi, Etadi, Cõpleſſioni E buona nell'Autunno, e nel Verno. & ſe ſi mangia con miſura e modo, gioua a tutte le compleſſioni, & etadi, eccetto che a' uecchi, perche gli accreſce il catarro.

DE' CIBI 3

HISTORIE NATVRALI.

I Fichi non nutriſcono quãto i grani, e la carne, ma piu de gli altri frutti, e piu preſto. Quando incominciano à maturare, moſtrano il latte; quando ſono maturi, il formento; e quando ſono maturiſſimi, il mele. Sono compoſti di ſeme, ſcorza, e carne. Il ſeme non nutriſce, anzi è di natura di pietra. La ſcorza è dura da digerirſi. Ma la carne nutriſce aſſai. Appreſſo loro ſi beue l'acqua freſca, perche ſono caldi, sì come appreſſo i frutti freddi ſi beue il vino. Ingraſſano, leuano il mal colore, giouano al coito; e quando ſono affatto maturi, ſono ancora del tutto ſenza pericolo. I ſecchi giouano alla toſſe, e perche ſono glutinoſi, ſi mangiano con le noci, ò con le mandorle, che coſì ſi fanno piu apperitiui, e piu ſani. Purgano le reni che ſono ſane, e non quelle che ſono vlcerate dalla viſcoſità, ma ſono alquanto ventoſi. Sono caldi nel ſecondo grado, e ſecchi nel mezzo del primo. A molti prouocano il ſudore, & generano pidocchi. Queſto arbore per la poca radice preſto inuecchia, & il frutto non ha neſſun'odore.

SI deue guardare l'huomo d'inghiottire la ſcorza, & i granelli, che ſono dẽtro l'vua, perche impediſcono la digeſtione, e tardano il deſcendere de gli eſcrementi. Nõ ſi ci beua appreſſo acqua che ſia con neue, perche genera dolori colici. L'vua bianca ſi loda piu della negra, perche è piu penetrabile; e ſe per alcuni giorni ſtarà colta, & appeſa, perderà la ventoſità, e diuerrà migliore. Quãto ella è piu matura, è anco di minor nutrimento. Che l'vua nutriſca ne fanno fede i guardiani delle vigne, che p un pezzo non mangiano altri cibi. Ella gioua ancora al petto, et al polmone. L'vua paſſa dolce ingraſſa il fegato che è ſano, ma nuoce a quello ch'è duro, e coſì alla milza: gioua allo ſtomaco, & a' dolori de gl'inteſtini, alle reni & alla veſica; apre l'opilationi, e ſtringe aſſai. Quella che ha dell'acerbo, nutriſce meno, e ſtringe il corpo. Quella che non ha granelli, è migliore dell'altre, & è ottima per il petto, e per la toſſe.

A 2

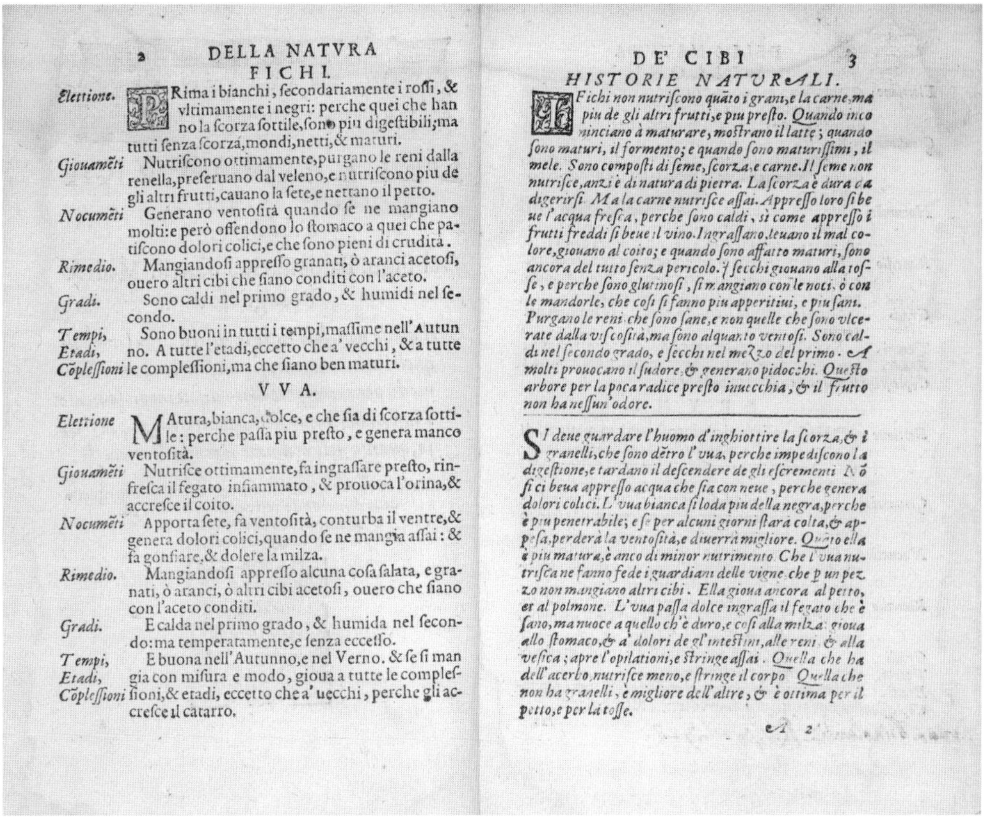

Fig. 1.3.

Like Boldo, Durante also included an alphabetic list of contents. In this way he produced a brief, straightforward, user-friendly guide which nonetheless also displayed its scholarly credentials through the use of the tabular or grid format, common among scientists.[55]

Many medical authors of regimens, and certainly the most successful ones, already had experience of the publishing world when they produced their first regimen. Durante's highly successful *Herbario* came out just a year before his *Tesoro*. It integrated many elements from Pietro Andrea Mattioli's 1544 herbal so this was yet again a text more innovative in form than in contents, thanks in particular to its rich visual apparatus.[56] Authors of regimens belonged to that large category of doctors who boasted a wide and varied body of academic interests, stretching from literature to philosophy, from

[55] Swan, 'From Blowfish', 122–8.

[56] Durante, *Herbario*. He was also the author of a treatise on food in Latin, two treatises on theological and religious subjects, as well as some poetry, and had rendered two books of the *Aeneid* in verse.

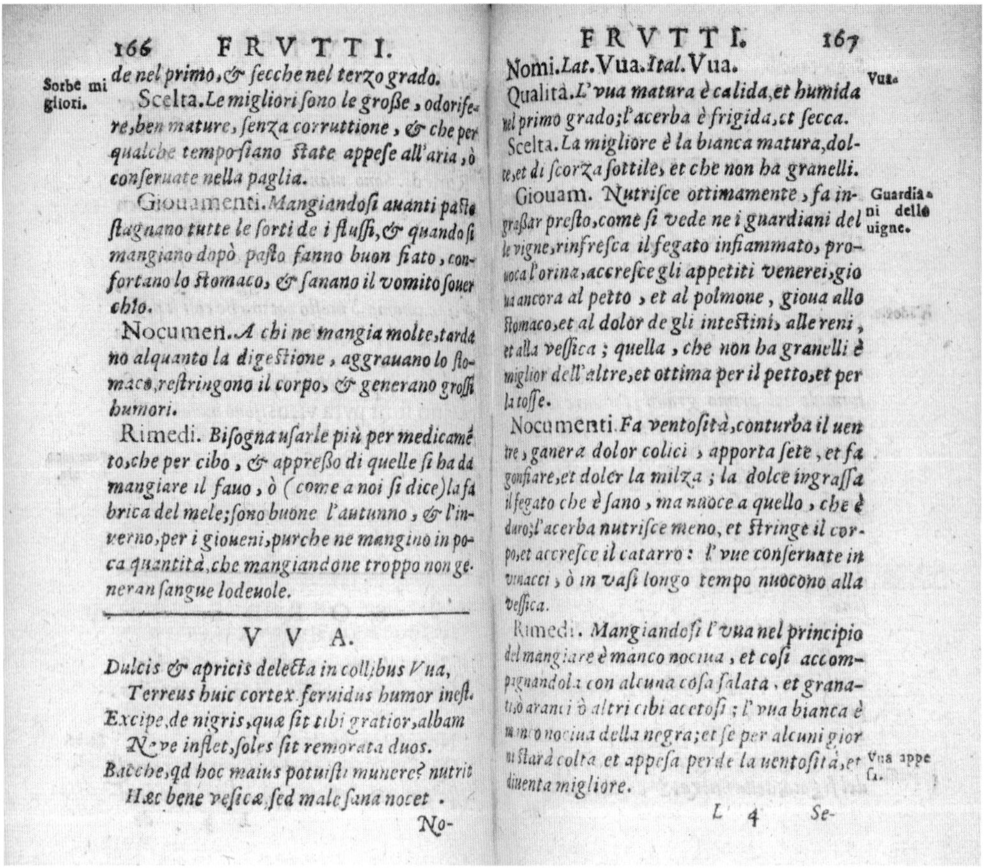

166 FRVTTI.

Sorbe migliori.

de nel primo, & secche nel terzo grado.

Scelta. Le migliori sono le grosse, odorife-re, ben mature, senza corruttione, & che per qualche tempo siano state appese all'aria, ò conservate nella paglia.

Giovamenti. Mangiandosi avanti pasto stagnano tutte le sorti de i flussi, & quando si mangiano dopò pasto fanno buon fiato, confortano lo stomaco, & sanano il vomito soverchio.

Nocumen. A chi ne mangia molte, tarda no alquanto la digestione, aggravano lo stomaco, restringono il corpo, & generano grossi humori.

Rimedi. Bisogna usarle più per medicame-to, che per cibo, & appresso di quelle si ha da mangiare il savo, ò (come a noi si dice) la fabrica del mele; sono buone l'autunno, & l'inverno, per i giovani, purche ne mangino in poca quantità, che mangiandone troppo non generan sangue lodevole.

V V A.

Dulcis & apricis delecta in collibus Vua,
Terreus huic cortex feruidus humor inest.
Excipe, de nigris, quæ sit tibi gratior, albam
Nive inflet, soles sit remorata duos.
Bacche, qd hoc maius potuisti munere? nutrit
Hæc bene vesicæ, sed male sana nocet .

No-

FRVTTI. 167

Nomi. Lat. Vua. Ital. Vua.

Vua.

Qualità. L'uua matura è calida, et humida nel primo grado; l'acerba è frigida, et secca.

Scelta. La migliore è la bianca matura, dolce, et di scorza sottile, et che non ha granelli.

Giovam. Nutrisce ottimamente, fa in-grassar presto, come si vede ne i guardiani del-le vigne, rinfresca il fegato infiammato, provoca l'orina, accresce gli appetiti venerei, gio-ua ancora al petto, et al polmone, giova allo stomaco, et al dolor de gli intestini, alle reni, et alla vessica; quella, che non ha granelli è miglior dell'altre, et ottima per il petto, et per la tosse. — *Guardia-ni delle uigne.*

Nocumenti. Fa ventosità, conturba il ven-tre, ganera dolor colici, apporta sete, et fa gonfiare, et doler la milza; la dolce ingrassa il fegato che è sano, ma nuoce a quello, che è duro; l'acerba nutrisce meno, et stringe il corpo, et accresce il catarro: l'uue conservate in vinacci, ò in vasi longo tempo nuocono alla vessica.

Rimedi. Mangiandosi l'uua nel principio del mangiare è manco nociua, et così accompagnandola con alcuna cosa salata, et grana-to, aranci ò altri cibi acetosi; l'uua bianca è manco nociua della negra; et se per alcuni gior ni starà colta, et appesa perde la ventosità, et diuenta migliore. — *Vua appe-sa.*

L 4　Se-

Fig. 1.4.

theology to history.[57] Some of them however, had also engaged with highly commercial titles in the fields of sensationalist literature and books of secrets. Pisanelli had not only published a plague tract in vernacular (1577), which included a section on secrets, and a commentary on Aristotle in Latin but had also penned two pamphlets on unusual meteorological events that had occurred in Rome: the appearance of a 'fire dragon' on the night of 29 January 1575 and that of a comet in May 1582. Basilio Paravicino, the editor and translator of Petronio's Latin regimen, was also author of some curious and erudite works in vernacular such as the celebrated *Discorso sul riso* (a discourse on laughter).

These observations suggest that the gulf separating medical authors from learned polygraphs who, as we have seen had been instrumental in the first wave

---

[57] On this composite profile of the 16th-century physician see Siraisi, *The Clock*; Maclean, 'Girolamo Cardano'; and, more broadly, De Renzi, 'Medical Competence'.

of propagation of health advice literature in vernacular, was no longer as wide as in the first decades of the sixteenth century. Like professional writers, many of our doctors were complex intellectual figures, their interests extending well beyond medicine to many fields of knowledge. Moreover, like the polygraphs, they were conversant with the economic logic of the book market and undoubtedly, the longing for the fame and financial rewards that publishing success could bring must have been a powerful motivation behind the decision to compile, translate, or edit a regimen.

Patrons, too, were not indifferent to the lure of print. Associating one's name with a successful regimen would have brought recognition to the sponsor of the work, as well as to the author. Although difficult to trace, the role of the patron was crucial in enabling the publication of a regimen. Unusually, this is illustrated in some detail in the dedications accompanying Viviani's regimen (1626). The unexpected death of his patron, Cardinal Orsini, while the book was at the press, led Viviani to seek instead the patronage of the deceased's brothers to support the promotion of the forthcoming book. At the same time he still wished to capitalize on the great man's favour and hence attached two letters received from the cardinal to the regimen. These gave an account of the process that led to its publication and from them we learn that the work had been commissioned (and presumably funded) by the cardinal and then read to him for approval before being sent to the press. Moreover, the cardinal had a say in the choice of the place of publication (Venice), on the regimen format (portable, 'to put in a bag') and on the style adopted by the work. The letters also reveal the dual motivation underpinning the cardinal's support. He was persuaded that the work would 'bring great acclaim' ('apporterá gran grido') to the author and in the meantime would boost his own reputation as an agent of a valuable cultural enterprise. Hence he was planning to donate a copy, fresh from the printers, to His Holiness the Pope, presumably hoping to impress the pontiff with the work of his protégé.[58]

THE READERS

Printed vernacular guides to healthy living were therefore a lively genre, and the increasing number of new titles and re-editions clearly reflected a widespread demand for preventive knowledge which regimens themselves in turn helped to stimulate. It is also quite evident that printed health advice was not intended for the specific complexion (individual balance of humours which determines one's predisposition to illness) of a named patron or dedicatee, as has sometimes been argued. Far from being rules *ad personam* the recommendations outlined in these works had a universal value. Indeed, as we have seen in the case of Cardinal Orsini, the motivations of the patron in promoting the publication of a regimen were related precisely to the expectation of a general appreciation of the work, which

---

[58] Viviani, *Trattato*, 2–3. Other texts that reveal they have been commissioned by a patron are Boldo, *Libro della natura* and the translation of Petronio, *Del viver*.

would also reflect positively upon the image of the patron. Savonarola's regimen, written in the mid-fifteenth century and dedicated to Lionello d'Este, is the only case we have come across which includes some references to the specific habits and needs of the dedicatee, possibly due to the fact that it pre-dates the age of print and was not intended for wide circulation. This work has been seen to be part of a broader genre of personalized regimens which developed in the court environment in the fifteenth century.[59] Even in this case, however, the references to Lionello's complexion are very few and marginal to the narrative and by and large this text, too, carries a universal value and aims to provide advice valid for a large audience.

Overall, the discourse on complexion shifts from being centred on the individual to being structured around particular categories in the early modern age. Valentin Groebner has traced a sixteenth-century shift away from an idea of complexion based on one's individual internal disposition, that only the doctor could identify, to a group-based definition of complexion. According to this view one's physical constitution and psychological temperament were revealed by one's physiognomy (how one looked), and determined by astrological specificities (when one was born), and environmental factors (where one was born).[60] Our study of printed regimens confirms the prevalence of a taxonomic approach to complexion, though it high-lights the role of class, age, and place, rather than physiognomy and astrology, as the main criteria that presided over the definition of various complexions. Our analysis also suggests that the spread of print and the subsequent possibility of reaching a wider audience may have been a factor in this shift of attention from individual to group constitutions. The wish to make preventive literature appealing to a varied reading public, with diverse needs, meant that ideas of individual complexion lost their prominence. They were overshadowed by advice that in some cases differenti-ated between social classes, in others between age groups, and which in most cases paid considerable attention to locality when prescribing specific preventive meas-ures and particular models of healthy lifestyles. Another separate category often singled out in regimens is that of scholars, thought to have a particularly delicate complexion and thus to require an especially sober and moderate lifestyle.

However, despite their stated intentions of universality, the great majority of regimens actually explicitly addressed a privileged audience, as betrayed by the many references to the types of dwellings readers are expected to inhabit, and the objects and clothes they are meant to use. The idea that paying attention to one's health was essentially an activity undertaken by the well-to-do and was a distin-guishing sign of the intelligence and learning typical of the nobility was increas-ingly emphasized. Hence the advice given targeted those deemed to possess the moral virtues necessary to make good use of it. Ficino for example excludes the possibility that the lazy, 'inert', and dissolute could follow his advice. Paschetti makes explicit the assumption that only some social categories were capable of looking after their health.[61] Promoting healthy living was therefore constructed in

[59] Nicoud, *Les Régimes*, 341–51; Crisciani, 'Histories', 308.
[60] Groebner, '*Complexio*/Complexion'.
[61] Ficino, *De le tre vite*, 29ʳ; Paschetti, *Del conservar.*

some regimens as a genteel pastime. In Paschetti's, every evening a number of gentlemen who have undertaken a journey together with their doctor (the author) sit down and talk about their health and the best way to improve it. Nonetheless, as we shall see in the course of our analysis, some seventeenth-century regimens rejected this paradigm, criticizing the unhealthy habits of courtiers and the life-styles of nobles, and demonstrating that they were addressing the concerns of a larger audience and were sensitive to class tensions.[62]

As well as being socially distinct, the audience addressed in regimens is by and large a male one. Only a very small number of regimens include occasional advice for women, and this is systematically related to the specific needs of pregnant women. The physiology of the female body was understood as being determined by women's reproductive functions and hence women had their own genre of pre-ventive advice literature, specifically tailored to managing women's health. These texts were organized entirely around the promotion of fertility and the health of mother and child during pregnancy and after childbirth. The advice given was, however, comprehensive and holistic, including the necessary information pertain-ing to all the Non-Naturals for any given 'female' disorders according to a woman's constitution. The first of these works was written by Doctor Michele Savonarola in the late fifteenth century but was only available as a manuscript. However, much of part III of Marinelli's very successful *Le medicine partinenti alle infermitá delle donne*, first printed in 1563, was drawn word for word from Savonarola's text.[63] It was structured in short question-and-answer style, rather like the popular regimen by Manfredi. Scipione Mercurio also published a similar guide to women's health and midwifery in 1596, *La commare*, which went through many editions.[64]

However, just as the appeal of regimens extended beyond the socially privileged groups represented in the text, so women may have been drawn to read them, which may explain why some were actually dedicated to noblewomen. Signifi-cantly, Durante dedicated his best-selling *Tesoro* to Camilla Peretti, sister of Pope Sisto V, suggesting that she should use the treatise under the supervision of her personal physician.[65] Moreover, it is possible that dedicating a book to a woman had the effect of encouraging others of her sex to read it, as some scholars have argued.[66] The involvement of a woman patron may therefore be seen as another strategic choice aimed at expanding the book's potential readership.

Although we lack direct evidence for the existence of a female readership of regimens, we can infer from the presence of these texts in many households that they were at least physically accessible to many women. In fact if we shift our attention from intended to actual readerships we observe that regimens feature among the books of a relatively large range of social groups. Indeed the evidence from the few surviving inventories of private libraries that include the titles of books points to a wide social distribution of owners of regimens—certainly wider

[62] See esp. Fonseca, *Del conservare* and Frediano, *Arca novella*.
[63] Marinelli, *Le medicine*. See Bell's discussion of the genre in *How to Do It*, esp. 93.
[64] Mercurio, *La commare*. See Bell, *How to Do It*, chs. 2–3.
[65] Some editions of Rangoni's regimen (see n. 32) and Salando's *Trattato* were also dedicated to women.
[66] Richardson, *Printing*, 218.

than the background of dedicatees and the declared targeted readers would imply.[67]
It comes as no surprise to find the regimen by the Paduan doctor Salando (1607)
and two contributions to the debate on the effects of cold and hot drinking (by
Meyden, 1608 and Cassiani, 1603) in the library of Vincenzo Giustiniani, a
nobleman and scholar. But a best-seller like Durante's regimen had a much wider
distribution, being found among the books of professionals (lawyers and notaries)
and administrative staff of the city of Parma, and even of humble parish priests,
at the turn of the seventeenth century.[68] Still in Parma, in the period 1623–80, we
encounter Durante once again and another best-seller, Pisanelli's tract on food, as
well as Savonarola's regimen and the more popular *Il perché* by Manfredi, amongst
the books owned by theologians, physicians, and other untitled citizens, of
unknown occupation. Two noblemen owned the regimen by Viviani (1626),
while the thick vernacular translation of Galen's *De tuenda sanitatis* (*Di Galeno*,
1549) is found among the very few books possessed by the Florentine apothecary
Mario Vetri in 1591[69]

   These examples of ownership also document the geographical spread of interest
in the preventive genre, which extended beyond the main sites of the printing
industry to provincial towns, something confirmed by the conspicuous presence of
vernacular regimens in the stock held by booksellers. Among the books on sale at
the Perin bookshop in Vicenza on 1 July 1596 we find 'Arnaldo da Villanova' (presumably the *Opera utilissima* attributed to Arnau); Manfredi's *Il perché*; Romoli's
work with Grospré's regimen appended; the ubiquitous Durante; and just one regimen in Latin (*De conservanda bona valetudine*).[70] As many as sixteen copies of a
book entitled *Del conservar la sanità,* about which we know nothing more, are
present in the shop inventory of the Verona bookseller Bochino, compiled in
1586.[71] In religious houses regimens are also common in smaller localities, where
the friars were perhaps a vehicle for the dissemination of the ideals of preventive
health: in the mid-sixteenth century for example, the library of the monastery of
Rivalta Scrivia (near Tortona) contained Manfredi's work.[72]

   Occasional annotations on the cover or back of regimens now preserved in public libraries confirm they were also possessed by common people, outside the circle
of nobles and the medical profession. A 1629 edition of Manfredi's *Libro del perché,* for example, bears on the first page the note 'today 4 August 1653, this book
belongs to Francesco Moni from Pistoia, husband of Lavinia'.[73] One of the two
copies of Bertaldi's regimen (1620) in the Turin National Library had three

   [67] Very rarely household inventories give book titles, more frequently they simply list the number
of books, sometimes classified broadly by subject.
   [68] Danesi Squarzina, *La collezione Giustiniani*, vol. i. *Inventari I*, 382: the inventory was made in
1638. Dallasta, *Eredità di carta*, 166.
   [69] Dallasta, *Eredità di carta*, 238–9 and 242; Perini, 'Libri'.
   [70] Mantese, *I mille libri*, 41.
   [71] Carpané, 'Libri', 218. Many of the books were not inventoried by title but by type; e.g. '49
books in 4° of different kinds'; '65 in 8°'; and 'Greek authors'.
   [72] Rozzo (ed.), *Biblioteche*, 179.
   [73] 'adi 4 di agosto 1653 Questo Libbro e di Francesco Moni di Pistoia Lavinia Conjux'. This is in
the Angelica Library in Rome, quoted in von Tippelskirch, *Letture*, 55.

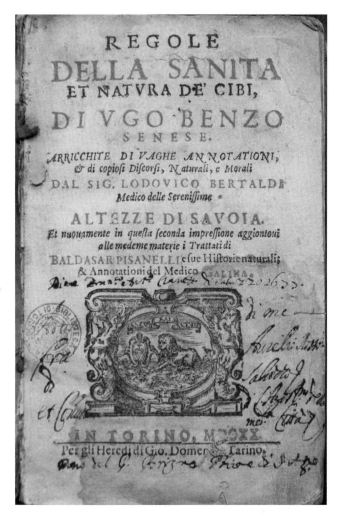

Figs. 1.5.–1.6. The long life of regimens is suggested by these three annotations to Bertaldi's (1620). There are two sets of handwriting on the frontispiece, which translate as: 'This belongs to Friar Aurelio Rosso from the friary of S. Augustine in Saluzzo, a gift from Father Brigna, Prior of S. Augustine, 1654', and: 'This belongs to Francesco Antonio Cravetto from Saluzzo, 1677' (Fig. 1.5). On the back cover we read: 'This book was given to me, Friar Aurelio Rosso from Saluzzo by Mister Gioachino Ganibaudi this year, 1654, on the 18th of June, to pray to God in his memory' (Fig. 1.6).

(possibly four) subsequent owners. One was an Augustinian friar from the small town of Saluzzo, who had been given it by the Father Prior of the same monastery in 1654, another was a common man, a certain Francesco Antoni, also from Saluzzo, who wrote his signature in it in 1677.[74] Then on the book's last, blank page we find

[74] 'Di me Frà Aurelio Rosso di Saluzzo e conventuale di S. Agostino della medesima Città, dono del padre Brigna Priore di S. Agostino 1654; Di me Francesco Antonio Cravetto di Saluzzo 1677'.

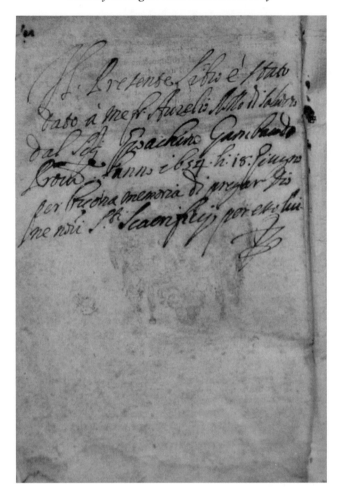

Fig. 1.6.

indication of a fourth owner, a layman called Gioachino Ganibaudi, who bequeathed the book requesting the beneficiary to pray for his soul (see Figs. 1.5 and 1.6).[75]

The dates of ownership inscribed on these copies also demonstrate the long life of these books. The first example shows that Manfredi's regimen, printed in 1629, was still circulating twenty-four years later, and the second, that Bertaldi's work was still changing owners and being donated or bequeathed fifty-seven years after it appeared in print. When we try to establish the extent of the readership for these books we should therefore bear in mind that they were not associated only with single, individual readers but often with several subsequent readers. We also find evidence of shared ownership—that is of multiple readers having simultaneous

---

[75] 'Il presente libro è stato dato a me Frate Aurelio Rosso di Saluzzo dal signor Gioachino Ganibaudi corr. anno 1654 li 18 giugno per buona memoria di pregar Dio nei nostri sacrifici per esso lui'.

access to the same book. Books, in fact, were often not owned individually but collectively, by groups of friends and colleagues. Angela Nuovo has drawn attention to the formula *et amicorum* that scholars penned on the frontispiece of their manuscripts in the fifteenth century, next to the signature of possession. The habit of collective book ownership reflected the humanist ideal of sharing knowledge that was perceived as the first duty of the true scholar; Nuovo suggests that the practice might have extended to the following century and to the printed book.[76] Indeed we have encountered an example of this in the copy of Ficino's regimen (1548) held by Cambridge University Library (see Fig. 1.7).

There was not only collective use of some regimens but use could be protracted over time. The numerous annotations, some of them dated, found on the copy of Lennio's regimen in the British Library, offer evidence of use by the same reader at different stages and over a very long stretch of time (1602, 1619, 1620, and 1641), suggesting that the book was still being read and commented on nearly eighty years after its first printing. The annotations include citations from Pliny, observations about the text, and pointing finger signs added on the margins signal elements of interest. Elsewhere the same hand makes a note of the pages where certain facts or subjects are discussed, showing that the reader wants to refer back to these passages. Long recommendations about how to prepare and use wine to preserve teeth, and health in general, are then added on the index page which notes the virtues of wine. Similar marks in the margins, page references, and observations are to be found in many other regimens still held in our libraries, revealing the very active reading to which these books were subjected (see for example Fig. 1.8).[77]

THE DISSEMINATION OF PREVENTIVE ADVICE: BOOKS FOR THE HOME

The vitality of this culture of prevention can also be gauged by the extent to which health advice was disseminated through a variety of ostensibly non-medical genres that became popular in this period: texts of a practical, technical nature that provided instructions for making things in the domestic environment (in particular remedies and recipes for meals); and various treatises that set out the rules for the regulation of different aspects of household management. In both cases we are dealing with texts that address the home and its inhabitants.[78]

A know-how genre that developed in close parallel with regimens is recipe books. In the Italian peninsula the first such texts were published in the 1520s, and some of them, such as the slim *Dificio di ricette* (1525) or the more substantial *Secreti del reverendo donno Alessio Piemontese* (1557), went through several editions.[79] Recipe

---

[76] Nuovo, '"Et Amicorum"'.

[77] See e.g. the copies of Paschetti's regimen at Cambridge University Library, of the 1558 edition of Cornaro's at the British Library, and of Pictorius' at the Turin National library.

[78] See Dennis's remarks in her 'Representing', 30–3.

[79] *Opera nuova intitolata Dificio di ricette* and Piemontese, *Secreti*. This was translated into six languages, including English, within a few years of its first appearance, and then frequently reprinted. On these texts, Tessa Storey, 'Italian Books'; and Eamon, *Science*, ch. 4.

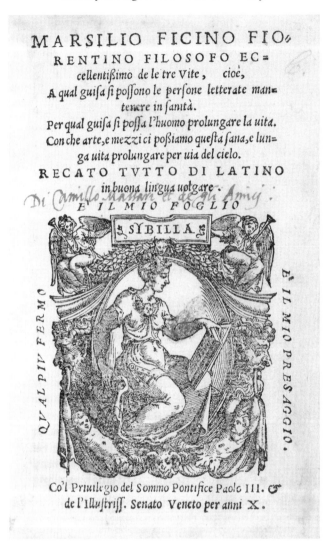

Fig. 1.7. The note: '*Di Camillo Massara et de gli amicj*' (This belongs to Camillo Massara and friends) on this frontispiece to Ficino's regimen is evidence of collective ownership.

books or books of secrets were collections of recipes for making both remedies for the treatment of a variety of health disorders and products for the daily care of the household and the body. While recipes for preserving food are also common, in the sixteenth-century Italian texts culinary recipes are notably absent. At first sight recipe books and regimens differed both in terms of authorship and form: the books of secrets were not written by doctors and did not include advice about healthy lifestyles, only practical instructions for producing various kinds of remedies and other, often health-related substances. Regimens by contrast are advice

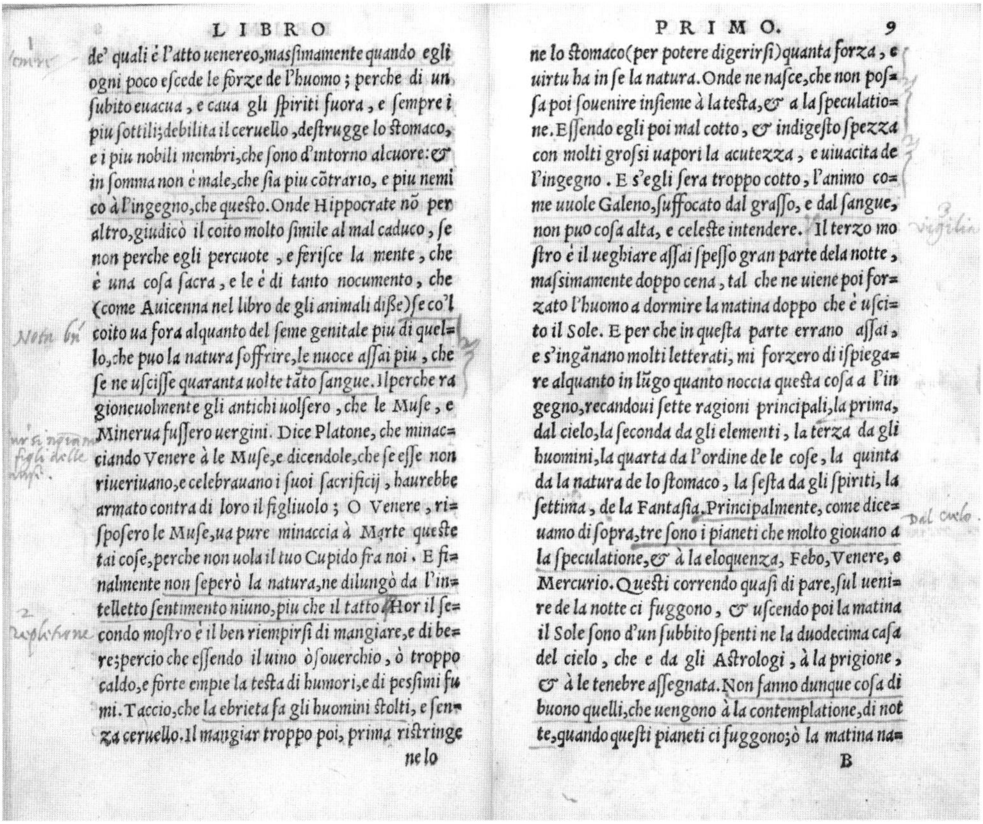

LIBRO

de' quali è l'atto uenereo, massimamente quando egli ogni poco escede le forze de l'huomo; perche di un subito euacua, e caua gli spiriti fuora, e sempre i piu sottili; debilita il ceruello, destrugge lo stomaco, e i piu nobili membri, che sono d'intorno al cuore: e in somma non è male, che sia piu cōtrario, e piu nemi co à l'ingegno, che questo. Onde Hippocrate nō per altro, giudicò il coito molto simile al mal caduco, se non perche egli percuote, e ferisce la mente, che è una cosa sacra, e le è di tanto nocumento, che (come Auicenna nel libro de gli animali disse) se co'l coito ua fora alquanto del seme genitale piu di quello, che puo la natura soffrire, le nuoce assai piu, che se ne uscisse quaranta uolte tāto sangue. Iperche ra gioneuolmente gli antichi uolsero, che le Muse, e Minerua fussero uergini. Dice Platone, che minacciando Venere à le Muse, e dicendole, che se esse non riueriuano, e celebrauano i suoi sacrificij, haurebbe armato contra di loro il figliuolo; O Venere, risposero le Muse, ua pure minaccia à Marte queste tai cose, perche non uola il tuo Cupido fra noi. E finalmente non seperò la natura, ne dilungò da l'intelletto sentimento niuno, piu che il tatto. Hor il secondo mostro è il ben riempirsi di mangiare, e di bere; percio che essendo il uino ò souerchio, ò troppo caldo, e forte empie la testa di humori, e di pessimi fu mi. Taccio, che la ebrieta fa gli huomini stolti, e senza ceruello. Il mangiar troppo poi, prima ristringe

ne lo

PRIMO. 9

ne lo stomaco (per potere digerirsi) quanta forza, e uirtu ha in se la natura. Onde ne nasce, che non possa poi souenire insieme à la testa, e à la speculatione. Essendo egli poi mal cotto, e indigesto spezza con molti grossi uapori la acutezza, e uiuacita de l'ingegno. E s'egli sera troppo cotto, l'animo come uuole Galeno, suffocato dal grasso, e dal sangue, non puo cosa alta, e celeste intendere. Il terzo mo stro e il ueghiare assai spesso gran parte dela notte, massimamente doppo cena, tal che ne uiene poi forzato l'huomo a dormire la matina doppo che è uscito il Sole. E per che in questa parte errano assai, e s'ingānano molti letterati, mi forzero di ispiegare alquanto in lūgo quanto noccia questa cosa a l'in gegno, recandoui sette ragioni principali, la prima, dal cielo, la seconda da gli elementi, la terza da gli huomini, la quarta da l'ordine de le cose, la quinta da la natura de lo stomaco, la sesta da gli spiriti, la settima, de la Fantasia. Principalmente, come diceuamo di sopra, tre sono i pianeti che molto giouano a la speculatione, e à la eloquenza, Febo, Venere, e Mercurio. Questi correndo quasi di pare, sul uenire de la notte ci fuggono, e uscendo poi la matina il Sole sono d'un subito spenti ne la duodecima casa del cielo, che e da gli Astrologi, à la prigione, e à le tenebre assegnata. Non fanno dunque cosa di buono quelli, che uengono à la contemplatione, di not te, quando questi pianeti ci fuggono; ò la matina na

B

Fig. 1.8. A reader's marginalia which draws attention to passages on the dangers of excessive sexual intercourse, overeating, and drinking.

books and although they occasionally include a few recipes these remain a marginal element in the texts. The only case of a real conflation of the two genres is represented by the highly successful *Breue compendio*, written by Domenico Auda, apothecary at the hospital of Santo Spirito in Rome (the book had at least twenty-one editions up to 1776). Here the recipes occupy two-thirds of the book, while 170 out of 336 pages consist of a very simple regimen.

Yet, despite their distinctive features, regimens and books of secrets to some extent shared similar concerns since the latter also contained recipes for making a range of preparations (ointments, elixirs, etc.) which were not aimed at treating specific ailments but at protecting the health and vitality of various parts of the body. This component has been overlooked in recent analyses of the genre that have largely focused on therapeutic remedies and culinary recipes.[80] Yet non-curative

---

[80] For a critique of this approach Cavallo, 'Secrets'. Research on this genre has been carried out especially in the English context. Among the many works, Leong and Pennell, 'Recipe Collection'; and the essays in Leong and Rankin (eds.), *Secrets*.

recipes were numerous. Less than a third of the 350 or so recipes that make up the first edition of Alessio Piemontese's frequently reprinted *I secreti* are therapeutic, and the others are largely concerned with the making of products relevant to the complex management of the early modern household and safeguarding its members' health.[81] The many recipes for purifying the ambient air or for perfuming bodies, clothing, and furnishings, and the dozen or so for maintaining and protecting skin, hair, teeth, and gums show that conserving health, and not just curing illness, lies at the heart of the collection and dissemination of Italian 'secrets'. Thus we find instructions for life-prolonging elixirs, for a powder that 'lengthens life', and another for a liqueur that 'conserves, strengthens, returns natural heat and energy, mak[ing] you vigorous of body, head, and mind, giving colour to the face and sweet breath, and keep[ing] you young and robust'.[82] More than has been acknowledged so far, therefore, books of secrets included secrets of healthy living.

Some of the preventive themes discussed in regimens are also dealt with in the cookery books that began to be published in the last decades of the fifteenth century. Even the title of the first cookbook printed in Italy: *De honesta voluptate et valitudine* (On Honest Pleasure and Health), indicates the concern for the impact of diet on health that was attracting growing attention in courtly environments in the fifteenth century. This collection of the culinary recipes by a famous chef, Martino from Como, was put together by the humanist scholar Bartolomeo Platina, curator of the Vatican Library and published in Latin in 1475, in the vernacular in 1478, and then reprinted several times in the following century. The text not only considers the effects of different foods on health but begins with ten short chapters of recommendations touching on how to choose a healthy place to live and on healthy ways of exercising the body, sleeping, eating, and having sex.[83]

The second important type of books that also contributed to the dissemination of the principles of preventive health is that of prescriptive literature. This category embraced a wide range of texts and fields of concern, from those outlining the rules that would regulate the correct running of the household and the management of servants, to those focusing on the duties expected of the male head of the family and of the young bride. The extraordinary development undergone by such books in the sixteenth and early seventeenth century was paralleled by the multiplication of treatises on domestic architecture that set out the principles for the construction of a decorous home. Though they have been discussed separately by scholars—as part of the history of food, the family, domestic service, or architecture—these treatises share to some extent similar purposes, testifying to the increased attention for the 'decorum' of the household as an organized and ordered hierarchical space. A well-regulated household was seen as a manifestation of the virtue of its head, capable of organizing his life and surroundings in a rational and harmonious way.

---

[81] Eamon, *Science*, 144–6.
[82] Piemontese, *Secreti*, 2 and 8, and *Dei secreti . . . Parte terza*, 5. The first edition only consisted of Part 1 of the work. Parts 2 and 3 were published in separate books in 1559, and Part 4 appeared in 1620.
[83] On this text Laurioux, *Gastronomie*.

An aspect that has so far been overlooked is that health occupies a significant place among the concerns expressed in these books, as they pay considerable attention to the salubriousness of the home and prescribe the hygienic and sanitary measures that should be adopted in everyday life. The well-run household is also a healthy household and prevention is among the duties expected of its members. This is certainly evident in architects' treatises, which, as we will see in Chapter 3, reveal the extent to which the professional vocabulary of this group and the design and location of houses were affected by health concerns.

Advice on conserving one's health is also a theme in the *libri dello scalco* or *del trinciante* (books of the steward or the carver) which flourished in Italy from the mid-sixteenth century for nearly a hundred years.[84] These are treatises on the rules regulating the preparation of food and table service compiled by stewards—the figures in charge of overseeing dining at the courts of popes, cardinals, and princes. As well as offering guidelines about choosing and preserving wine and food, the allocation of duties amongst kitchen staff and those serving at table, and the organization of banquets, these books provide dietary advice which is imbued with health concerns. Hence they discuss the effects of particular foods and recipes on the various humoral complexions, suggesting that, at least on paper, health considerations played a role in the design of menus. Some of these texts also contain sections on other Non-Naturals, in particular on the relationship between eating, exercising, and sleeping. For example, *Refugio over ammonitorio del gentiluomo*, which was written by Francesco Colle, the *scalco* of Duke Alfonso of Ferrara in 1533, includes advice about the health-giving qualities of certain foods and types of air, the benefits of certain kinds of exercise and ways of sleeping.[85] The subject of exercise, together with that of baths and frictions, is then developed in complete chapters and in greater detail in some editions of *La singolare dottrina*, authored by Domenico Romoli, *scalco* of Cardinal Ridolfi and then of Pope Paul III.[86]

The compilation of such books arose from the experience of serving at the flourishing princely courts of northern Italian rulers such as the Gonzagas, the Sforzas, and the Estes during the quattrocento, as well as at the increasing numbers of cardinal courts in Rome in the last decades of that century. By 1500 the cardinals' courts were already employing anything between 150 to more than 300 staff. This expansion brought with it the need for a rationalization of their tasks, and from 1550 the books of the *scalco* provided an apt medium for codifying the conventions of domestic service.[87] The circulation in printed form of this corpus of rules also met the demand generated by the Italian nobility more broadly. As an elite group in the process of defining an appropriate lifestyle for itself, it was eager to draw on court models and was starting, for example, to employ the services of the *scalco* and their staff in its banquets.

---

[84] On this genre Faccioli, 'La cucina'.   [85] Colle, *Refugio*.

[86] This is the same treatise which was published with an appended regimen of health by Robert Grospré. See n. 29.

[87] Fragnito, 'La trattatistica', esp. 137.

This quest to appropriate court ceremonial was also the driving force behind the development of another type of treatise, which dealt not only with the management of courtly dining but more widely with the rules which presided over the everyday running of a cardinal's court. Written by and for the *maestro di casa*, the official who oversaw the work of all the domestic staff in the household, these handbooks specified in minute detail the duties of the various employees, the salaries and food portions they were entitled to, and their expected physical and moral characteristics. In the process they conveyed notions of healthy living in various ways: they explained the hygienic precautions to be adopted by those in charge of cooking and serving meals; they warned the steward about harmful foods, encouraged him to devise diets that matched the complexion of his master, and praised the effects of exercise, recommending that the lord take it regularly. They even stipulated that the household physician should prescribe a rule of healthy living that would take into account not just their master's complexion and age but also the local climate.[88]

From the late sixteenth century onwards, the rules outlined in these tracts were no longer restricted to the environment of the cardinal's palace but directed—even in the wording of their titles—to any household of quality. The principles of healthy living promoted by these texts were therefore intended to reach a wider public of gentlefolk keen to organize their households according to the models codified at the courts of princes and cardinals.[89] And in fact the high number of re-editions of these handbooks, usually published in portable editions, suggests they were read and used well beyond the circle of cardinals' courts.

These texts on the ordered running of the court were complemented by books of instructions about the prudent management of the household directed to the paterfamilias—the *oeconomica* genre. Though the first treatises of this type appeared in the fifteenth century, penned by humanists, their production intensified after 1550, when they also acquired a different and broader meaning. While in the earlier period *oeconomica* texts could be seen as an aspect of the wider discussion on ideal political forms, from the mid-sixteenth century they appear to have been closely connected with the debate on what constituted nobility—a controversy of special significance in a period that witnessed a process of aristocratization of the urban patriciates. Hence, while in the first examples of the genre the household was perceived as a microcosm of political organization, and its correct ruling a metaphor for the health of the polity, in the following century a well-regulated household became an indication of the noble quality of its master and an expression of civilized behaviour.[90]

Books of household management cover many topics, from domestic economy to agronomy—an indication of the interest that urban patricians were now taking in increasing the profits from their landed properties.[91] But above all they aim to

---

[88] See e.g. Timotei, *Il cortegiano*, 101.
[89] On this literature and its audience see Fragnito, 'La trattatistica', 140, 180–2, and 171.
[90] Frigo, *Il padre di famiglia*, ch. 2; Romano, *Housecraft*, 3–21.
[91] Casali, '"Economica"', esp. 555–6.

define the responsibilities of each member of the family and household—husband, wife, children, and different ranks of servants—and how they should behave towards one another. Special attention is also given to manners and attitudes appropriate to the social standing, age, and gender of the person, including correct physical deportment or the clothes they should wear. These recommendations extend to preventive health prescriptions; for example, to the exercises most suitable to the different age groups and genders, reflecting the same distinctions we find in regimens.[92] But they also contain practical advice on how to make a house salubrious by orienting the building correctly as regards sun and wind, and through the layout and size of the rooms and windows.[93]

Sometimes the recommendations on wifely duties or the proper upbringing of offspring are conceived of as separate tracts. Treatises on the education of children in particular underwent a considerable expansion in the late sixteenth century. At this point, moreover, these handbooks appear to be increasingly imbued with Counter-Reformation values, so that the care of the soul acquires a central position and parents and tutors are depicted as spiritual guides whose primary duty is to teach children and subordinates to live according to the principles of the Catholic faith.[94] This religiously-inspired household management literature was penned by ecclesiastics—bishops or members of the regular clergy—but from the turn of the century even lay authors, like Lombardelli, increasingly subscribed to the ethos of what Silvano Razzi defines as 'Christian domestic economy' (*economica Cristiana*). One of the consequences of this transformation is that these texts appear to address a wider social audience than their predecessors, an audience now also made up of people of little means and ill-educated.[95] Lombardelli's aim, for example, is explicitly to address those who learn an 'art' or profession and attend a school or a workshop, while Antoniano's text was ordered to be read to parishioners in all Catholic churches in northern Italy.[96] These handbooks thus became yet another tool through which the post-Tridentine Church pursued its policy of Christianization.

However, physical health was not ignored; on the contrary, the care for and control of one's body was seen to fit the wider disciplinary programme promoted by the Counter-Reformation. This is manifest especially in the first tracts of this kind, which maintain a significant practical component, whereas in later works the care of the soul becomes so dominant that it occupies the majority of the treatise.[97] Several texts include sometimes very detailed recommendations about the management of emotions, hygiene routines, and desirable sleeping habits that are justified in health terms as well as moral terms, and closely follow the principles outlined in regimens.[98] Some authors, like Frigerio and Meduna, even

---

[92] For e.g. Piccolomini, *De la institutione*, III. 13 and X. 5; Paleario, *Dell'economia*, 64.

[93] e.g. Caggio, *Iconomica*, 57–8; Lanteri, *Della economica*, 35–9.

[94] Casali, '"Economica"', 557–9.

[95] Some, like Carroli, *Instrutione*, 563–71.

[96] Lombardelli, *De gli vfizii*, 210–15; on Antoniano, English, 'Physical Education', 236.

[97] Casali, '"Economica"', 559.

[98] On recommendations about hygiene Lombardelli, *De gli vifizii*, 150, 157, 159, 162–3, 210, 216–17, and *Il giovane studente*, 23; about sleep, Frigerio, *Arte*, 23–4, 32, and 39.

incorporate a mini-regimen in the script, which at several pages long is a summary of the basic prescriptions regarding all six Non-Naturals.[99] From the late sixteenth century, therefore, Counter-Reformation policy gave a significant boost to the dissemination of a preventive culture. Framed within a narrative of spiritual discipline and conveyed by authors who carried the moral authority of the Church, the message was now effectively reaching a wide and diverse social audience.

INSTRUCTIONS FOR THE ASPIRING GENTLEMAN

Another broad category of books that transmitted the ideals of preventive health were the manuals for the training of young gentlemen. In the sixteenth and early seventeenth centuries it was these texts which elaborated new codes of genteel life by describing in minute detail the behaviour and physical qualities that made a man noble. Simply by his appearance and conduct a gentleman was supposed to express the distance which lay not just between himself and manual workers but also between himself and the figure of the knight at arms with whom notions of chivalry were associated. These new codes of gentility boosted the growth of a culture of prevention in many ways. The focus on the physical characteristics of the gentleman brought with it renewed attention on the care the body required in order to appear to be perfect and glowing with health. Well-being was a precondition of gentility.

The reasons for the development of these new models of conduct for the gentleman are to be found in the profound social changes taking place in Italy during this period. The life of the nobility was undergoing a revolution, 'a real anthropological mutation' in Amedeo Quondam's words, which transformed the aspirations, values, physical appearance, and conduct and gestures associated with gentility.[100] Starting from the 1520s but with much more vigour after 1550—as the work of literary scholars has demonstrated—we see the development of a flourishing literature that elaborated detailed new codes of behaviour in all spheres of noble life. These treatises, which dealt with issues as varied as chivalric games, sports, conversation, duelling, letter-writing, playing cards or dice, dancing, and *villeggiatura*, contributed to forging a common noble identity and a class ideology for a group that was in actual fact heterogeneous because of the varied ways in which nobility was acquired in Italy. For a long time, in fact, in the states of northern and central Italy, rather than being a juridical condition nobility was defined by the exercise of power. Here a ruling class often defined by a trade, banking, or tax-farming background rather than by inherited rights and feudal property was regarded as 'noble' on the grounds of their political and civil status and of the moral and intellectual qualities demonstrated by involvement in public office.[101] Nor was the nobility a military class now that Italian society

[99] Frigerio, *Arte*, 122–4; and Meduna, *Lo scolare*, 48–53.
[100] Quondam, 'Elogio del gentiluomo', 19.
[101] Donati, *L'idea*, chs. 3–4.

was completely demilitarized. The largely mercantile urban elites had soon extricated themselves from military involvement (much earlier than the aristocracy in other European countries), and were happy to decide on and to finance wars, preferring however to use mercenaries rather than fight themselves.[102] Moreover, fearful of revolts, the ruling class had encouraged the disarming of urban militias by the early sixteenth century.[103]

This peculiar noble identity was challenged in various ways after the severe military defeat suffered in the Italian wars of the early sixteenth century and the development of dynastic powers in a number of states. At least at the level of ceremonial, these developments gave some impetus to the cultural models of the chivalric and feudal nobility common in the rest of Europe. The urban patriciates underwent a process of aristocratization: access to administrative offices and magistracies became hereditary and the number of gentlemen who received a stipend to participate in court life increased substantially. Institutions specifically devoted to the education of young nobles were created by the Jesuits. Any involvement in manual work and trade was disdained while financial investments in landed property, a tribute to the traditional association between the nobility and the land, grew considerably. Having time to kill became a value and the habit of spending long periods in the *villa* during the warmer weather was an imperative. Hence there was a need, paradoxically felt in Italy more than in the traditional strongholds of the feudal nobility, to codify in detail what it meant to live nobly through an extensive production of prescriptive texts.[104]

The long controversy about what constituted true nobility engaged writers for more than a century and created a synthesis between the humanistic ideal of civil nobility, based on moral and intellectual characteristics, and the aristocratic and military model imported from outside. Italian nobles became more similar to their European counterparts but also maintained distinctive qualities: nobility could derive from birth but should in any case be associated with virtue.[105] Though ideas of nobility as a natural condition that predisposes one to virtue were becoming more acceptable, these continued to be tempered by the uninterrupted polemics against noblemen who lived without purpose. Hence the importance of proving true noble status through a set of habits and attitudes in which grace, courtesy, agreeable manners, discretion, and measure in all domains figure highly. The defining qualities of the true nobleman were expressed through adherence to codified behavioural rules, and the display of discipline over the body and the emotions. In other words, the new definition of being noble placed considerable weight on physical manifestations of nobility, putting the body at centre stage: good health,

[102] Chittolini, 'Il "militare" ', 67–79.

[103] Chittolini, 'Il "militare" ', 67–79. The employment of mercenaries, common throughout the peninsula, was then a structural element in the Papal States, on which this study focuses. The reasons for the marginal involvement of Roman noblemen in the army are outlined by Brunelli, 'Identità'. See also his *Soldati*.

[104] For a specific example, Boutier, 'Le nobiltà del Gran Ducato', 213–17 and 221–4. More broadly see Donati, *L'idea*, chs. 4–5.

[105] Donati, *L'idea*, 151–74.

pulitezza in the triple sense of politeness, decorum, and cleanliness, and firm control of passions became instrumental in proving the quality of the person and his ability to manage his body rationally.

CONCLUSION

From the first decades of the sixteenth century onwards, more and more people came into contact with rules of healthy living articulated by printed vernacular texts. Advances in book distribution and the increased accessibility of regimens in terms of book format, cost, and presentation of contents were key factors in the growing popularity of this genre. Publishers and editors alike clearly regarded texts of this kind as highly marketable, aware that a large demand existed for preventive advice at all levels of society. Hence the genre soon differentiated its forms and styles of communication, providing basic as well as complex and scholarly instructions for a socially and intellectually diverse public increasingly anxious about its well-being. The contemporary success of recipe books that enabled people to produce their own recipes both for the treatment of the sick body and the maintenance of the healthy one, is another sign of the attention that laypeople were increasingly devoting to the care of their bodies and to creating healthy surroundings. After some hesitation, therefore, doctors abandoned their misgivings about vernacular medical writing and took on the role of protagonists in the authorship and editing of health-advice texts. The best-sellers within the genre were indeed penned by physicians, who often acquired their fame precisely thanks to the publishing success of their regimens. In a period in which people were becoming more proactive in their attempts to live a long and healthy life, doctors saw active participation in the preventive genre as a way of displaying their indispensable knowledge and reaffirming their authority in guiding patients to the correct way of taking care of their health. Hence they enthusiastically embraced the role of pedagogues that classical texts had attributed to physicians. By fashioning themselves as health advisers they participated in the growing economy of commercial medicine, not through selling remedies but through selling advice.

Besides medically authored works, however, various other types of texts appeared, imbued with the principles that regimens were disseminating in a more systematic way. Health advice very similar to that found in the specialized preventive literature was scattered in recipe and cookery books, in the handbooks for the organization of domestic service and for household management, and in conduct manuals—all genres that, like regimens, enjoyed significant publishing success especially in the second half of the sixteenth century and the early decades of the seventeenth. Initially aimed at the world of the court, these texts were increasingly directed to a larger stratum of noble and affluent householders as their popularity and expanded readership testify. Preventive knowledge was therefore reaching a wider range of social strata. The transformation of cultural models for the nobility and of genteel lifestyles that was taking place in Italian society was a driving force in the democratization of these genres. The increased attention to the appearance of the body that characterizes new models of gentility boosted the demand for healthy living advice, while the management of one's immediate environment, according to the prescriptions laid out by doctors, came to be seen as yet another sign of the superior rational faculties that a gentleman naturally possessed in large measure. These developments, however—and in particular the rise of a culture of leisure in which great attention was paid to physical appearance—also provoked the reactions of moralists, especially from within the ranks of the Counter-Reformation Church. A moral discourse emerged that increasingly pervaded advice literature in its various manifestations, and this had the effect of tempering the excesses to which indulgence in vanity may have led, promoting instead values of restraint and sobriety and a culture of well-being in which health remained important but was seen as an expression of self-discipline and inner harmony—in other words as a reflection of spiritual health.

2

Practices of Healthy Living: The Sources

The popularity of regimens certainly proves that readers were avid consumers of preventive advice. But were the recommendations put into practice? Is there any evidence of how deeply ideas about preventive health penetrated late Renaissance Italian society? And did suggestions about how to create a healthy domestic environment have any impact on homes and daily life—at least amongst the upper echelons of society? In this chapter we discuss the sources which we have used to explore these questions, starting by presenting a family from the seventeenth-century Roman elite, the Spada-Veralli family, and discussing their correspondence which we use extensively in our exploration of practices. A very recently ennobled family, the Spadas, and their network are representative of the kind of genteel society to which many authors of regimens addressed their texts, and of the backdrop of values and customs they had to take into account when they composed their rules of healthy living. The family's ascent from the ranks of provincial lords to the status of civic patricians and later to that of urban nobles, with significant positions at the papal court, exemplifies a trajectory of social mobility that was common at the time and proves yet again the fluidity of what constitutes nobility in early modern Italy. The ideas of gentility they embody were shared therefore by a larger stratum of the population, outside the ranks of the nobility, who aspired to achieve similar status or were brought into contact with the lifestyle of the elite through sociability and their professional activities. As we have seen, these groups—clergymen, property agents, scholars, professionals, and government officers—were keen to acquire health advice, since attending to one's health had become yet another sign of refinement.

In the second half of the chapter we turn to a discussion of our study of material culture and the role assigned to objects in the effort to maintain one's health. Regimens are filled with references to the health significance of a range of household objects, and the chronology of their appearance and disappearance from use in the home may be seen as an indication of the dissemination of preventive ideas in health-related practices. The classical sources for the study of domestic goods have been household inventories and these documents have represented an important resource for our study. But as many have illustrated, and as we will outline in what follows, the value of the evidence they provide has many limitations. Hence household listings have been used in this study in conjunction with material and visual sources. We will argue that surviving museum pieces and various kinds of contemporary images may add new elements which substantiate or balance the archival evidence about the impact of medical discourse on the material culture of the home. At the same time, as well as playing a complementary role in our analysis, material and visual sources can in themselves stimulate new insights into contemporary health-related practices.

THE SPADA-VERALLI FAMILY: FROM RURAL LORDS, BANDITS, AND TAX FARMERS TO LEARNED GENTLEMEN

To what extent did physicians' advice influence their readers' behaviour and daily lives? The relationship between the concerns of doctors and lay health conduct has troubled medical historians for many decades now.[1] To try to grasp the extent to which patients recognized the doctor's authority and bowed to his superior knowledge, scholars have turned to documents produced directly by the patients (diaries, autobiographies, and correspondence) as straightforward indications of lay responses to disease. In spite of its methodological shortcomings, this literature has contributed a great deal to illuminate the patient's perspective.[2] But the focus has been on how people coped with disease, whether through self-medication, resort to the care of irregular practitioners, religious healing, or the prescriptions of a physician. Preventive concerns and activities are only discussed in passing in these works; the so-called 'ego documents' have not been approached from this perspective. Yet we know from recent studies of letters that advice concerning the precautions to be adopted to keep in good health was regularly given by anxious mothers to their offspring, and that private letters, in particular those exchanged by family members, frequently discussed issues of healthy living.[3]

To explore the relationship between preventive medical advice and lay practice we have identified a significant corpus of private letters exchanged by members of two noble families, the Spadas and the Verallis, who settled in Rome in the early seventeenth century and became related through marriage in 1636. The letters considered stretch from the 1570s to the 1670s and therefore cover a good portion of the period examined in this study.

Like many other Roman families in the seventeenth century, the Spadas were new to Rome. They originated in Romagna, in the Papal States, and more precisely in the small town of Brisighella, in the Faenza region. Their fortune and ennoblement were recent. The architect of the family's social mobility at the end of the sixteenth century was Paolo (see Fig. 2.1).

His father was already in the Pope's service as governor of the town of Brisighella when Paolo, a coal merchant, was nominated treasurer to Pope Clement VIII for the Romagna region. As was often the case with this kind of office, Paolo accumulated enormous wealth thanks to his role as a tax farmer—though not always through orthodox means—as well as gaining significant protectors in Rome.[4] These influential social

---

[1] This trend was given impetus by Roy Porter's 'The Patient's View'.
[2] See e.g. Beier, 'In Sickness'; Lane, ' "The Doctor" '; and Nicoud, 'L'Expérience'. For a critique of medical historians' usage of letters, Ruberg, 'The Letter'.
[3] See e.g. Daybell, *Women*, 179; and Zarzoso, 'Mediating', 116.
[4] Visceglia and Fosi, 'Marriage', 211.

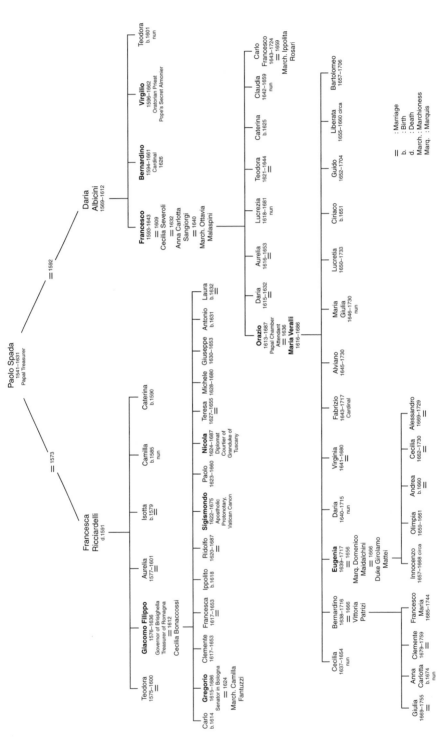

Fig. 2.1. Family tree of the Spada family, signalling, in bold, the characters frequently mentioned in our story.

relationships played a key role in supporting his ambition to gain a place at the Papal Curia for two of his sons from his second marriage, Bernardino and Virgilio. Paolo was probably aware that as the Pope was consolidating his secular power, the status of a family in the Papal States was increasingly associated with prestigious ecclesiastical careers more than any other honour. In the early seventeenth century, the two boys therefore received an academic education, being sent to study philosophy, theology, and law at Jesuit colleges in Rome and Bologna. While the family's landed properties went to their elder brothers, Francesco and Giacomo Filippo, who remained based in Romagna, Bernardino and Virgilio undertook religious careers and settled in Rome: the former was made a cardinal in 1626, while Virgilio, an Oratorian priest since 1622, served as secret almoner under two different popes in the 1640s and 1650s.

Paolo had invested considerable capital to settle Bernardino (Plate 2) in his curial career, and soon the latter took over the role of promoting the family's social ascent.[5] The numerous daughters of Bernardino's brothers were crucial to his strategy to raise the prestige of the Spada house.[6] One aspect of this entailed establishing important matrimonial alliances with the city's urban patriciate that would raise this family of recently enriched provincial notables from its obscure past and secure its inclusion among the ranks of Bologna grandees. As persuasively argued by Casanova, these marriages thus carried a political rather than an economic significance.[7] But the jewels in the crown were the marriages arranged for two of the male nephews, Gregorio and Orazio, who had been virtually adopted by Bernardino since childhood. While Gregorio was promised to Camilla, daughter of Marquis Fantuzzi, from one of the most influential and prestigious senatorial families in Bologna, Orazio (see Plate 3) was married to Maria Veralli in 1636. Although hailing from a family of the lesser nobility she was the sole designated heiress not only of the extensive feudal domains of Castel Viscardo but also of the estate left by her uncle, Cardinal Fabrizio Veralli.

Unlike the other marriages concluded by Bernardino, the appeal of this match did not lie in the (modest) status of the bride's family which was, furthermore, tainted by the infamous reputations of two of her close relatives. Maria's widowed father had conducted a scandalous liaison with a woman of low rank which eventually led to the birth of three illegitimate children. Her uncle was a gentleman bandit who had guided a feudal rebellion against the fiscal demands of an increasingly powerful papacy.[8] The attraction of this marital alliance, which united the grandson of a tax collector with the descendant of waning feudal landlords, was not just economic. Maria also brought with her a unique network of family relationships

---

[5] An expensive office as chamber attendant was purchased for him before he was appointed nuncio to France; Visceglia and Fosi, 'Marriage', 211.

[6] What follows is based on Casanova, 'Le donne'.

[7] Admission to the circle of the civic nobility was secured by the marriage of five of his nieces (daughters of his brothers Francesco and Giacomo Filippo) into families that held hereditary rights to municipal offices such as the local Senate. Casanova, 'Le donne', 64–5.

[8] On Giovan Battista and his brother-in-law Ramberto Malatesta, husband of Geronima Veralli, D'Amelia, 'Una lettera'.

with significant connections with the Papal Curia. She counted as many as three cardinals among her uncles and another four among her more distant relations. Through her maternal line she was even related in the fourth degree to a pope: Urban VII. The marriage therefore significantly reinforced the political position of the Spada clergymen, who were not noble and were new to the Curia.[9]

The second element of Bernardino's ambition for the family entailed ensuring that his nephews received an education suitable to the status of refined gentlemen, capable of fully engaging with the life of the academy, the court, and the salon.[10] To this end, as already mentioned, Bernardino had taken responsibility for the education of some of his nephews from an early age. In 1624, aged 9 and 11, Orazio and Gregorio followed him to Paris where he was papal nuncio for three years, then to Bologna where he was apostolic legate, and finally to Rome. After the death of his brother, Giacomo Filippo, Bernardino was also made legal guardian of Gregorio's two younger brothers, Nicola Bali and Sigismondo. Remarkably, military and physical training occupied only a marginal place in the education imparted to the young Spadas in the early seventeenth century. They acquired notions of jurisprudence and philosophy as well as of geometry and architecture so that they would be able to supervise the family's building projects.[11] Gregorio, on whose education we have more specific details, graduated in law and theology but he had also received training in the range of activities that defined a gentleman of his time: equitation and fencing, drawing, dancing, and playing various instruments. His uncle also had lists set up in the courtyard of their palace so he could practise his jousting skills since, like other noble youths, he participated in public tournaments in his teens.[12] Orazio and Nicola Bali, who had been familiar with court life since childhood, became court employees. Nicola was first made page and then *cameriere* of the Grand Duke of Tuscany. Orazio held the ceremonial role of *cameriere d'onore* of three popes and then of the Queen of Sweden. Gregorio had a more turbulent life but nevertheless his interests were largely humanistic. The diary of his grand tour in 1635 reveals his interest in monuments, artworks, and the pleasures of worldly life rather than military activities.[13] Later, he was renowned for his passion for music and theatre and held literary meetings in his house in Bologna. He shared with other members of the Spada family a special interest in architecture, and architectural drawings by himself and his cousin Orazio have survived (Fig. 2.2).[14]

Both uncles Bernardino and Virgilio on the other hand shook off the marks of their modest origins by cultivating broad scholarly interests and adopting the

---

[9] Visceglia and Fosi, 'Marriage', 213.

[10] This shift in ideals of masculinity is traced by Renée Baernstein in relation to another Roman family in her 'Reprobates'.

[11] Tabarrini, *Borromini e gli Spada*, 5–7.

[12] Neppi, *Palazzo Spada*, 137.

[13] Tabarrini, *Borromini e gli Spada*, 6–7.

[14] After the death of the uncles, Orazio was also engaged in various building and renovation projects of the family property in Rome, Castel Viscardo and in other locations. Tabarrini, *Borromini e gli Spada*, 8; and Neppi, *Palazzo Spada*, 207–8.

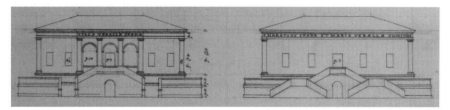

Fig. 2.2. Orazio Spada's mid-seventeenth-century drawings for the restructuring of the Villa Serpentara.

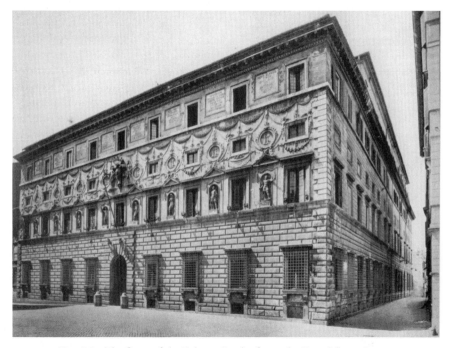

Fig. 2.3. The front of the Palazzo Spada, formerly Capodiferro, Rome.

lifestyle proper of the urban aristocracy. As testified by their libraries and the works they commissioned, their intellectual pursuits raged from astronomy to mathematics, geography, and architecture.[15] Bernardino settled in Rome in 1632 and set out to create a residence for himself and the family which was appropriate to his position. He bought the Capodiferro palace and over nearly two decades radically transformed it (Fig. 2.3), employing famed architects of the calibre of Maruscelli and Borromini, and turning it into the residence of his adopted nephews and of the newly wed Orazio and Maria.[16]

[15] Neppi, *Palazzo Spada*, 126.
[16] On the palace works Neppi, *Palazzo Spada*, 134–74.

He commissioned the ceiling fresco of the Meridian in one of the galleries of his palace in Rome in 1644 (Plate 4) and was a patron of optical studies in particular, as revealed also by the illusionistic paintings he ordered for the garden facades of the Spada palace and the celebrated forced perspective corridor designed by Borromini for its courtyard.[17]

It was especially during the long periods spent at the Spada villa in Tivoli that Bernardino pursued his intellectual interests. Even in the last year of his life Bernardino was said to have brought with him to Tivoli as many as twenty-two boxes of books for a study of the Tuscan historians he was planning to complete.[18] However, these moments of scholarly study were often broken by social visits. Letters reveal how the villa was not only a place of relaxation and study in late spring and summer but also of learned conversation. It was known in particular as a meeting place for members of the celebrated Academia dei Lincei. Here Bernardino could enjoy the company of other learned men, including doctors. Indeed he had established a particularly strong intellectual relationship with Giacomo Gibbesio (originally William Gibbes), a figure who epitomizes the broad intellectual interests characteristic of medical men in this period, including, as we have seen, the authors of regimens. An English doctor and poet who had converted to Catholicism, Gibbes settled in Rome in the 1650s, where he became university professor of rhetoric and also practised medicine at the hospital of Santo Spirito.[19] Bernardino was one of his patrons, exchanged regular scholarly correspondence with him, and even had a room permanently reserved for him in the Spada palace. These frequent social and intellectual exchanges between elite men and medical professionals represented the ideal context for the circulation of ideas of healthy living.

Villa life was also regarded as relaxing and salubrious, both for the body and the mind, and Maria and the children—in particular—moved to Tivoli for several months every year—from late spring to early autumn.[20] In the 1640s much money was invested in the renovation of the two buildings, Palazzo Cesi, and the smaller villa, Casino Cesi, that constituted the property, and above all in the expansion and transformation of its gardens. The acreage was quadrupled, creating parkland for animals, fountains, and other 'delights' (*delizie*) as well as a series of *viale*, ideal for taking walks (increasingly regarded, as we will see, as the preferred form of exercise), without being seen from the outside. Moreover the landscaping opened up a huge vista over the garden, woodlands, and a valley, offering great psychological benefits to the viewer. The cardinal, as his brother Virgilio testifies, would enjoy this from the antechamber where he usually took his meals.[21]

This building programme is in line with the changes that villas in general had undergone starting in the late sixteenth century. While villas and *villeggiatura* had already featured in the lives of the affluent in the previous century, country houses

---

[17] Vicini, *Il collezionismo*, 21.   [18] ASR, FSV, B.463, cap. XXXII.
[19] Tabarrini, *Borromini e gli Spada*, 62–3.
[20] The Spadas also used the Serpentara villa for daily outings. It was very close to the city but was relatively run down and belonged to Virgilio. After Virgilio's death, Orazio set out to renovate it (see Fig. 2.4).
[21] Neppi, *Palazzo Spada*, 290; and Tabarrini, *Borromini e gli Spada*, 184.

were formerly modest buildings and performed a double function as retreats from the duties and cares of urban life and as productive farms—hence the definition *vigna* (vineyard), common in the fifteenth century for these establishments.[22] Over the next two hundred years they became increasingly lavish and extravagant, surrounded by great architectural gardens rather than by farmed countryside. From the late sixteenth century, the country estate was no longer a source of food and income but a pleasurable place where the classical idea of *otium*, as a period devoted to contemplation and intellectual pursuits, merged more and more with an intense programme of social gatherings, feasts, and banquets.

The Spadas participated fully in these and in the other rituals of genteel life that had become fashionable amongst their peers. Through a shrewd policy of matrimonial alliances accompanied by the widening of their intellectual interests, the patronage of both the arts and the sciences, the building of suitable residences, and the learning of refined courtly manners from an early age, they had forged a new identity for themselves. Attention to health, as their letters reveal, was one of the prerogatives of their newly acquired noble status.

LETTERS

In the central decades of the seventeenth century, Palazzo Spada in Piazza Capodiferro was home to Cardinal Bernardino, his nephew Orazio, the latter's wife Maria Veralli, and their numerous children.[23] The sickly and crippled Giulia Veralli, Maria's only sibling, also lived with the Spadas until her death in 1643. The married couple were extremely prolific: as was customary among the aristocracy, Maria was pregnant every year. As Bernardino proudly commented in a letter to a friend written in January 1656, after twenty years of marriage, and aged 41, she had eleven living children, besides nine dead or miscarried, and was currently nine months' pregnant (see Plate 5).[24]

The life of this extended family seems to have been a relatively happy one. Bernardino was very fond of his great-nephews and -nieces and also of Orazio and Maria. The numerous letters Bernardino wrote to Maria during the frequent periods in which one of them was away from Rome demonstrate both his affection and the esteem in which he held her judgement. Their epistolary exchange shows how they consulted one another on many decisions concerning the running of the household—including plans for the renovation of the palace and issues of property—as if they were husband and wife. Renata Ago has noted that this configuration was typical of the families of high prelates in Rome. Thanks to the status enjoyed by cardinals in Roman society the clergyman was the real head of the family and ran the household in close cooperation with the wife of the married brother or, as in

---

[22] Coffin, *The Villa in Rome*, 11–15, 69, 86, 232, 252, 336, 367.

[23] Some rooms were also kept for nephews Sigismondo and Nicola Bali, who did not reside in Rome.

[24] Cited in Neppi, *Palazzo Spada*, 128 n. 32.

this case, of the nephew.[25] This state of affairs might have been a contributing factor in Orazio's decision to spend much of his time at the landed estate of Castel Viscardo (see Plate 6), supervising its running.

But Maria was also away for months at a time when she moved to the villa with the children. One way and another, the three characters were often apart and these separations generated a rich correspondence that largely survives in the well-kept family archives.[26] Their letters, as well as those written by another three members of the family (discussed in the next paragraph), offer a wealth of detail about the ways in which health was experienced and dealt with in everyday life and the extent to which the definitions of health hazards outlined in the advice literature were shared by laypeople. Of course we do not find evidence about every aspect of healthy living in letters; some areas of behaviour, such as personal hygiene, are simply not recorded. On the other hand, private letters are concerned with spheres of life not dealt with in regimens. For example, while guides to healthy living are in the majority gender- and age-specific, being written with the adult and male body in mind, letters provide precious information about the precautions taken during pregnancy and to preserve the health of children.

As well as the letters exchanged between Maria and her husband Orazio, and between Maria and Uncle Bernardino, we have considered letters written by another three women of the family: those by Orazio's mother, Daria Albicini, to her husband Paolo, the papal treasurer, in the years in which he was spending most of his time in Rome whilst she was based in Brisighella; those written at the turn of the seventeenth century by Giulia Benzoni (Maria Veralli's father's first wife) to her husband, and finally, a sizeable group of letters that Eugenia Spada, eldest daughter of Orazio and Maria, sent to her parents.[27] Eugenia moved to Viterbo in 1656, following her marriage to Marquis Maidalchini, and from then on, for a period of thirty years, she kept up an intense correspondence with her mother until the latter's death.[28] Letters were written at a rate of one every three to five days, sometimes even more often, and regularly included requests for guidance in every aspect of life, from childcare to choice of clothes, from how to govern servants to how to deal with her mother-in-law.[29] The letters she wrote to her father are less frequent but intensified after the death of her husband, when Eugenia needed advice on how to handle the difficult relationship with her in-laws in matters of property, the tutorship of her children, and finally her remarriage to the wealthy Duke Mattei.

---

[25] Ago, *Carriere*, 68–71.
[26] We have considered the following: ASR, FSV, B.491, letters of Cardinal Bernardino to Maria (1635–61); B.619, letters of Maria to uncle Bernardino (1640–61); B.607, letters of Orazio to Maria (1658–66); B.618, letters of Maria to Orazio (1678–9).
[27] ASR, FSV, B.459, letters of Daria Albicini to Paolo Spada (1601–12); B.449, letters of Giulia Benzoni to Giovan Battista Veralli (1590–1610).
[28] ASR, FSV, B.410, letters of Eugenia to Maria (1656–7); B.1115, letters of Eugenia to Maria (1658–72), and to Orazio (1664–72). We have not considered the letters written from 1672 to Maria's death in 1686.
[29] On the relationship between Maria and Eugenia as revealed by their letters, see D'Amelia, 'La presenza'.

The epistolary sources we have used are therefore largely authored by women. As many have demonstrated, letter-writing was an important area of female activity among the affluent in the early modern period.[30] Although a large proportion of a seventeenth-century noblewoman's correspondence consisted of courtesy letters (condolences, giving thanks, congratulations on appointments, engagements, births, recoveries, etc.), it was also their unspoken duty to keep in touch with the various members of the family and then inform the others of how everyone else was doing. It is these letters of a more personal nature that interest us. The art of writing letters was certainly culturally constructed, and by this time, thanks also to the influence of letter-writing manuals, it was a highly conventional literary form. There was still however a considerable difference between women's personal and ceremonial letters. For a start, the former were normally written by the woman herself and therefore created by her, notwithstanding the presence of a secretary in most noble houses.[31] Moreover, though they also included news about events of general interest, personal letters captured minute details of domestic life and everyday routines, providing precious insights into people's habits, concerns, and cultural assumptions.

Health maintenance figured prominently in women's family letters. It seems to have been a woman's role to remind her relations about the rules of healthy living, hence recommendations about what they should and should not do to keep healthy were often included. Accounts of the state of health of various members of the household, other kin, and acquaintances were also a regular feature of the letters, and these accounts also mentioned the servants, whose physical condition was always discussed in considerable detail. Hence some of the letters, especially those by Maria, who was clearly regarded as a medical expert, are veritable health bulletins. To give just one example, a letter to her husband in Castel Viscardo, dated 16 March 1678, first discusses the snowy weather, giving recommendations about the importance of keeping warm so that he does not catch a cold as this is a dangerous condition when one is no longer young. Maria also describes the items of clothing she is sending to Orazio to protect him from the cold weather. Then she updates him on the fragile health of the elderly servant Bona, who in fact died a few months later. Having taken *manna* (a mild laxative), Bona 'was able to relieve herself very easily' ('la scaricò assai bene'), and is now feeling better. Maria goes on to inform him about the state of her own catarrh and the medicine she has been obliged to give to her 26-year-old son. She then adds the good news that another son, Cardinal Fabrizio, is recovering from fever and now eats well, but concludes on a worrying note with news of another sickness in the household—that of their young grandchild Annuccia, daughter of their older son, who has had a slight fever since the previous evening; the doctor suspects rubella, though she is in good spirits and has a good appetite.[32] Later in the year other letters provided intimate

---

[30] See e.g. Daybell (ed.), *Early Modern*; Daybell, *Women*; and Couchman and Crabb (eds.), *Women's Letters*. On Italy, Zarri (ed.), *Per lettera*.

[31] See D'Amelia, 'Lo scambio'. Secretaries were busy serving the male master and had little time to spare for women's correspondence.

[32] ASR, FSV, B.618, 16.3.1678.

accounts of the servant Bona's state of health and of the treatment she receives from Maria and the surgeon.[33] Bona, who has been with the family for thirty years, is certainly the focus of special attention, but over the years Maria takes care of the ailments of many other members of her domestic staff, from the *maestro di casa* to the maids, from the secretary to the children's tutor, administering remedies and summoning the doctor or the barber when their condition is serious. Litters are even hired to take them to Rome when they fall ill at the villa.[34]

So although the Spada correspondence relates to a noble household, the attention paid to servants' physical conditions, the fact that the treatment they receive is not so different to that administered to members of the family, and that their ailments are described in similar terms, all indicate that the definitions of healthy and unhealthy found in letters and the responses enacted to prevent or cope with ill health were not confined to a restricted social group but had wider currency. Like her mother, Eugenia demonstrates familiarity with the physical and psychological afflictions of her servants, especially her *donne*—the circle of maids that shared so much of a noblewoman's day, assisting her in all the duties related to housekeeping and childcare. In her letters Eugenia regularly informs Maria of their ailments, and discusses the causes of their psychological distress with her, such as Marta's anxiety about her family in Rome in time of plague or Camilla's melancholy and her dislike of Viterbo and even of its bread.[35]

The close relationship that developed within the palace between the noblewoman and her *donne* was reinforced by their long acquaintance. With the exception of the *donna di faccende* (woman of all chores), who was local, Eugenia's maids were not strangers but had moved with the young spouse to Viterbo from Rome, where they were already employed in the service of her family. And in later years, when new maids or wet nurses were recruited, they were not unknown to Eugenia but were nieces or daughters of current or former servants of her family of origin, with whom regular contact had been maintained. Letters also suggests that the maids were often present when Eugenia writes to her mother for they send messages to the marchioness and her *donne* in Rome and likewise receive messages that are read out to them. And when Eugenia is unwell it is the faithful Camilla who takes up the pen and informs Maria about her daughter's health and the other occurrences in the household.[36] Members of the lower classes within the noble household were therefore regularly exposed to the discourse on health that permeated these letters and health concerns and vocabularies were widely shared, creating a common language of the body and its preservation. The palace was then another terrain for the dissemination of the medical culture and principles of healthy living popularized by vernacular regimens.

---

[33] ASR, FSV, B.618, 30.11.1678.
[34] e.g. ASR, FSV, B.491, 3.7.1638; B.619, 21.10.1659; B.618, 19.2.1678, 4.5.1678, and 9.10.1679.
[35] ASR, FSV, B.410, 2.7.1656, 29.7.1656, 11.2.1657, and 4.3.1657.
[36] ASR, FSV, B.410, 22.7.1657 and 2.9.1657.

Maria Spada, in particular, was a source of expertise and advice in health matters. It is well known that medical knowledge was widespread in early modern
societies but some figures undoubtedly stood out as medical experts in the family
and community. Maria embodies the characteristics of the medically informed
aristocratic lady that historians have identified in different European countries.[37]
As the letters indicate, Eugenia regularly turned to her for advice about healthy
lifestyles as well as on what line of treatment to adopt in case of ailments and
entirely relied on her recommendations. Maria was also a regular supplier of ointments, medicinal waters, and oral remedies for the various medical needs of her
daughter's family. These remedies were partly commissioned or purchased from the
apothecary and partly domestically produced—a number of medicinal recipes
against headache, 'ethic fever', and for the eyes are also found among the culinary
and household recipes preserved in the Spada archives.[38] Her authority even
extended to medical practitioners: she corresponded with the surgeon and doctors
in charge of Eugenia's health, discussing the proposed treatment, and at times also
contesting the prescribed cures; in one case she even persuaded Eugenia to take a
medicine of Maria's choice 'without telling the doctor'.[39] Maria also offered explanations of the causes of certain ailments: for example, in a letter to her husband,
clearly surprised that his haemorrhoids are troubling him despite the cold weather,
she expertly comments: 'I am not surprised that you suffer from haemorrhoids
more when it is cold than when it is hot for they proceed from internal heat, not
external, and sometimes walking too long makes them come back.'[40]

What interests us, however, are the observations in her letters about what constitutes a healthy lifestyle and the recommendations she provides regarding health
maintenance. She dispenses advice about the impact of certain foods and drinks on
the body, the appropriateness of going out and taking exercise, and even on how
frequently Eugenia should wash her hair while pregnant. Maria also advises on the
religious rituals her daughter should perform at different stages of her pregnancy
and after childbirth to ensure the good health of her child. In matters of medical
treatment, too, Maria combines natural and supernatural remedies. Hence she
sends her daughter and son-in-law *horationi* to be recited when particular diseases
strike a member of the family, and specific relics to be placed near the sickbed
alongside medicinal substances or compounds. Moreover, her pharmacopoeia
presents elements of natural magic as she believes in the healing and preserving
power of stones to be worn on the body.[41] She is therefore active in prevention and
cure through religious and talismanic means as well as medicinal remedies, showing

[37] See e.g. Pollock, *With Faith*; Leong, 'Making Medicines'; Rankin, 'Becoming'.
[38] ASR, FSV, B.448, 320–4 and other unnumbered pages.
[39] 'Piglierò l'agro di cedro come VS Ill. mi dice senza dir niente al medico'; ASR, FSV, B.410, 18.10.1656.
[40] 'Non mi meraviglio che si risenta dille moroide più nil freddo che nil caldo, perchè procedono da calore interno, e non dall'esterno, et alle volte il caminar troppo le fa risentire.' ASR, FSV, B.410, 22.7.1657.
[41] ASR, FSV, B.1115, 20.8.1662. For another example of this belief, ASR, FSV, B.449, 3.10.1599.

that a century after Trent, a family of the elite, closely connected to the top hierarchies of the Church, heartily believed in the action of what scholars have sometime described as 'folk remedies' characteristic of a popular, non-learned culture. Nor was the employment of religious or magical remedies pursued only when the cause of illness was supposed to be preternatural, as has sometimes been suggested.[42] The three types of remedies were used contemporaneously, though relics, especially, were employed only in the most serious cases.

Despite Maria's authority in health matters, doctors were frequently consulted by the Spadas for both preventive advice and medical treatment. The family's relationship with medical practitioners does not conform to the model according to which the doctor was called in only when self-medication had failed.[43] Resorting to doctors certainly came after domestic diagnosis by the woman carer (rather than by the sick person itself as often suggested), and normally took place when there was suspicion that the affliction might develop into something serious, namely fever. Signs such as sweating and 'alteration' of the body temperature were particularly alarming as fever was perceived as a threatening condition from which recovery was not guaranteed.[44] The decision to summon the doctor therefore largely depended on the diagnosis made in the household rather than on the outcome of domestic treatment.

Throughout the period, the doctor's advice was also held in great esteem in matters of prevention. The physician was consulted on issues of travelling and the timing of going to the villa, as moving to localities with a different type of air was thought to be possibly harmful.[45] It also transpires from letters that patients treasured their doctor's opinion on the advantages of drinking certain types of wine and on the health benefits of going to the spas.[46] This had become a fashionable activity among the elites of late Renaissance Italy for both preventive and curative purposes and Bernardino Spada was an eager follower of such fashion. But his decision to take the waters was based on specific explanations of the nature of such waters and how these worked on the body, supplied by his doctor.[47] Moreover, once at San Casciano he continued to send for his Roman physician's 'approval' (*approvazione*) on the procedure to follow when taking the waters and on whether mud baths were also advisable.[48] Similarly, while submitting himself to the treatment known as 'taking the marc' (*prendere le vinaccie*) in Frascati he was anxious to check with the family doctor that the method employed was correct, 'so that if any error has been made we can get it right'.[49] The doctor's advice was also blindly followed by Eugenia when her child's wet nurse was ill and it was a matter of urgency to decide

[42] Gentilcore, *Healers and Healing*, 12–17 and 22.
[43] Gentilcore, *Healers and Healing*, 6.
[44] Among the many examples ASR, FSV, B.491, 1.7.1655. On the scaring effect of fever see the account of Bernardino's death; ASR, FSV, B.463, cap.XXXII.
[45] ASR, FSV, B.618, 7.12.1678. See also further examples in Ch. 3.
[46] ASR, FSV, B.491, 7.7.1655.
[47] ASR, FSV, B.491, 4.9.1642.
[48] ASR, FSV, B.491, 13.9.1642.
[49] 'ació che se ci fosse qualche errore lo possiamo correggere'; ASR, FSV, B.491, 22.10.1638.

whether the health of the suckling child was at risk of being affected by her milk and a new *balia* should be found.[50]

The doctor was regularly approached for his knowledge of preventive medicine and he was clearly considered a health adviser rather than just someone to be called in the case of a serious illness. While the treatment of the sick was often the result of the combined efforts of the doctor and the patient's family, who frequently interfered with and modified the physician's prescriptions, it would seem that the physician's opinion in matters of health maintenance went largely undisputed. Laypeople seem to have been overawed by his knowledge of the properties of foods, drinks, air, and water. To what extent such advice was then followed, adapted, or manipulated, is another matter that Chapters 3-8 will explore in detail.

The fact that doctors were considered to be health advisers can undoubtedly contribute to explaining the success that regimens enjoyed in this period. Not many households could afford the luxury of employing a personal physician always available for consultation as was the case for noble families like the Spadas, and so the health-advice literature was there to address similar needs among less prosperous sectors of society. For at least twenty years from the 1640s, the Spadas employed a doctor named Gabriele Fonseca, of Portuguese origins. His name recurs frequently in the letters though occasionally we find that the family turned to another doctor, Giangiacomo, for treatment. Fonseca's family and professional history might have made him particularly sympathetic to ideas of healthy living. Curiously, he was in fact the nephew of the renowned Doctor Rodrigo, the author of a health regimen, *Del conservare la sanitá*, published in Pisa in 1603, as well as of other works in Latin. Rodrigo had also been directly involved in the professional education of his nephew: Gabriele graduated from the University of Pisa, where his uncle was professor of medicine and also started his career in the same city.[51] We can speculate that Gabriele absorbed from his uncle a sense of the importance of lifestyle in preserving health and that this knowledge and sensitivity for preventive issues informed his professional practice.

THE MATERIAL CULTURE OF HEALTH

One of the ways in which we explore the penetration of health advice into daily life is by probing whether there is a relationship between the development of a preventive medical discourse and the appearance and disappearance in late Renaissance homes of objects whose use was directly related to the implementation of this advice. Our starting point for this focus on material goods was the regimens themselves. These gave increasingly detailed instructions about the particular objects required for the creation of a healthy environment (such as leather wall hangings or wood panelling), or for the performance of health routines (such as the combs and towels needed for rubbing the head every morning). This specificity drew our

---

[50] ASR, FSV, B.1115, 6.8.1662.
[51] Volpi Rosselli, 'I portoghesi', 128, 131–2; and Marangoni, 'Un medico portoghese', 209–15.

attention to the preventive possibilities inherent in domestic material culture and the frequently overlooked health significance of objects. Drawing on sources such as inventories, images, and letters we have sought to track the presence and use of such objects in daily life, to consider ways in which these objects facilitated and even prompted people's practices of healthy living, following what one scholar has described as a 'material culture route to lived experience'.[52]

The quest for healthy living also seems to have been accompanied by innovation in domestic material culture. Authors often intimate that certain objects were relatively unknown, and offer instructions on their uses and how this affects health. For example in the mid-sixteenth century Rangoni explained what windows could be made out of, and how and when to open and shut them in order to minimize the dangers posed by the air.[53] Others even offer their own prototype objects, reinforcing our sense that there was a dynamic relationship between the world of material goods and the world of medical ideas. For example, in the mid-seventeenth century Panaroli, presumably aware that his readers may not have been familiar with, nor had the wherewithal to purchase, a perfume burner, explained how they could make a perfectly operational burner at home using a pan and a piece of pierced parchment.[54] This innovative relationship between physicians and the material culture of health is made even more explicit in Persio's 1593 tract in praise of 'hot drinking'. This offered both designs and meticulous instructions for the construction of what may have been the first 'table water heater'; a kettle in modern English.[55] As an object it was clearly intended not only to facilitate the healthy practice of hot drinking, but to conform to notions of decorum at the table. In time, such innovations may themselves have been an agent for change, possibly facilitating the spread of a subsequent fashion for drinking hot drinks such as hot chocolate and coffee.

Many of the objects we discuss here are, for the most part, 'everyday objects'— things like hats, pillows, glasses, or combs, and as such have recently been the focus of scholarly interest.[56] As Hamling and Richardson explain, although such objects were used 'as part of everyday activities' they were not necessarily 'common' or associated with 'popular' or 'low' culture. They might have been luxury items in themselves, but none the less 'formed part of everyday experience', particularly for the elites or middling classes.[57] The examples we have chosen from museum collections are even less likely to be 'everyday' versions of these objects, given that the very fact of their survival tends to be by virtue of their aesthetic or financial value. Nonetheless, they are objects which, as Daniel Miller has argued, by their very commonness and 'everydayness' are rendered invisible to the user, fading into the background as trivial details, and often, consequently, virtually absent from historical records. He argues that these objects are important precisely because 'the

---

[52] Harvey, *History*, 7.   [53] Rangoni, *Consiglio*, 11.
[54] Panaroli, *Aerologia*, 86–7.
[55] See Ch. 7.
[56] On 'everyday' objects see Hamling and Richardson (eds.), *Everyday Objects*. Also Fumerton and Hunt (eds.), *Renaissance Culture*; and Pennell, 'Mundane Materiality'.
[57] Hamling and Richardson (eds.), *Everyday Objects*, 12–14.

less we are aware of them, the more powerfully they can determine our expectations by setting the scene and ensuring normative behaviour'.[58] Following this line of argument we could suggest that many of the objects discussed here, such as reclining chairs and foot-warmers, had a certain 'agency' in daily life as their presence reminded their owners to take day sleep in the correct position, or to warm their feet; likewise even the layout of gardens, with their shady walkways, prominent fountains, and rows of citrus trees could have constantly 'nudged' their owners towards entering them, and thereby engage in healthy living practices.

In our discussions of objects we seek to add a new medical perspective to previous explanations for the presence and diffusion of objects, or for their evolution. Our intention is to highlight the importance of medicine in giving meaning to everyday objects which were closely connected to the body and its functions. In some cases we are building on observations by previous scholars who have broadly identified the purpose of objects without being aware of the complexity of the medical ramifications. It has often been noted for example that bed curtains and canopies kept out the cold, but this has not been specifically linked to medical discourse on protecting the head, nor to issues of darkness, silence, and the importance of good sleep for health. In other cases our linkage between objects and specifically medical issues is entirely novel, such as our observations on the appearance of the daybed and prescriptive advice on day sleep, in Chapter 4. Likewise it seems as if hitherto there has been no awareness of the health-related explanations for the shape and size of drinking glasses and wine flasks or for their lids.

Inventories are often the first port of call for historians researching material culture, and we have drawn on them here as a way of gauging the absence or presence of objects in homes in later sixteenth- and seventeenth-century Rome, and as indicating the chronology of their appearance and the extent of their social diffusion. Rome was not only home to the papal court, but to as many as fifty cardinals' courts and their 'families', 200 high-ranking prelates, as well as the families of the Roman elite.[59] As such it had a vigorous consumer culture and recent scholarship on material culture in general and that of Renaissance Italy in particular has provided the background against which we have framed our questions.[60] In order to explore the presence of health-related objects we selected ninety inventories, covering the period from 1553 to 1692. Fifty-nine are from the archives of Roman notarial offices, which includes three from the Spada-Veralli family archives, selected to complement our study of the family letters. A further thirty-one inventories came from the Archive of the Vicar of Rome, drawn up in 1605–6 to record and value the possessions of women who, having renounced prostitution, were entering the convent for converted prostitutes.[61]

---

[58] Miller, *Materiality*, 5.

[59] Delumeau, *Vie économique et sociale*, 37–8.

[60] e.g. Ajmar-Wollheim and Dennis (eds.), *At Home*; O'Malley and Welch, *The Material Renaissance*; Musacchio, *Art, Marriage, and Family*; and Lindow, *The Renaissance Palace*.

[61] We have 15 for the period 1550–99; 25 for 1600–49 (or 56 with the *convertite*); and 18 for 1650–1700.

As a source, inventories have been subject to much debate, centring around questions of reliability and about what can be inferred from often deceptively complete lists of goods.[62] Chief amongst their many drawbacks is that of their 'silences' and omissions. In the case of many of the inventories, for example, we do not know the profession, social status, wealth, or social or material context of the owner of the goods. Of sixty inventories from the notarial archive, we only know the professions of twenty-four: five were members of the nobility; eight were educated professionals, such as a lawyer, priest, or surgeon; and the remaining eleven were artisans (a goldsmith, a cobbler), shop owners (including a greengrocer), and servants. Several were widows or apparently single women. Given that our motive for looking at these inventories was to provide a snapshot of the possessions to be found across the social hierarchy from these inventories alone, the vagueness of the social status of many owners makes it hard for us to generalize about the presence of these objects amongst all but the most elevated social groups. This said, familiarity with a range of Roman documents and the work of other scholars enables us to 'place' these documents to a certain extent. In particular a recent study into the material culture of the middling ranks of professionals, merchants, and Roman elites in the seventeenth and early eighteenth centuries has provided a context for our study.[63] The length of the inventory, the number of rooms in the house as well as the proportion of 'old', 'worn', new, and 'used' goods in any given document, plus subtle distinctions in the materials from which they are fashioned, all contribute to give some indication of the specific economic circumstances of the individual concerned.[64] Overall poorer sectors of society are proportionately much less well represented in the archive than the comfortably-off and the wealthy, just as women are less visible than men. For this reason we chose to include three inventories drawn up inside a hospital—as only the poor died in hospital—and the sample of thirty inventories relating to former prostitutes from the Vicar General's archive as representing the poorer, female-headed households in the city.[65]

Perhaps the most frustrating absence from inventories for our purposes is that of small, economically insignificant objects. This is particularly the case with the inventories of the wealthy, who have so many high-value goods that the notary does not take the trouble to note them down. Or faced with a poor household he might group together a dilapidated assortment of kitchen implements under the generic heading 'of little interest and value'. Since some of the objects which particularly interested us were of this kind, such absences are extremely disappointing. For example, of all our inventories we find only one which records soap. This was owned by a former prostitute and was worth a mere 10 *baiocchi*; roughly the price of dinner in a hostelry.[66] It seems very unlikely she alone should have had soaps,

---

[62] See e.g. Cowen Orlin, 'Fiction'.

[63] Ago, *Il gusto*. For her study she draws on about 80 inventories, 100 wills, and 20 account books.

[64] On these subtle distinctions Ago, 'Gerarchia' and *Il gusto*.

[65] The documents relating to the *Convertite* can be found in ASVR, MCI, vol. 198, 1605–6. For a fuller discussion of prostitutes, their wealth and possessions, Storey, *Carnal Commerce*, 20–2 and 162–212.

[66] ASVR, MCI, 198, Beatrice de Mendoz Hispana, 5.4.1605, 7ʳ.

given how little these were worth. Presumably they were noted down because there were four of them in a small box, which perhaps indicates that they were unused, and therefore constituted a viable record in the inventory of a poor woman. However, it may be that soaps, having touched the skin of the owner, had no resale value on their own.

Combs and brushes for the body are another comparatively rarely mentioned object—although combs used for work in the textile trade, for combing/carding wool and linen, appear frequently. Yet, it is hard to imagine that women, at least, never used them. Indeed, we do find a few belonging either to the very wealthy or to former prostitutes. The absence of hats and head coverings is equally perplexing, given that in almost every image of men that we see from the period, ranging from expensive portraits to popular prints, men always wear hats or caps. Again, their invisibility is probably due to a combination of factors, ranging from the scarce resale potential of the more pedestrian examples to the fact that as with soaps, their proximity to the scalp, with its diseases, parasites, and excrements, probably rendered them unsellable.

Despite these inconsistencies and absences, however, used appropriately, inventories are still an extremely valuable and rich source of information in many ways, more than compensating for what they cannot tell us. This is particularly the case when they are combined with other sources. For example, just by giving us a sense of the kind of objects which were to be found in homes across the social spectrum, such as commodes, bed-warmers, and towels, we are given a glimpse of the diffusion of health-related practices. But there are other more specific advantages. For example, their detail can illuminate multiple uses for objects. This versatility is something which the regimens alert us to as they suggest ways in which particular objects may be substituted by other more readily available items. For example, an entry in the inventory of the magnificent Ludovisi palace from the late seventeenth century shows that despite the presence of two painted, gilded, and elaborately carved daybeds, there was also a wooden chest which the inventory notes 'serves as a daybed'.[67] Why such a wealthy family had not troubled to buy another purpose-built object is intriguing—perhaps it was used by servants—but at only 3 palms wide and 8 palms long, it was hard and not well suited for comfortable sleep; ideal for the kind of light rest considered safe by physicians after lunch. Daybeds feature in very few inventories, yet if this 'doubling-up' of furniture was acceptable even in such a wealthy household, it may well have been the norm elsewhere; so we can only speculate as to how many other households did take day rest, or use objects to promote healthy living, but left no material traces of these practices, since they merely used alternative domestic goods.

The detail given about objects in inventories and the varied nomenclature can also alert us to the subtleties of the distinctions between objects made at the time which have been lost over the centuries. Indeed, sometimes it is thanks to the inventories that we actually become aware of the existence and diffusion of certain objects.

---

[67] ASR, TNC, Uff.10, vol. 284, Duchessa di Sora, Villa Ludovisa, 27.3.1685, 157ʳ–183ʳ.

For example, *fiaschi da neve* (snow flasks) appear in inventories, are absent from museum collections, but probably correspond to objects described in the regimens for chilling water and wine. These were long-necked flasks specially designed to be placed into a basin filled with snow or ice for the chilling of water, since it was thought by many to be healthier to drink cold wine and water than to drink it at room temperature (see Plate 20).

VISUAL SOURCES

Although historians have long since adopted images as historical sources, recent decades have seen a more wholehearted and complex engagement with them, often referred to as 'the visual turn' in history. This has been accompanied by wide-ranging discussions on the difficulties of using them since no image is an unproblematic 'illustration' of reality.[68] Whether they are adopted as ways of documenting or exploring historical objects or events, they come with a set of caveats recently summarized by Peter Burke into ten 'rules' for historians.[69] Broadly, these remind us that in all cases there is a need to pay attention to questions such as why an image was created; the broader social context in which it was intended to be viewed; the visual conventions of the period; and the conventions of the genre itself. In particular here we adopt what Burke describes as the 'eyewitnessing' approach—by which he means seeking out things which are either literally or metaphorically in the background, on the basis that the further into the background a given detail can be found, the more reliable it is likely to be 'precisely because the artist was not using it in order to prove something'.[70]

In a few cases we do use images purely as illustrations, as in the contemporary portraits of the Spada family, the paintings of their palaces, and the genre scene showing a bookshop in Plate 1. Or we use them to illustrate a particular kind of object, such as the reclining chair in Fig. 4.1 and Plate 11 or the sedan chair in Fig. 5.1. When possible we have corroborated the accuracy of these images with surviving material objects.[71] Images can also document contemporary social practices, which is how we approach Giovanni Battista Falda's celebrated engravings of late seventeenth-century Rome (Figs. 5.5, 5.6, 5.8, and 6.5). These panoramic views celebrate the reconstruction of a magnificent 'new Rome' under the Counter-Reformation papacy, portraying its buildings in an almost theatrical manner.[72] As part of this, Falda was seeking to convey an ideal of the orderly, uncluttered spaces, where the Roman elite 'acted' out their public lives. However, into these

---

[68] There is now an extended bibliography on this subject. For a recent survey of the scholarship see *Cultural and Social History*, 7/4 (2010) which has several articles dedicated to the topic with an overview by Behr, Usborne, and Wieber, 'Introduction'. See also Burke, *Eyewitnessing*.

[69] Burke, 'Interrogating'.

[70] Burke, *Eyewitnessing*, 32 and 'Interrogating', 439.

[71] These are not always shown, given limitations on space, lack of availability of suitable images, and licensing restrictions.

[72] On G. B. Falda see the entry by Tozzi and Margiotta in *Dizionario biografico*.

otherwise very sterile images he injects some animation, in the form of genteel activities which were associated with urban and villa life. Although the images are undoubtedly idealizing, such details are clearly intended to 'have a connection' to the kind of activities which took place in these spaces, showing us what were considered appropriate and desirable activities for a villa garden.[73] At the same time the fact that boules, *pallamaglio* (pall-mall), and water games are included in such carefully choreographed images draws our attention, as historians, to the social importance of these games, an importance we might otherwise have missed.

Other much cheaper kinds of printed image served a range of functions. Very often they had a moralizing intent, some aiming also to amuse. The one shown at Fig. 3.5 is taken from a seventeenth-century sequence of twelve pictures which formed a comic-strip style narrative warning men of the dangers of consorting with courtesans.[74] So-called 'popular' prints in general were designed to appeal to a broad public, using details which would situate the characters and events so as to be easily recognizable by all. In this context, we read the appearance of something such as a window fitting or a foot-warmer (see Fig. 3.9) as implying that they must have become relatively common objects in order to have been visually relevant to the intended range of viewers and thereby testifying to the social diffusion of specific health-related material objects within the home in that period.[75]

Another quite different image which tries more self-consciously to capture the social reality of the lower echelons of society is that known as the *Well-Laid Table* (Plate 20), painted in the early seventeenth century by an unknown follower of Caravaggio. Using the 'genre' tradition it aimed for a certain naturalism of style and content, partly through the careful choice of objects used to create the overall 'mise-en-scène' of an inn or *osteria*.[76] Given this, the presence of a glass cooling flask, a snow flask (*fiasco da neve*), and a wine cooler (*rinfrescatore*)—in such a carefully set scene of 'everyday life' suggests that they were by then commonplace objects such as one would find in an inn or *osteria*, underlining for us the extent to which cold drinking practices had extended down through the social hierarchy.

In general paintings are more problematic images for the historian, given the complexity of symbolism, classical quotations, and the internal conventions of different genre. For example, all the images of daybeds we have found show them in an *all'antica*, classicizing style which corresponds to the mythological and erotic nature of the subject matter.[77] On the one hand, a late seventeenth-century inventory from a Roman palace does confirm that they could be extremely elaborate objects, but unable to track down a surviving Italian example, we cannot corroborate the available images. Over the Channel, surviving English daybeds suggest the

---

[73] On idealizing portraits see Retford, 'Thomas Bardwell's', 502, 506.

[74] The seminal text on narrative prints is Kunzle, *The Early Comic Strip*. For a detailed discussion of this particular genre see Storey, *Carnal Commerce*, 25–56. On moralizing prints more generally see Matthews Grieco, 'Pedagogical Prints'.

[75] On representations of the domestic interior see esp. Aynsley and Grant, 'Introduction'.

[76] On genre painting, its subjects, and the picaresque in Italy see Porzio, 'Aspetti'.

[77] e.g. Giulio Romano's *Wedding Banquet of Cupid and Psyche*, Palazzo Te, Mantua (1523–4), and the *Venus and Cupid* by Lambert Sustris (c.1560), at the Louvre.

evolution of two distinct styles—one wider, more comfortable, and elaborate; the other narrow, harder, and more portable—but whether these had anything in common with those in use in Italy is at present unknown.

In her observations on religious painting in Renaissance Italy, Flora Dennis explains that many artists added 'visual power and resonance' by setting religious scenes in a contemporary context, thereby reaffirming the normality of the scene, and 'bridging the gap between Renaissance audiences and the biblical events of a historically and culturally remote…past'.[78] We draw on several such paintings here, which frame biblical accounts of births within the home, and in so doing depict contemporary beds. Facilitated by Thornton's meticulous study of the history of Renaissance furnishings, in Chapter 4 we have been able to suggest a relationship between changing styles of bed and bed hanging and evolving medical injunctions to protect sleepers from draughts and the cold. In particular, it was the weight and fullness of the drapes on beds in later sixteenth-century paintings which prompted speculation about the increased attention to the thermal properties of hangings.

In another such religious painting, Allori's *Birth of the Virgin* (Plate 7), the focus of our interest is a portable brazier used to warm both baby and swaddling clothes. Whereas we interpret the presence of a foot-warmer in a popular print as hinting at their wider social diffusion, the fact that Allori was an extremely successful painter working for the Florentine elite leads us to a different set of observations. The same is true of Plate 21, known as *Preparations for a Banquet* by a German artist (1658–1722) about whom little is known other than that he settled in Rome in the late seventeenth century and resided for three years with the Marquis Pallavicino as well as being patronized by the Pope.[79] Although probably painted just a couple of decades after our time frame, the carefully placed collection of different-sized and -shaped glasses bears a close resemblance to some seventeenth-century examples from the Victoria and Albert Museum. Both Allori and Berentz used objects as elements in a carefully constructed display of the paraphernalia of elite life as a way of 'endorsing their client's social distinction'.[80] By adding an inscription to the brazier Allori may have intended to draw attention to it; whilst the glasses in Berentz are arguably part of the central focus of the painting. Yet, as we show in Chapters 3 and 7, both these apparently everyday objects had a health significance which has generally been overlooked, and their centrality in both paintings encourages conjecture about the relationship between the role they played in promoting health and their fashionability and social importance at that time.

A last group of images have been selected because of the physical, medically beneficial impact they were believed to have on the viewer and his or her 'animal spirits', which governed the intellect, sense perceptions, and above all, 'the passions', as discussed in Chapter 6. Whether in tapestry or paint, these—and other

[78] Dennis, 'Developing', 24.
[79] Berentz was born in 1658 in Hamburg and died in 1722 in Rome.
[80] Dutch artists would often include fashionable objects in their paintings of interiors, Loughman, 'Between Reality', 90.

similar idealizing views of gardens, illustrating the delights and pleasures of villa or country life—functioned in a number of ways to promote the health of the spirits (see Plates 18 and 19). The intricate details and pleasant subject matter provided stimulation and good cheer for the spirits of the intellect whilst the predominance of green was thought to soothe the spirits of the eyes. Indeed, gazing on such an image was understood to be just as effective for the health of the passions and spirits of the eyes as seeing a real one. Although painted fruit and flowers could not have a smell, like the carved details of flowers on fireplaces, those in the painted image recall the sweet air of gardens inciting at least the memory of scents, whilst depictions of songbirds or musical instruments comforted and cheered the spirits of the ears.

CONCLUSION

Letters, paintings, inventories, and objects all present their own problems to the historian seeking insight into the practices and attitudes of those other than published authors. Nonetheless, each source ultimately also has much to offer, particularly when used in combination with the others. Each, in different ways, corroborates, complements, and adds new perspectives to what we learn from the regimens, greatly enhancing our understanding of the many ways in which health was pursued in daily life, the objects which enabled it, and the attitudes surrounding this quest for longevity. In Chapters 3–8 we will draw on all three sources in our exploration of the six 'Non-Naturals' which underpinned healthy living, facilitating our attempt to balance prescription and practice, as well as enabling us to shed new light on how early modern people attempted to keep themselves healthy and enjoy a 'long and healthy life' in the face of the uncertainties and difficulties of daily living.

3

Worrying About the Air

'Nothing is more necessary to life than air, since without it we couldn't live for even a moment,' stated the author of one health regimen in 1603.[1] Although the importance of the air to one's health had always been understood, we will argue in this chapter that it assumed increasing significance over the sixteenth century. 'Good' air promoted longevity and vitality, and 'bad' air accounted for a huge range of serious illnesses and long-term decline. Late medieval regimens had varied in their approach to discussions of air; with some ignoring certain issues altogether and most treating the matter quite briefly.[2] By the mid-sixteenth century a gradual shift in emphasis in the genre as a whole meant that in some cases the chapters on air simply became much longer; in others, entire volumes were devoted exclusively to this element.[3] This was achieved both through more extended discussions of traditional topics and the appearance of entirely new themes. For example, greater attention is paid to bad air, particularly cold air, and to the impact of such air on the body. Certain areas of the body, such as the head, hands, and feet, are also singled out as being especially vulnerable to cold air. Another characteristic of the late sixteenth-century regimen is a focus on the relationship between local climates and health, with special interest in the properties and health significance of winds, particularly local winds. With this came a heightened awareness of the need to protect oneself from various environmental conditions, which entailed far more detailed advice on how to locate and design a healthy home so as to minimize the impact of temperature and winds. This was accompanied by the multiplication of references to practices and objects which could be used within and around the home to protect the body from bad air and the extremes of the climate. Likewise if we look at architectural treatises, household management advice, or the correspondence between members of the lay elite, we find that the air was a constant source of concern, influencing not only precepts, but also practices to a striking degree. In this chapter we will outline the medical explanations given for the effects

---

[1] 'Niuna cosa è alla vita piú dell'aria necessaria poi che senza quella né certo un momento potiamo vivere.' Fonseca, *Del conservare*, 118.

[2] Marilyn Nicoud's study of late medieval regimens shows how much diversity there was within the genre: *Les Régimes*. This continues to be true of early modern regimens.

[3] For example, while Fonseca, *Del conservare* (1603), Durante, *Il tesoro* (1565), and Viviani, *Trattato del custodire* (1626) have 7 to 13 pages on air and breathing, Frediano, *Arca novella* (1656), devotes about 70 pages to it and Pietragrassa, *Politica medica* (1650) wrote a 400-page volume on air. However, there are still authors who ignore the topic altogether, e.g. Auda, *Breue compendio* (1652), and others, like Anguillara, *Vaticinio* (1589), who make just a passing comment.

of air on one's health and the key recommendations made by doctors as well as offering some explanations for this rising tide of anxiety about the air. We will then look at the way in which ideas about the air affected the principles governing the design, management, and even furnishing of a healthy home, and consider their impact on the domestic lives of the elite.

THE MEDICAL ADVICE

When early modern authors wrote about the air they had a number of qualities in mind which had a variety of effects on health. A key concept was that of the 'temperament' of the air—whether it was hot, cold, wet, or dry. This was associated largely with night and day, seasonal change, and, after the mid-sixteenth century, with the winds. Broadly speaking, hot air had a 'relaxing' effect on the body—opening the pores and rendering it flaccid. Humid air softened and dampened the body both within and without. Cold air constricted, closing the pores and hardening the body, whilst dry air had a desiccating effect. Whether these attributes of the air had a positive or negative effect on the body depended partly on the individual's constitution and age but also on whether they were to be expected for the time of year. This was because the individual body was considered to be used to the seasonal weather and diurnal cycles associated with its native region, so any unseasonal weather or unusual changes in air temperature represented a considerable threat to the body.

Air was also described as 'good' or 'bad'. Following criteria established in Avicenna's *Canon*, good air was 'temperate', therefore neither too cold, too hot, too dry, nor damp; it was also light, thin, bright, clear, sweet-smelling, and moved gently. It was found high up, without being too exposed. Generally however there was more detail about how to identify bad air, which was blamed for a wide spectrum of bodily disorders. Instead, the focus was on specific identifiable qualities which produced 'bad' air and their effects on the body. Foul-smelling air, for example, was described in terms such as *fetido*, *corrotto*, and *pestilente*, and was feared as 'corrupting' the body. Its sources were usually things such as sewers, carcasses, and certain plants such as box, yew, nuts, figs, and cabbages.[4] Foul air rising from within the body was also dangerous, whether a product of undigested food in the stomach, rotting teeth, or rotting gums. Although there was much continuity in these definitions of bad air, there was also change. Most significantly, although 'putrid' bad air is clearly an ongoing concern, it is not at the centre of discussions, whilst the term 'miasma' is used rarely, if ever, in health regimens. In her overview of the topic Hannaway notes that scholars view miasma and corrupt air as having remained the predominant explanation for plague and disease until well into the nineteenth century.[5] However, what we find in the regimens is a clear shift of emphasis from the dangers of putrid or miasmatic air to the dangers represented by cold or damp air. Cold air was feared for its rapid and detrimental effects on the

---

[4] Many of these were cited in Avicenna's *Canon*.
[5] Hannaway 'Environment and Miasmata', 295, 296, 304.

body, particularly by closing the pores, whilst damp air was envisaged as being literally thicker, heavier, and more dense, thereby blocking the pores, again with severe negative consequences. Thus night air, fogs and mists, airless valleys, or closed houses were all suspect. Sea air was not traditionally well regarded. It was viewed as dangerously thick, hot, and damp, although some late sixteenth-century authors writing panegyrics to coastal cities like Venice and Genoa found circumstances in which it could be a more positive influence.[6] And just as air which was too cold and damp was bad, so was air which was excessively hot, particularly if it was humid.

Winds also played an increasingly crucial role in discussions of air quality. Although the characteristics of at least one or two winds had usually been mentioned in medieval regimens, by the mid-sixteenth century lengthy discussions of their influence on air quality had become a regular feature in most regimens. Broadly speaking north and east winds were understood as cool and drying with east winds as the healthiest. West winds tended to be damp, whilst south winds, combining damp and hot air, were invariably considered the worst of all for health. However, their initial qualities could be exacerbated by many factors; winds which had travelled over battlefields, swamps, and marshes were dangerous for example, those passing over clay picked up excess humidity, whilst passing over trees was beneficial. In later regimens the number of winds discussed also increased from four to as many as twelve or sixteen, with explanations of their respective qualities. We can take as a comparison an early Renaissance and an early seventeenth-century regimen. The former, written in 1480, gives the most 'essential' information: to avoid southern winds, and to ensure one's winter home is protected by mountains from north winds in particular.[7] The latter devotes eighteen pages to a discussion of the winds and their qualities, focusing on twelve named winds and the kinds of ailments associated with them.[8] Given the complexity of the advice, coupled with the importance of understanding the qualities of the air and winds, we can see why a short verse was included in a late seventeenth-century household advice manual which encapsulated the major points for its readers.

> He who desires in life to keep himself healthy
> Flees the air from the West and the *Occaso*
> From the corrupt mists and the *Pantano*
> Stinking reason for adverse fortune
> The rising sun generates purer air
> And if Boreas (the north wind) blows, it is much safer.[9]

Just as air was 'bad' in different ways, so it had differing effects on the body and as the role played by air in health gained in importance, so too did accounts of its power to harm. These shifted from the simple explanations of the dangers of an

---

[6] Gropretio sees it as damaging in *Un breue et notabile trattato*, 367. In Paschetti, sea air is both heavy, *caliginoso*, and damp, but the riviera of Genova is 'pure and healthy'. *Del conservare*, 128.

[7] Benzi, *Tractato utilissimo*, 2.

[8] Paschetti, *Del conservare*, 126–44.

[9] 'Chi brama in vita mantenersi sano | Fugga l'aria fra' l'ostro e fra l'occaso | Da le nebbie corrotta, e dal Pantano | Puzzolente cagion d'averso caso | Genera il sol nascente Aria piu pura | E se Borea vi spira e piu sicùra.' Tanara, *L'economia*, 5.

overheating heart or suffocation by 'fumosities', to lengthy lists of ailments, such as that penned by one late sixteenth-century author who noted pessimistically:

> Because such airs weigh on the head, [they] offend the animal spirits...relax the joints...block the pores, prohibit the movement of animal spirits...Shadowy thick airs darken the heart, trouble the mind, harden the body, slow down concoction, and speed up old age.[10]

Explanations of the dangers focused on three areas of the body in particular: the heart, the brain, and the pores. The heart was immediately affected by the quality and temperature of incoming air, and it was thought that its temperature should be kept stable. Breathing in hot air was therefore dangerous, since the heart might overheat, whilst damp hot air was believed to suffocate since it was heavier and pressed in on the body.[11] Another concern was that breathing in corrupt or pestilential air could 'corrupt' the vital spirits produced in the heart, leading to a rapid temperature change and grave illness.[12]

Particularly noticeable was the heightened sense of the brain's vulnerability to cold air. This can be explained by the early sixteenth-century revival of interest in Galenic and Hippocratic views over Aristotelian teachings, exemplified after the 1550s by frequent references to the authority of Hippocrates. Aristotle, who had held greater sway in medieval scholastic thought, had emphasized the role of the heart over the brain. The brain was viewed traditionally as a cold and watery organ, and Aristotle maintained that because it was bloodless it could not contain the 'animal spirits' believed to carry heat and vitality around the body, and therefore could play no role in sensation and thought.[13] Hippocratic teaching held, on the contrary, that 'man's head is the root of all ills'. Hippocrates had taught that intelligence and sensation were brought into the brain in the air, transmitted by the animal spirits, and that the brain therefore acted as mediator between the external world and the soul. This was interpreted as meaning that to conserve its health one should ensure that nothing altered the brain's temperature, since this had a rapid knock-on effect throughout the body.[14] And given that it was a cold organ, anything which made it even colder or damper, such as the passage of cold air via the nose to the brain (cold, damp night air was particularly feared) should be avoided. This was thought to damage the animal spirits, thereby making one's responses and intellectual functions sluggish.[15]

---

[10] 'Perche tal'Aere grava la testa, e offende gli spiriti animali...rilassa le gionture...perche entrato nel corpo, opilando i meati, prohibisce il transito de gli spiriti animali....L'aere tenebroso, e grosso, offusca il cuore, conturba la mente, aggrava il corpo, ritarda la concottione, e accelera la vecchiezza.' Durante, *Il tesoro*, 3.

[11] Petronio, *Del viver*, 7.

[12] [Maineri], *Opera utilissima*, ch. 2, echoed by Manfredi, *Il perché*, 148; Lennio, *Della complessione*, 32; and Viviani, *Trattato del custodire*, 130.

[13] Rocca, *Galen*, 64.

[14] Citing Hippocrates, Traffichetti writes: 'Il capo dell'huomo é radice di tutti li mali,' and he cites Galen repeatedly; *L'arte di conservar*, 171–3, 178.

[15] *L'arte di conservar*, 172–3. See Rocca, *Galen*, 26–7 on Hippocratic understandings; 28–31 on Aristotle; and 60–4 on Galenic views.

Impure air—whether from external or internal sources—also damaged the functions of the brain. Authors described the effects of these fumes variously, with one explaining that they 'thickened' the animal spirits, which either cast a 'shadow' on the brain, thereby 'rusting' it, or that these 'thicker' spirits then obstructed the pores of the skull.[16] This then prevented respiration and the escape of unhealthy vapours from within the head. These dangers to the brain assumed particular importance for those whose profession or status made them reliant on their intellects. Marsilio Ficino, who addressed the concerns of such men in his late fifteenth-century regimen for elderly scholars, returns time and again to the dangers posed by impure and cold night air to the brain, but many of the regimens were implicitly or explicitly addressing a readership whose social position rested on their intellectual powers.[17]

Although there was also some danger to the head from hot air, the vulnerability of the brain was particularly evident when making a transition from a hot or cold environment to its opposite. Doctors feared that if the pores of the head were opened excessively wide as a result of great heat, and one moved suddenly to a cold environment, the pores were left wide open, ready to receive a blast of cold air which could cause 'lesions' to the brain and lungs.[18] Thus writing in 1592 Petronio even admonishes those doctors who unbind wounds on the head in the morning when the air is still dangerously cool since the 'cold morning air bites into them endangering the brain'.[19]

Concerns about the winds and the brain's vulnerability seem to have intersected in later sixteenth-century thought. Worries about the brain focused both on where the head was positioned, high on the body and thus exposed to the impact of winds, and on the various 'entry points' for air located on the head. It was again Petronio who explained that the head was particularly vulnerable to air because the head is 'concave, resting on the top of the body like a cupping glass...so that winds then fill the head...and passing first through the brain' leave their strength there.[20] He used this model to explain why Romans were so susceptible to head ailments. Another likened the head to a 'chimney placed high up on the body through which pass the smoky vapours rising from the fire below'.[21] Theories about the damage to the brain were even more sophisticated by the mid-seventeenth century when one writer described how the sutures on the skull also permitted the entry of air to the brain, exposing it to 'alterations'.[22] Hence his exhortation to his readers that 'above all one must save and defend the head'.[23] One of the simplest

---

[16] 'Ingrossa l'intelletto...adombra e circonda a guisa d'una rubigine tutte le virtù dell'anima.' Benzi, *Tractato utilissimo*, 2ᵛ and 4.

[17] For Ficino see *De le tre vite*, 13ʳ and 56ʳ. A traditional concern in regimens as can be seen in Arnau de Villanova's regimen written for the King of Aragon in the early 14th century. Paschetti also stresses that 'administrators of the Republic' should maintain their health; *Del conservar*, 5.

[18] Paschetti, *Del conservar*, 133–4.

[19] Petronio, *Del viver*, 7.

[20] 'Perche è concava, e sta appoggiata sopra il corpo, come se fosse una ventosa...La testa adunque si viene ad empire dall'aere...quell'aere passa prima al cervello.' Petronio, *Del viver*, 202.

[21] 'Assomiglia a un camino, al quale ascendeno le fumosità, e vapori che dal fuoco si levano.' Traffichetti, *L'arte di conservar*, 178.

[22] Frediano, *Arca novella*, 47.   [23] Frediano, *Arca novella*, 46.

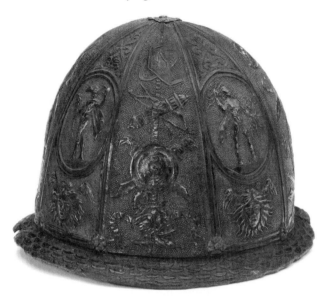

Fig. 3.1. Hats of this shape became popular in Italy in the second half of the sixteenth century (Levi-Pisetzki, *Storia del costume*, iii. 155). Made of thick pieces of leather they would have kept the head and brain warm and protected them from damp air—increasingly perceived as a major threat to health. The classically inspired imagery and decorations suggest a ceremonial use (h. 18.5 cm, d. 24.5 cm). (M. A.-W.).

ways in which the head and brain could be protected was simply by wearing some form of cap and numerous writers recommend a variety of headgear (see Fig. 3.1). One goes to the extent of pointing out how many things can be used to 'defend the head from external injuries by the air', listing berets, hats, and caps, even including a complicated discussion for their use according to the weight of the hat, and the density and porosity of each individual's scalp![24]

The pores—whether of the skin or skull—were another area of the body crucially affected by air quality and temperature. Since they were 'the windows of breath' and 'the roads of perspiration' through which the body breathed and transpired, according to most writers the key to a healthy body lay in keeping the pores open to just the right degree.[25] Temperature extremes endangered the body by either closing or opening the pores inappropriately. Cold air made the pores close, whilst damp air could obstruct them, in both cases blocking the passage of cool clean air into the body, and the exit of excess heat and other superfluous waste products out of the body.[26] In the case of hot air, the subsequent widening of the pores could allow the *fumeés* and spirits to leave the body too quickly, or let cold

---

[24] 'Al qual uso di diffendere la testa dalle estrinseche ingiurie dell'aere.' Traffichetti, *L'arte di conservar*, 173.

[25] 'Le finestre del respiro' and 'Le strade della perspirazione'; Traffichetti, *L'arte di conservar*, 14–15.

[26] Traffichetti, *L'arte di conservar*, 15–16.

air rush in unhindered. We can see how these understandings of the pores influenced contemporary explanations of the causes of illness and death in an account of the death of Cardinal Aldobrandino, in February 1622. He was reported as having left Ravenna and travelled by day and night for three days in an attempt to arrive in Rome in time for the beginning of the conclave that would elect Gregory XIV. However, this reckless behaviour had led to his death 'because the cold had made his pores narrow and his blood had frozen'.[27]

Interestingly however, although we find mention of the dangers of inhaling 'corrupt' air through the mouth, or of cold air damaging the brain, we find barely any references to the idea that penetration of the body by noxious or pestilential air via the pores represented a particularly serious threat, or that the pores should be kept closed against insalubrious external air. This flies in the face of established scholarship on hygiene which has emphasized the idea that by the mid-sixteenth century, open pores represented a danger to health, particularly in the context of bathing, due to fears that pores widened by the heat were then penetrated by pestilential air.[28] Possibly this concern with the danger of open pores was quite specific to plague literature or was more specific to the French medical context. If anything, Italian regimens are more concerned with the danger already mentioned, of inhaling pestilential air through the mouth which travels straight to the heart, and which, either by altering its temperature or suffocating it and the vital spirits, leads to sudden death.[29] And whilst any imbalance was potentially dangerous, contemporary Italian regimens seem above all to have been concerned with the danger which *closed* rather than *open* pores represented to the body.[30]

THE SOURCES OF NEW IDEAS ABOUT AIR

How can we account for this increased anxiety about 'bad' air in all its forms? We might expect a significant contributing factor to be the long-term impact of plague on people's perceptions of health. According to classical medical authors the plague was prompted by the corruption of the air which caused those whose body was already distempered to become ill and these time-honoured theories continued to be revered. It is true that contagionism—the idea that disease could also be transmitted through direct contact with the sick or via intermediate objects—was increasingly gaining currency amongst public health authorities and members of the medical profession. Even this new approach, however, assigned considerable

---

[27] Cited in D'Onofrio, *La Villa Aldobrandini*, 77.

[28] This was first highlighted by Georges Vigarello in *Concepts of Cleanliness*, 9, citing sources dealing principally with fears of the plague in the context of steam baths and bathing.

[29] Echoed by Manfredi in *Il perche*, 148; Lennio, *Della complessione*, 32; and Viviani, *Trattato del custodire*, 130.

[30] Pietragrassa is the exception; nonetheless, he still concluded that the main danger was that of obstructing the entry of air as a result of excessively narrowed pores; *Politica medica*, 194, 197–202.

importance to the air as the main vehicle of disease.[31] It has recently been shown also that Fracastoro's contagionist theory, far from radically breaking with tradition, acknowledged the key role of overheated and damp air in determining the putrefaction of the imperceptible particles that compose the body and are then transmitted to another body.[32] Cohn has recently brought to our attention examples of those voices which, in the last quarter of the sixteenth century, challenged the assumption that plague derived from poisonous air created by remote causes such as planetary injunctions and earthquakes. However, his conclusion that these ideas equated to a rejection of the importance that the Galenic-Hippocratic paradigm attributed to air quality, is ill-founded. Some doctors took great pains to demonstrate that in some cases the air was not corrupted when the plague first made its appearance, and that in these specific cases the disease was more likely to have derived from contagion from infected goods and peoples than from the air. In other words their arguments relate to defined episodes of plague and did not aim to question the role of air in disease in general, as Cohn concludes. On the contrary, their detailed analyses of the atmospheric conditions when the epidemic broke out—for example the observations that this was crisp and dry, never foggy and misty—seem to confirm continued adherence to the established classification of air as either healthy or unhealthy.[33]

Hence repeated outbursts of plague during the period must have heightened preoccupations about the quality of the air. And although the regimens were not overly concerned with plague, we are probably witnessing generic fears about the dangers of pestilent air embedded in their advice.[34] For example, the 'French Disease'—as the disease we know as syphilis was termed—had first appeared in the 1490s and had ravaged sixteenth-century Europeans. Although links were made between transmission of the disease and physical contact, pestilent air—whether generated by the stars, the weather, or other factors—also loomed large in people's explanations of the underlying causes.[35]

On the other hand one should not overemphasize the role of epidemics in the increased concerns about air we notice in regimens. The publication of new healthy living guides in the vernacular grew from the late 1540s onwards and remained steady in the following decades, a period that witnessed a respite from the plague—with only sporadic appearances in certain localities of northern Italy before the violent generalized outbreak of 1575–8.[36] This also means that the genre was already well established when the publication of plague tracts soared, as a result of the pandemic of 1575. As recently demonstrated by Cohn, almost half of the plague-related texts published in the sixteenth century appeared in the two peak

---

[31] See e.g. how Gerolamo Mercuriale reconciled the two conceptual frameworks in his interpretation of the plague of 1575 in Venice; Palmer, 'Girolamo Mercuriale'.

[32] Pennuto, 'La natura dei contagi'.

[33] Cohn, *Cultures of Plague*, 192–202, esp. 200–1.

[34] Del Panta, *Le epidemie*, 117–78.

[35] For a comprehensive survey of the discussions surrounding syphilis amongst medical writers see Arrizabalaga, Henderson, and French, *The Great Pox*, 113–44, 234–51.

[36] The relationship between these two genres is discussed in Ch. 1.

years of this plague.[37] The continuous interest in healthy living guides from the 1540s to the last quarter of the seventeenth century thus appears to be relatively independent from the chronology of the plague and of writings about the plague in Italy.

Since increased attention surrounded in particular the effects of cold weather on the body it is worth considering whether this could have been prompted by an actual change in the climate. There is some consensus amongst climate historians that between the mid-fourteenth and the nineteenth centuries there was a 'mini-ice age', thought to have been at its most severe towards the end of the sixteenth and into the seventeenth century. This was marked by a drop in average temperatures, and longer, colder winters with more rain and snow, as well as many extreme climate events.[38] Certainly developments in Italian regimens can be seen to follow the outlines of this chronology, as the 1560s saw a new focus on the effects of temperature and of winds on different parts of the body, along with discussions of a range of material objects which can be used to minimize the impact of the cold.

We have already seen how increasing familiarity with Hippocratic medical texts had influenced concerns about the effects of cold on the brain, and it was also one of the driving forces behind the new regard for the relationship between the body and local environmental conditions—particularly the effects of winds. This is not to say that earlier generations of doctors had been entirely ignorant of Hippocratic teaching on the air, but the attention paid to it in the Arab/Greek tradition was extremely varied. In medieval regimens the focus had been principally on seasonal change and this was continued in early modern regimens.[39] However, the 'rediscovery' of a key Hippocratic text, *Airs, Waters, Places*, first made widely available in a printed Latin translation in 1525, gave the discussions on environment a new focus.[40] It was also a text which 'more than any other Hippocratic treatise, seems likely to have appealed to Renaissance readers beyond, as well as within, the medical community'.[41]

In *Airs, Waters, Places*, Hippocrates, taking seasonal change as a given, had placed greater emphasis on the ways in which specific local climatic conditions affected the dwellers of a given region. Thus in the normal course of events a body was used to its local climate, as prevailing winds and local weather patterns determined the

---

[37] Cohn, *Cultures of Plague*, 26 and 77. Interestingly, on the basis of the bibliography of plague texts provided by Cohn, only Marsilio Ficino and Bartolomeo Traffichetti appear to have written both kinds of vernacular tracts.

[38] This is explained most fully and recently in Behringer, *A Cultural History of Climate*, 85–90. Also, Pfister, 'Weeping in the Snow'; Kamen, 'Climate and Crisis', 369–76.

[39] See Arnaldi, *Regimen sanitatis*, 111.

[40] Nicoud mentions that the Galenic commentary on *Airs, Waters, Places* was 'known throughout the high Middle Ages' in a Latin translation; Nicoud, *Les Régimes*, 157. Nancy Siraisi is not at all convinced about the extent to which they were known prior to the 16th century. See her *History, Medicine*, 73. Both Nutton and Siraisi document the increased importance of Hippocratic teachings and knowledge of *Airs, Waters, Places*, in particular after the mid-16th century: Siraisi, *History, Medicine*, and Nutton, 'Hippocrates in the Renaissance'.

[41] Siraisi, *History, Medicine*, 93–4.

kinds of illness to which the body was predisposed throughout the year in that specific place. Indeed, the impact of local climates on the body was considered to be so significant that it was also used to explain the physiognomy, character, and morality of different racial groups. Hence doctors were expected to have detailed knowledge of the local climate and weather patterns for the area in which they lived.[42]

An eloquent example of the influence of Hippocrates on sixteenth-century medical thought emerges from the editorial alterations introduced in a late sixteenth-century edition of the fifteenth-century regimen by physician Michele Savonarola. In the re-edition by Boldo not only is new material on air added, but direct reference is made to Hippocrates' advice that long-term illness is best cured through a change of location, and hence of air. Moreover he exhorts the reader to read the full text for himself: 'So that you can really understand the importance of changing places, it is necessary for you to diligently read that which Hippocrates wrote in the book *Airs, Waters, Places*.'[43]

It was surely as a direct consequence of this emphasis on place and health that regionalism became one of the distinctive features of the mid-sixteenth-century regimen, as we see a growing desire to relate health advice to the specific local environment in which people lived.[44] There is not only a marked increase and detail in the advice on where to locate one's home and how to orient it as regards winds, but a new subgenre emerged which offered people tailor-made advice for their individual cities. The first city-specific regimen in Italian was authored in 1565 by Tommaso Rangoni. Asserting that the site of a city or home is the primary constituent of health, the book is structured around ten points which affect the climate of Venice.[45] These include consideration of the 'aspect' of the city or house, the height and air quality of specific districts, the influence of the soil, the sea and lagoon, the prevailing winds, and the effects of nearby mountain ranges. These appear to have been intended to help readers choose where to site their homes or recognize the health problems associated with their chosen neighbourhoods. The genre was evidently popular, as evinced by the publication of a regimen for Romans which appeared first in Latin in 1582, then in Italian in 1592, and one for Genoa in 1603 by Paschetti. Nearly a century later in 1691, Rangoni's text on Venice was republished, whilst another short regimen for Romans appeared by Ciccolini in 1697.[46]

It is in conjunction with this interest in localism that we witness the rise of a new interest in winds noted earlier. This trend was even more marked in the city-specific regimens, which paid attention to local prevailing winds, even discussing

---

[42] See his advice for doctors moving to a new place in *Airs, Waters, Places*, 148–9. Galen also summarized the Hippocratic emphasis on environment; De Lacy (ed.), *Galen on Hippocrates*, 517.

[43] Boldo, *Libra della Natura*, 213.

[44] Although Nicoud notes that some medieval regimen made references to distinctive local foods and factors; *Les Régimes*, 167, 171.

[45] Rangoni, *Consiglio*.

[46] Petronio, *Del viver*; Paschetti, *Del conservar*; Ciccolini, *L'oro della sanità*. Lennio has a 4-page discussion on environment and national character and physique; *Della complessione*, 11–15.

physical features which affected their qualities or deviated their course, such as hills or city walls. Thus Rome was deemed to have very bad air because of its exposure to damp southerly and westerly winds, exacerbated by the humidity rising from the many underground water sources, and winds coming in over the Pontine Marshes. The many hills were thought to complicate the picture, sheltering some areas from dangerous winds, in others preventing winds from blowing through them and cleaning out the thick and heavy air.[47] This interest in local winds culminated in publications for doctors specifically on the winds of a particular city. A treatise on winds and 'that which a doctor ought to know and on the site of the city of Pisa' was published in 1628 by Doctor Cartegni.[48] Fourteen years later, in 1642, two publications appeared by Doctor Domenico Panaroli. *Aerologia* (The Science of Winds) is a discussion of many winds and their effects on health in Rome, intended to be the first in a multi-volume work on the Non-Naturals, which was never completed. *L'aria celimontana* (The Air on the Caelian Hill), although not a regimen, is a defence of the air on the Caelian Hill, evidently as a rebuttal to contemporary views which opined that it was an unhealthy place in which to live.

This increased interest in the relationship between local climate and health cannot be explained purely with reference to Hippocratic medical texts. Two areas of classical learning in particular affected those writing regimens: natural history and architectural theory. Pliny's *Natural History*, which contained references to the winds and health, appeared in fifty-five editions between 1469 and 1600.[49] Ptolomy's *Tetrabiblos* was also popular, and contained references to the planets, the atmosphere, winds, and the impact of climate on different races, whilst his *Geography* (or *Cosmographia*), which was introduced in a Greek edition by Erasmus in 1533, included discussions of the air, the elements, planets, stars, and climate zones.[50] Furthermore, the voyages of discovery, circumnavigation of the globe, and the development of overseas trade resulted in encounters with new races and cultures during the late fifteenth and early sixteenth centuries which added impetus not only to this fascination in the natural sciences, but also to the interest in climate-based explanations for the cultural and physical differences between different races. Furthermore, cosmography (the study of the universe and what is now termed geography) became an increasingly prestigious and popular subject, particularly in Rome.

Another key influence on contemporary thought was the Renaissance revival of interest in Greek and Roman architecture. References to ideas about the relationship between buildings, locations, and healthy airs were scattered throughout classical genres, as for example the extremely influential letters of Pliny the Younger. He included precise descriptions of his country villas in his correspondence which, according to one contemporary, circulated as 'bedtime' reading

---

[47] Petronio's introduction to the winds of Rome covers 4 pages, and he returns to it repeatedly throughout his regimen, *Del viver*, 10–14.

[48] Cartageni, *Trattato de' venti*.

[49] For a discussion of the circulation of these texts and ideas see Findlen, 'Natural History', esp. 439 for the editions of Pliny.

[50] On geography see Vogel, 'Cosmography'.

amongst fifteenth-century humanists.[51] However, the crucial influence on six-teenth-century architecture were *The Ten Books of Architecture* by Vitruvius writ-ten between 80 BC and AD 15. First printed in Latin in 1486, there were further editions within two years and Italian editions by the 1520s and this text was vital to debates on healthy building practices. Early on in his treatise Vitruvius clarifies the importance of medicine for architects, commenting that any architect worth his salt

> Should know the science of medicine, as this depends on those inclinations of the heavens which the Greeks call climates, and know about airs, and about which places are healthful and which disease ridden, and about the different applications of water, for without these studies no dwelling can possibly be healthful.[52]

Consequently, substantial sections of the treatise are dedicated to how to choose a suitable location for one's home or city and how to orient these with regard to the local air quality, climate, and winds, so as best to preserve health, following the principles laid down by Hippocrates.[53] Some of this advice on sites had already been transmitted to Renaissance Italy in the late medieval regimens by, for exam-ple, Aldobrandino da Siena.[54] Broadly, they suggested that one's home should be relatively high up so as to be open to breezes and the warmth of the sun, but not so high as to be exposed to strong winds and the biting cold. One should avoid proximity to any buildings, mountains, walls, or cliffs which might block the pas-sage of air or the sun's drying and warming rays. Generally speaking a house should rely on ventilation and windows facing the north or east, since winds from these directions were considered cool and drying, always preferable to hot damp winds. What the translation of Vitruvius brought into the arena was far more detail about the orientation and layout of buildings (see Fig. 3.2).

This was advice which, although already known amongst fifteenth-century humanists, was seized and greatly elaborated upon by Leon Battista Alberti in his *De re aedificatoria* (On Architecture) written in 1452, first printed in 1485, and first published in Italian in 1546.[55] This has been described as being 'perhaps the most significant contribution ever made to the literature of architecture', even though it was written 'for a circle of humanist patrons desiring a set of criteria for their building projects' rather than purely as a manual for architects.[56] Importantly, Alberti took Vitruvian principles of healthy building very much to heart, discuss-ing matters relating to choosing a healthy site or city in five chapters of book I, and another chapter in book IV.[57] Throughout the following two and a half centuries the advice imparted in Alberti was reiterated over and over again. We see it starting

---

[51] De la Ruffinière du Prey, *The Villas of Pliny*, 21.

[52] Vitruvius, *Ten Books on Architecture*, I. 23.

[53] Vitruvius, *Ten Books on Architecture*, I. 17–31.

[54] Albeit simpler and more general rules. See Aldobrandino, *Le Régime du corps*, 12 and 66–7; and for where to live in times of plague, [Maineri], *Opera utilissima*, 104.

[55] We refer to the 1546 edition, published in Venice by Vincenzo Valgrisi.

[56] Kruft, *A History of Architectural Theory*, 49, 44.

[57] Alberti, *Art of Building*, I, chs. 3–7; and IV, ch. 2.

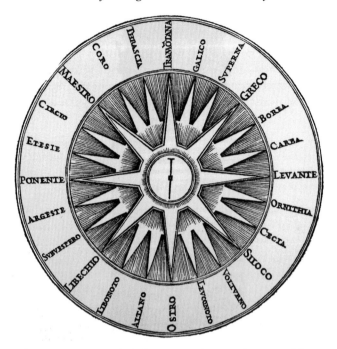

Fig. 3.2. Wind compasses were included in most architectural treatises following the example set by Vitruvius, as in this 1590 version by Giovanni Antonio Rusconi.

with the late fifteenth-century manuscript treatises by architects such as Francesco di Giorgio Martini and Filarete and, by 1537, Serlio notes in the introduction to the manuscript of book VI of his treatise that there is no need for him to write about how to site and orient a house 'because Vitruvius and Alberti have discussed this at such length that there is nothing to add'.[58] By 1615 when the architect Scamozzi published his treatise 'on the idea of a universal architecture' he didn't take his reader's memory of Alberti for granted however, taking instead sixty pages to cover more or less the same ground as his predecessor, including an updated account of the different climates and winds to be found in all the principal cities of Italy.[59] In a treatise from 1627 we are given a sense not just of the continuity of the discourse on health and architecture, but its circularity. In his chapter on selecting a location and respecting the climate, Zanini cites not only the Roman authors Vitruvius, Cato, and Varro but also the Persian Avicenna and, interestingly, Castor

[58] Filarete, *Trattato di architettura*; Martini, *Trattato di architettura*; Serlio, *Architettura civile*, 44. Although circulating in manuscript the inclusion of these ideas nonetheless demonstrates how familiar contemporaries were with them. Myra Rosenfeld considers that, although unpublished, bk. VI was 'one of the most influential of his writings' and known to later architects presumably through the manuscripts; Rosenfeld, *Sebastiano Serlio*, 17.

[59] Scamozzi, *L'idea dell'architettura*—a reprinted facsimile of the edition published in Venice in 1615.

Durante, the author of the most popular contemporary health regimen.[60] And judging from the publication in 1726 of a late seventeenth-century treatise by Giovanni Biagio Amico, in which two chapters are devoted to choice of site and the air, little had changed. In the preface, the editor notes that the author has drawn on the doctrines of the 'ancient architects, since nothing new can be invented'.[61]

The composition of many sixteenth- and seventeenth-century regimens, as well as the building or restructuring of the palaces and villas of the Italian elite, must therefore be placed in the broader intellectual, social, and cultural framework of humanism with its overarching quest to recover all forms of knowledge from the classical past and, where possible, to apply it to the contemporary context. So our ambitious physicians were writing their regimens in a milieu in which wealthy patrons of the arts read Pliny and Alberti when planning their palaces, architects read healthy living guides when writing their treatises, and all around them was a growing fascination with natural history and geography. This was also a society in which there was undoubtedly much overlap between what we now regard as separate professional spheres, with much contact between members of the educated elite, whether centring around the papal court, the academies, or the less formal social gatherings known as *conversazioni* held by cardinals, now considered to be precursors to the later eighteenth-century salon.[62] In this environment men of the nobility—whether laymen or clergy—as well as doctors, architects, and artists immersed themselves in the latest developments in the sciences and the arts. For example, the head of the Spada family, Bernardino, made cardinal in 1626, was interested in astronomy, mathematics, geography, the sciences, and architecture and commissioned the astrological ceiling fresco of the Meridian in his palace in Rome in 1644 (see Plate 4).[63] He opened his palace and villa to members of the academies, and in the summer his villa in Tivoli was known as a kind of alternative meeting place for members of the celebrated Academia dei Lincei.[64]

WHERE TO BUILD A HEALTHY HOME

The diffusion of the new architectural principles coincided with a period of rapid economic growth which was accompanied by a dramatic surge in palace building across Italy. In Rome this was led by the papacy, cardinals, and baronial families on the definitive return of the papacy from Avignon in the mid-fifteenth century. New palaces were required to house the cardinals, ambassadors, and nobility drawn to the new capital of Christianity and the ancient baronial roman families rapidly followed by establishing themselves in the city. Twelve new palaces were erected in

---

[60] Zanini, *Della architettura*, II. 120.

[61] 'Che da gli antichi architetti ci sono state insegnate, non potendosi sopra ciò rinvenire cosa di nuovo'; Amico, *L'architetto prattico*, 1. See also Capra, *Nuova architettura civile*—a reprint of a 1678 text.

[62] See Madignier, 'Sociabilité informelle'.

[63] Vicini, *Il collezionismo*, 21.

[64] On the cardinal's sociability and supervision of his architects, see Tabarrini, *Borromini e gli Spada*, 3–7, 135–6.

the fifteenth century—mostly in the last quarter of the century—and fifty-five were built in the sixteenth century, as well as the many old palaces which were remodelled entirely.[65] Throughout this fervour of building activity, which continued into the mid-seventeenth century, there is every indication that the Vitruvian principles of healthy building, which were reiterated by doctors in their regimens, underpinned the location and design of palaces and villas.[66]

Advice on the importance of the location of one's home for one's health was taken up by medical and lay writers with gusto. One explained, for example:

> I would like this habitation to enjoy lively Air...I believe that one must insist more on the goodness of this air, than any other thing; because on this one's health depends, and this conserves it, it clarifies the spirits, and the blood, cheers the heart and mind...prolongs life and delays old age.[67]

It was not only printed works which espoused such views. When Marquis Vincenzo Giustiniani wrote to a friend, between 1615 and 1620, advising him about the site and construction of a private house and garden he likewise emphasized these themes. A wealthy banker and art collector, he, like many of his class, had been involved in the planning of his palace and villas. He was drawing on personal experience when he recommended in particular that 'One should choose a site which is high rather than low, so that the building will stand out; it should be exposed to healthy winds and protected from harmful ones'[68] (see Fig. 3.3). And judging from the comments of the French essayist Montaigne, who travelled to Rome in 1581, the Romans were indeed punctilious in observing this kind of health recommendation when it came to the location of their homes. They were so aware of the way different areas in the city could affect their health at different times of the year that apparently they

> Make a distinction between the streets, and quarters of the town, even parts of their homes, out of respect for their health. Such that they change their homes by the season, some renting out two or three palaces at great expense, in order to rehouse themselves appropriately each season, according to their doctor's advice.[69]

His surprised comment that they even changed the home used according to the season 'out of respect for their health' may suggest that this concern about healthy buildings was particularly Italian. Judging from the extent to which architectural and medical ideas had converged in Italian regimens, it was certainly a common Italian preoccupation and many patrician families solved the problem by owning

---

[65] Delumeau, *Vie économique*, 275–6.

[66] See e.g. Coffin's discussion of the late 15th-century Villa Belvedere in relation to the Pope's health; *Magnificent Buildings*, 66–9; and on Cortesi's recommendations for a cardinal's palace, see Weil-Garris and d'Amico (eds.), *The Renaissance Cardinal's Ideal Palace*, 53–4. Also Russell, 'Girolamo Mercuriale's *De Arte gymnastica*'.

[67] Tanara, *L'economia*, 4.

[68] 'Ma si deve eleggere unsito piuttosto altro che basso, che sia spettabile; esposto a venti salutiferi, e riparato da'maligni.' Bottari, *Lettere*, vi, Letter 23: Vincenzo Giustiniani, Marquis of Bassano to the lawyer, Teodoro Amiden, 104.

[69] Our translation of Montaigne, *Viaggio in Italia*, 216.

one or more country villas to which they repaired in late spring and stayed until the early autumn. This was a solution which had been advocated by Pliny and subsequently by Renaissance architects and medical writers and, coupled with the desire to emulate the lifestyles of the ancient Romans, there were the many obvious health advantages. Indeed the contrast between life in towns and life in the country became something of a contemporary polemic; in towns for example the air was 'imprisoned' by the many buildings and narrow streets; this made it stagnant and potentially harmful. But also 'lazy city folk' whose rich diet and lack of exercise meant they failed to digest their food properly were more likely to emit dangerous 'dense exhalations', even though the many fires and the sound of bells were believed to 'rectify' city air.[70] Villas, on the contrary, could be sited in clean pure air, away from the noise and stench of the city such that a character in a 1550 dialogue on the pleasures of country life argues: 'We should not be surprised if the inhabitants of the villa are always healthy, robust, of vigorous appearance, and if on the contrary those in the city are squalid, lean, short-winded and of shorter life'.[71]

Even so, there were potential drawbacks to having a country villa. The flat countryside just around Rome and Genoa had 'thick' air on windless days whilst villas located in the shadow of hills lacked healthy breezes.[72] Villas could become too warm, since they had no other buildings to shade them, and there were dangers from the proximity of 'peasants, because with dirtiness and the dung of the stalls the air is made imperfect'.[73] One result of these varied observations about villas was that the regimen tended to advise readers on how to adapt to life in their country villas, such as avoiding the dangerous hot vapours rising from the burning earth which can trigger respiratory problems by taking only slow walks in the evening when the sun has set.[74] One author considers that villas should in fact not be used in the summer but only in spring and autumn, when the air is lighter, without vapour, and caressed by breezes.[75]

Despite these caveats, villas certainly proved immensely popular with sixteenth-century elites across Italy. Around Rome for example, over twenty new magnificent villas were built between 1470 and 1600 with a further nine in the nearby hills, and this is only counting the most significant amongst them.[76] The years between 1540 and 1620 were the high point of this revival, and the popes chose Frascati as their rural seat.[77] Whilst to the modern reader, the emphasis placed on the healthiness of the sites may appear to be merely part of the rhetorical tradition, read in the context of lay accounts and building plans, the air was clearly a crucial factor in the

---

[70] 'Ci sono esalazioni dense...perchè gli habitanti delle città di rado sono famelici, tardi digeriscono, hanno i sensi non molto purgati, sono di piena e quadrata corporatura e fatti molto pigri al moto.' Pietragrassa, *Politica medica*, 388.

[71] Gallo, *Le dieci giornate*, 142–3.

[72] Petronio, *Del viver*, 301; Paschetti, *Del conservar*, 127–8.

[73] Tanara, *L'economia*, 4.

[74] Paschetti, *Del conservar*, 130.

[75] Pietragrassa, *Politica medica*, 407–8.

[76] Delumeau, *Vie économique et sociale*, 277–9. For a recent study of the villa life around Rome see Ehrlich, *Landscape and Identity*.

[77] Ehrlich, *Landscape and Identity*, 1.

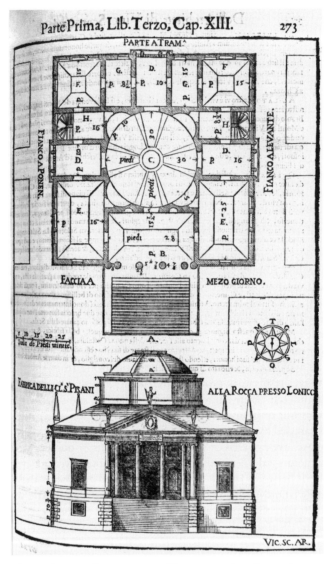

Fig. 3.3. In his architectural treatise, in addition to a lengthy section on the winds, Scamozzi specifically noted that healthy air confers health on the body and 'mirth' on the soul. This shows his plan and elevation for Villa Pisani alla Rocca near Vicenza, built high on a rock between 1576 and 1578. In the accompanying text he emphasized that the windows face one another across the building because this helps 'to purify the air'.

choice of a site. The architect Domenico Fontana who designed the Villa Massimo in the 1570s for Cardinal Montalto, later Pope Pius IV, explained that he had chosen the site, on the highest hill in Rome, because of 'the healthiness and sweetness of the air in this place'.[78] And a late sixteenth-century description of the villa at Tivoli owned by Cardinal Hippolito d'Este stresses that it was a location 'famed for the goodness of its airs. Thanks to the distance from the marshes, and the height of the hill, the site is clean [*netto*] of every bad vapour, and continually purged by northern and western winds.'[79] Furthermore it appears that prior to taking the villa the cardinal had consulted his doctor about whether the air at Tivoli was beneficial for his health, and they had agreed that it would be 'useful and beneficial for the nature and being [*essere*] of the cardinal'.[80] There are also traces of what the cardinal himself thought about the air. In a letter to his brother in July 1555 he wrote: 'I have withdrawn to Tivoli, as I had intended, where in effect you can feel a notable difference in the air from Rome, and I hope soon that my health will benefit from it, with God's grace.'[81] (see Fig. 3.4).

Whether building in the city or countryside, this emphasis on elevated sites so as to benefit from the healthiest airs also affected perceptions about the height of buildings and the use of rooms. We are accustomed to linking the height of a building with displays of magnificence. What this perspective misses is an awareness of the association which was made between health, the height of a home, and status. Whilst Serlio had recommended that the houses of merchants or citizens could be raised by 3 feet above the ground 'for greater magnificence *and* healthiness' (our emphasis),[82] a mid-sixteenth-century regimen on Venice directs that houses and palaces 'should go to the sky with their height', and that one must live 'sufficiently high so as to take airs when needed', though whether this was to rise above the damp air from the canals is not specified.[83] Certainly, advice for those living in Rome warned that basement or ground-floor rooms were made unhealthy by dust in summer and the 'density, heaviness, and thickness' of the air in winter, which was exacerbated by vapours from the river, ground water, and the narrowness of streets which imprisoned the cold damp air.[84]

---

[78] Massimo, *Notizie istoriche*, 41.

[79] 'Tivoli…è celebratissima per la bontà dell'aere, il quale oltre che per la lontananza dalle palude et per la rilevatura del sito è netto d'ogni cattivo vapour e anco continuamente purgato dai venti di Settentrione et di Ponente.' From the *Descrittione di Tivoli*, written in about 1571 to accompany French engravings of the villa, cited in Coffin, *The Villa d'Este*, 142–3.

[80] 'Et si vedeva per consolta di medici che l'aria della citta' di Tivoli si ritrovava utile et giovevole alla natura et essere del Cardinale.' Cited in Barisi, Fabiolo, and Madonna (eds.), *Villa d'Este*, 16.

[81] Letter from Ippolito d'Este to Ercole, Duke of Ferrara, 1550, cited in Pacifici, *Ippolito II d'Este*, 270, 349, and 420.

[82] '*Per magiore magnificenzia et sanitade*' Serlio, *Architettura civile*, 51, 54.

[83] 'Che le case, abitazioni e palagi vanno al cielo con la loro altezza', and 'Da eleggere di altezza sufficiente, che possa prendere aere quando conviene, percioché il molto aere s'altera come il puoco'; Rangoni, *Consiglio*, 7 and 27.

[84] 'Piu grassa, piu densa e piu grossa.' Petronio, *Del viver*, 7–9 on dangers of low accommodation, and 209. See also Durante, *Il tesoro*, 6–7.

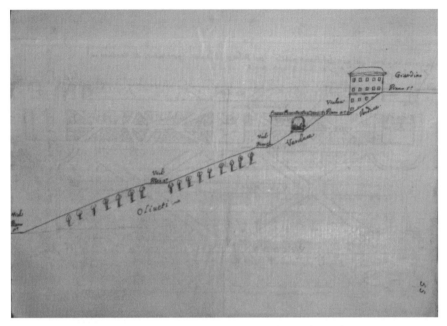

Fig. 3.4. This anonymous drawing from the Spada archives shows the Casino Cesi, just outside Tivoli, probably drawn up in connection with Bernardino's plan to extend the property around 1641. It was used as a villa and was ideally positioned on top of a hill, with formal garden and olive groves below.

Although some authors worried that living on the top storey could cause undue exposure to violent winds, Petronio was not one of them.[85] In his regimen for Romans, first published in 1582 and dedicated to Pope Gregory XIII, he advised living 'when possible, in the highest place in this city', in rooms which were 'open to the sun' and permitting through-passage to winds.[86] Known to have followed his physician's advice closely, the Pope appears to have taken these injunctions very much to heart, having a structure known as 'The Tower of the Winds' built above the Vatican palace between 1578 and 1580.[87] According to a contemporary account this was 'exposed and open on all sides to all the winds', and was intended as a place 'in which he can retreat sometimes for pleasure and

---

[85] On violent winds high up, see Scamozzi, *L'idea dell'architettura*, 222. Pietragrassa says to use the ground floor for summer and upper floors for winter whilst the middle floors are always suitable; *Politica medica*, 410–11.

[86] 'Habitar quanto si può, nel più alto luogo di questa Città…che non si fermi molto nelle più basse parti della casa.' Petronio, *Del viver*, 209.

[87] On the pope's adherence to Petronio's advice Andretta, 'Les Régimes de santé des papes'. For a study of the tower and its decoration Courtright, *The Papacy*, 28–9. Note also that the construction and design were influenced by Ignazio Danti's 1581 *Trattato dei venti*, reproduced in Courtright's book.

to take a breather from business'.[88] We can perhaps even imagine the 80-year-old pope putting Petronio's early morning 'transpiration' routine for elderly men into practice up in his tower. 'It will be useful', notes Petronio, 'when a man dresses, after sunrise, for him to stop for a while at one of those windows, looking either north or west, though taking care to close the other ones: and *so in this manner, having opened all the pores by this time, he will pull the purest of airs towards him*' (our emphasis).[89]

INSIDE THE HEALTHY HOME

As we have seen from Montaigne's comments on the way Romans used different areas of their homes according to the season, internal layout was also key to healthy living. Alberti and his successors had given detailed advice on the orientation and placing of rooms with respect to the sunlight, the changing seasons, and the prevailing winds as regards their effects on temperature and humidity. For example, rooms used during the summer should face north, to avoid scorching heat and benefit from cool evening breezes, and those used in the winter should face south to gain as much benefit from the sun which could 'rectify' the cool damp air. Summer rooms were airy, higher, with more windows, whilst those intended for winter use were to be smaller with lower ceilings to prevent the accumulation of damaging cold vapours and to conserve heat. Rooms used in the evening, such as bathrooms and dining rooms, were to face west so they would be warmed and lit by the evening sun when in use. Rooms most used in the morning such as bedrooms, studies, and libraries were to face east so the early morning sun could dispel any dangerous damp vapours which had accumulated during the night.[90] The author of a regimen published in Pavia in 1650 was so particular that he devoted a good two pages of detailed instructions to conveying such matters to his readers, even specifying three ideal locations for dining rooms; facing west during the winter, east or north during the summer, and east during the unstable weather of spring and autumn.[91]

Architects also agreed that storerooms must be placed so as to ensure that fabrics, tools, or foodstuffs were kept away from damp air which might rust them, or encourage pests, even though they disagreed on where exactly the ideal place

[88] 'Per ritirarsi alle volte a diporto, e respirare da' negotij; in una di esse la più eminente, et che d'ogn'intorno é esposta e apertissima a tutti i venti.' This comment was made by a contemporary architect about the tower; Giovanni Antonio Rusconi, in *Della architettura*, 18. This usage contrasts with Courtright's suggestion that it was used for papal blessings, but fits better with her observation that it resembles a classical *diaeta*, which was traditionally intended as a retreat. Courtright, *The Papacy*, 63.

[89] 'Sará utile, quando l'huomo si veste, dopo che il sole e' levato, se si fermara' alquanto ad una di quelle fenestre, che risguardino, o verso Tramontana, o verso Ponente, con avvertire però, che le altre siano chiuse, poi che a questo modo, havendo in quell'hora aperti tutti li meati, tirara' a se l'aere più puro.' Petronio, *Del viver*, 301.

[90] Alberti, *Art of Building*, 23, 28–9, 32, 140–2, and 145–53.

[91] 'Camere e cenacoli nella primavera and autunno, aperti verso levante.' Pietragrassa, *Politica medica*, 412–13.

was.[92] Alberti, aware of the dangers of temperature changes, took the issue of moving from hot to colder environments very seriously, suggesting some form of transitional space 'to avoid the eventuality that the inhabitants, when leaving a cold environment, enter straight into a warm one, or from such a one to one exposed to frost and winds...which would gravely damage the health of every organism'.[93] Another requirement of the healthy home—particularly in a city—was open spaces in and around the building, particularly 'lovely gardens' which would permit the flow of clean air and allow the family to walk, exercise, and play games, all activities deemed of great advantage to health. Alberti recommends a courtyard in the heart of the house, atriums with balconies, and porticoes carefully situated according to the aspect, so that one can look outside, and 'stay in the sun or the fresh air' according to the season.[94] This was particularly important in city houses.

Patricia Waddy's meticulous analysis of a number of seventeenth-century Roman palaces observes that these principles of 'climate control' were widely implemented. Palaces were indeed oriented in accordance with health recommendations, although particularly as regards the movement of the sun rather than the wind, possibly because the close proximity of city walls and other buildings mitigated the effects of winds.[95] Furthermore, she observes that whilst palaces built in the fifteenth century had the rooms built in a sequence—often around a courtyard—as was recommended in the early Renaissance treatises—a different solution to temperature control known as the double apartment was found by the late sixteenth century. This was a double (parallel) row of rooms of which the external ones, benefiting from winds and tending to be airier, were used in the summer, whilst the more sheltered inner ones were used in winter (or maybe vice versa), according to the position of the room.[96] And judging from the comments by a contemporary writer in 1612, this ability to vary one's accommodation according to the season, like considerations of height, entered into concerns of status and decorum. He noted that in Rome 'He who does not have various apartments on one floor with many rooms on each, to change according to the season, does not live decorously.'[97]

Another example of the strong correlation between ideals of healthy architecture and contemporary practices can be found in structural alterations made to Palazzo Spada in the early seventeenth century by Cardinal Bernardino Spada, a man who had many changes made to the building whilst he lived there, several of which were undertaken with a view to making the palace healthier. His main rooms for summer use, for example, faced north; these were a study, library, and bedroom,

---

[92] Alberti favoured the southern and eastern parts of the house. Martini however explained that winds from the south and west brought 'putrid vapours and encouraged pests'. He favoured east-facing storerooms as did Pietragrassa. Alberti, *Art of Building*, 153; Martini, *Trattato*, 39; Pietragrassa, *Politica medica*, 436.

[93] Alberti, *Art of Building*, 23, 146.

[94] Alberti, *Art of Building*, 418, 432–4.

[95] Waddy, *Seventeenth-Century Roman Palaces*, 16–23. These issues are also considered by Lillie, *Florentine Villas*, 198–9.

[96] Waddy, *Seventeenth-Century Roman Palaces*, 16–17.

[97] 'E chi non ha vari appartamtenti ad un piano di molte stanze l'uno, da mutare secondo le stagioni, non abita con decoro.' Tassoni, *Pensieri e scritti preparatori*, 879.

which would have kept them cool in summer as well as giving even light and dry air, which were good for storing books.[98] Then, in 1632, he had a large south-facing room at the back of the palace, which gave onto a garden, divided into four smaller rooms with a terrace for use in winter. It must also have had a lower ceiling put in, as he wrote that 'the low ceilings do not suffocate during the winter but are pleasing [*danno gusto*], defending one from the rigours of the season'.[99] These alterations would have reduced the amount of damp cold air as well as making them easier to heat and as a contemporary observer later noted: 'The cardinal has lived and slept in these rooms for many years, well protected from the cold and benefiting from several hours of sun after midday.'[100] Interestingly, his brother later commented that when, after a lapse of many years, the cardinal subsequently reconverted these rooms back into two large ones, he had sacrificed health for splendour, 'such that they cannot be lived in at all'.[101] In addition, in 1633 when planning to raise the level of the garden and to lower the level of the alleyway beside the palace, Bernardino cited amongst other reasons that 'By lowering it [the alleyway] the rooms on the lower floor would have become healthier, becoming further from, and raised above, the earth.'[102] Concerns about keeping the palace airy, and protecting the residents from damaging winds, also emerge in accounts of how in the same period he transformed the atrium into 'a more airy vestibule', and covered a particular loggia with glass to give protection from sea winds—even though this apparently ruined the looks of the vestibule.[103] These examples serve to clarify the strong correlation between medical and architectural ideas in this period and the impact they had on actual practice. Given contemporary understandings of the profound interrelationship between the built environment and one's health, at a time when so many of the elite were engaged in building or rebuilding their palaces and villas, it should not surprise us to find that doctors, architects, and other commentators should have sought to emphasize the importance of creating an ideal domestic environment for their wealthy patrons and readers. This is a factor which has not always been given due consideration by architectural historians, who have tended to focus more on issues of status, luxury, and wealth than health when discussing the design of historical buildings.

HEATING AND 'RECTIFYING' THE AMBIENT AIR

We have seen that choosing the ideal site and building according to healthy criteria was a fundamental way of defending oneself from bad air. But not everyone was

[98] Neppi, *Palazzo Spada*, 136–7.   [99] Neppi, *Palazzo Spada*, 137.

[100] 'Il cardinale per molti anni ha habitato e dormito d'inverno in detti camerini assai riparati dal freddo, e che godono doppo mezzo dì più hore di sole.' Neppi, *Palazzo Spada*, 165.

[101] 'Quali non si possono habitare in modo alcuno.' Neppi, *Palazzo Spada*, 289, doc. 47.

[102] 'Del sudetto sbassamento le camere del piano da basso sarebbono diventate tanto più sane, o sollevate dal terreno.' Neppi, *Palazzo Spada* , 269, doc. 21.

[103] Neppi, *Palazzo Spada*, 137 for the atrium and 269 for the loggia.

able to build a house anew and even those who did might still find they had bad air. Luckily, according to the health-advice books, there was still much the house-holder could do to improve and manage both the temperature and quality of the air. During the period under scrutiny the procedures and objects which could be employed in the home were described in an increasingly detailed fashion in regimens. Not only did their instructions become more specific but they mentioned a variety of domestic fixtures, furnishings, and objects—from fireplaces to wall hangings, from perfume burners to hand- and foot-warmers—that were regarded as playing a role in improving the air. It would seem that these artefacts were increasingly understood to be multifunctional, seamlessly combining the demands of domestic decorum and comfort with the requirements of healthy living. Window-panes for example were a relatively new addition to the burgeoning domestic material culture of sixteenth-century Italy which related to health concerns. They provided a means for reducing the cold and blocking the passage of unhealthy winds, although evidently they were not something which the authors could take for granted. A mid-sixteenth-century doctor advised his readers to have windows of transparent glass, or linen or paper, and explains when to use them: 'Close these when it is opportune, and open them to allow winds to enter and exit,' adding that they should be opened also to allow the sun to enter and rectify the air.[104] These instructions suggest that whilst glass panes might have been common amongst the wealthy, the author was presuming a degree of unfamiliarity with window fittings amongst his readers—which is borne out by other sources. When the French essayist Michel de Montaigne travelled through Italy in 1581/2 he noted of his accommodation that 'The rooms, lacking glass and shutters at the windows, are not very comfortable.'[105] Fifty years later another regimen by Doctor Fonseca reiterated that the key to maintaining a temperate environment lay in the use of fires, glass panes or parchment at the windows, and wall hangings.[106] A comparison of the furnishings found in Palazzo Capodiferro, later Palazzo Spada in Rome, in 1565 and 1663, reflects this transition from waxed textiles to glass. Whereas in 1565 most rooms had several frames for *impannate* and some had glass windows, by 1663 neither kind of window fitting is mentioned, which suggests that by then they were all glass, permanently fixed to the structure rather than being moveable goods.[107] Meanwhile, we continue to find mention of cheaper waxed textile blinds known as *gelosie* in the household inventories of the less well-to-do, including those of former prostitutes, up to 1656 (for example see Fig. 3.5).

The third element identified by Dr Fonseca as necessary for temperature control was wall hangings, and they were used to draw in the dampness from the air

---

[104] 'Serrarsi in tempi opportuni e aprirsi accomodate per l'entrare e uscire de venti.' Rangoni, *Consiglio*, 11.
[105] 'Le camere, mancando di vetri e d'imposte alla finestre, sono meno commode.' The comment is made after staying at Rovigo, but is intended as a general observation. See also for Rovereto, Montaigne, *Viaggio in Italia*, 123, 93.
[106] Fonseca, *Del conservar*, 123.
[107] ASR, FSV, vol. 264, 'Inventario di Bernardina di Capo di Ferro', 1.8.1565, 371–2; vol. 269, 'Inventario di Virgilio Spada', 21.5.1663, 195.

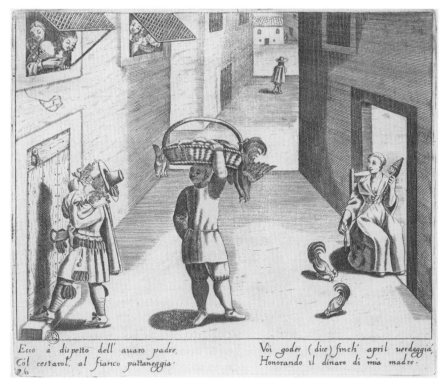

Ecco a dispetto dell' auaro padre,
Col cestarol, al fianco puttaneggia·
2.6

Voi goder (dice) finch' april uerdeggia,
Honorando il dinaro di mia madre·

Fig. 3.5. Detail from a mid-seventeenth-century moralizing print showing a window fitting which allowed people to adjust the flow of air and sunlight into rooms. Windowpanes are also visible in Plate 1.

since, as we saw earlier, damp air represented a great danger because it could block the pores. Unadorned walls were therefore discouraged, and if a room was not panelled, wall hangings were recommended—especially in the low-ceilinged mezzanine apartments where even patricians resorted to living in the cold season.[108] But wall hangings could be changed with the season. For winter authors recommended those made with thick wool because they tempered the coldness of the walls, particularly if made of a 'shiny' colour like purple, 'which creates a certain domain of heat'—an interesting comment, suggesting that the health value attributed to an object was also meant to be conveyed by its aesthetic features.[109] In summer, the same author recommends silks 'because they don't impede the small amount of fresh exhalations which are exuded by the porous surfaces of the walls'.[110] Wall hangings however were not a cheap

[108] Paschetti, *Del conservar*, 132–3.   [109] Pietragrassa, *Politica medica*, 412.
[110] 'Non impediscono quell poco di fresca esalazione che esce della superficie porosa delle pareti.' Pietragrassa, *Politica medica*, 412.

commodity, if in good condition, particularly given the quantity of skins or drapes required to cover whole rooms, which is how they were used. Roman inventories show that their presence was confined to the homes of the more prosperous, and that the gilded and embossed leather hangings known as *corami* were far more common than those in damasks or silks. Indeed, the homes of patricians were crammed with hangings. In 1563 in Palazzo Capodiferro every room was equipped with hooks for hanging *tappezzerie* and *paramenti*, of different materials. A hundred years later we find the walls could be covered in huge numbers of brilliantly coloured wall hangings, whether made of *corame*, damask, or wool. Some of these were hanging and others were stored away, presumably awaiting the change in season.[111] It was more common lower down the social hierarchy to have just one room furnished with wall hangings, as did Beatrice de Mendoza Hispana in 1605, who possessed one 'room' of new red and yellow gilded *corami*, comprising no fewer than 260 panels, which were worth 52 *scudi:* a princely sum for a woman who had survived through prostitution before entering a convent for converted prostitutes.[112]

Fire was obviously a primary weapon against the cold, but it was also believed to 'rectify' and purge the air by making it 'mobile, dissipating it, thinning and clarifying it' thus eliminating corrupt vapours and the damaging heavy particles in damp air.[113] Scented substances used in conjunction with fire 'rectified' malignant air by altering its temperament, whether making it cooler or hotter, drier or damper, according to the complexion of the herbs, wood resins, and animal substances used. They could also counter the dangerous effects of putrid air and were therefore a crucial element in the armoury against the power of noxious air, hence the physician Tomaso Rangoni's recommendation in 1565 that in winter a fire of 'praiseworthy woods should be lit, so as to rectify the air'.[114]

An analysis of fireplaces provides interesting evidence of perceptions of the role performed by fire and perfumes in preserving health within the household. From the late fifteenth century, as the prominence and popularity of fireplaces within domestic interiors increased, we see how often motifs carved on fireplaces centred on the themes of fire, heat, or flowers, thereby visually reinforcing their perceived healthy effects. Writing in the 1460s, the architect Filarete had supported the connection between form and function and provided some further guidelines on the materiality and design of fireplaces: they should be made of beautiful stone, able to conduct the heat, and include a frieze of a subject which alluded to fire, such as Vulcan, the god of fire (see Fig. 3.6).[115]

---

[111] ASR, FSV, vol. 264, 'Testamento di Bernardina di Capo di Ferro', 1.8.1565, 44ʳ, and her 'Inventario' at 371ʳ. See ASR, FSV, vol. 269, 'Inventario di Virgilio Spada', 21.5.1663, 195, 206ʳ, and 213ʳ for the *arazzi*.

[112] ASVR, MCI, vol. 198, 5.04.1605, 6ʳ. See also Storey, *Carnal Commerce*, 192–4 for a discussion of *corami* in the homes of prostitutes.

[113] Hence the belief that the many 'fires' in cities improved the air quality; Panaroli, *Aerologia*, 86.

[114] Rangoni, *Consiglio*, 11: 'Habbia il camino comodo che non spande, il fumo dove s'accende il fuoco di legna lodevole che rettifichi l'aere il verno come fanno le rugiade fresche d'estate'.

[115] Filarete, *Trattato d'architettura*, I. 267–8.

(a)   (b)

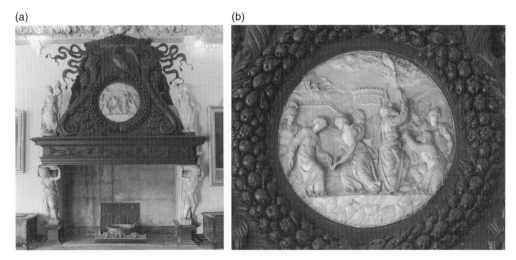

Fig. 3.6a–b. The medallion on this chimneypiece in the Palazzo Doria, Genoa, *c*.1533, depicts Prometheus giving fire to humankind, possibly intended to reinforce the sensation of actual heat given out by the fire (M. A.-W.).

These depictions would not only fulfil Renaissance notions of decorum—whereby theme and purpose of an object would go hand in hand—but reinforce its purpose. Many examples of sixteenth-century fireplaces embody these principles. The ability of the fire to purify—both literally and metaphorically—is encapsulated by the Latin inscription carved on one early sixteenth-century fireplace: 'SORDIDA PVRGAT' ('it purges dirty things') (see Fig. 3.7).

Other ornamental features typical of fireplaces were candelabra and vases from which exuberant foliage sprouted, while illusionistic garlands of flowers were often suspended across the lintel below, all evoking the healthy, comforting scent of these substances, particularly as they came into contact with fire (see Fig. 3.8).

Unlike the age-old centrally positioned open hearth, the fireplace made spaces relatively smoke-free and therefore more salubrious. By the late sixteenth century its exclusive association with the elite interior was declining, and even the homes of the less well-off could be seen to have a fireplace. Household inventories also document the ubiquity of a complex material culture related to fire during this period, with firedogs, pokers, tongs, and bellows featuring by the fireplace to ensure that the fire would burn brightly and efficiently, and chests were made in which to keep spent ashes.[116] The gaping hole of the fireplace also represented a potential source of draughts and smoke, and architectural treatises made suggestions as to how to minimize these, stressing the importance of designing the

---

[116] For fireplaces in the homes of Roman prostitutes, see Storey, *Carnal Commerce*, 191. For Europe generally see Sarti, *Vita di casa*, 137–8.

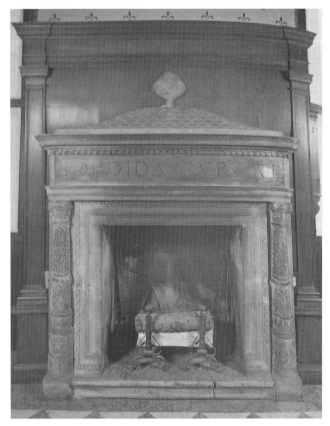

Fig. 3.7. The inscription ('it purges dirty things') on this mantelpiece from northern Italy alludes to the power of fire to purify the air (M. A.-W.).

chimneypiece in such a way that harmful smoke would be swept away from the room.[117] The Venetian humanist Alvise Cornaro, writing in the 1550s, extolled the virtues of a fireplace designed so that 'one can sit by the fire, and the heat does not affect the head'.[118] Alternatively one could use a fire screen, made of wood and waxed textile, like that used by Cardinal Virgilio Spada.[119] One danger associated with the effects of fires on the body was in fact that of excessive heat. Approaching a fire too swiftly particularly after meals was bad, given that it dried the body out quickly, but likewise overheating the body was dangerous. A mid-seventeenth-century regimen describes how this could happen, and in the process we learn something about the portable objects used within the home to warm the air. He

[117] Martini, *Trattati*, I. 96: 'per alcun modo nuociar non possa'. For Alberti on advice on locating fires, *Art of Building*, 147–8.

[118] Quoted in Attardi, *Il camino veneto*, 31: 'con poche legna, et poco fuoco si fa gran calore' and 'si può stare al fuoco, che il calor non può dar alla testa'.

[119] ASR, FSV, vol. 269, C195, 21.5.1663, 209ʳ.

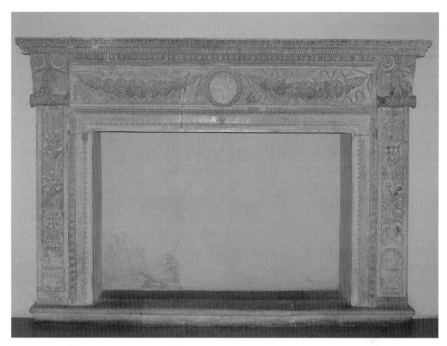

Fig. 3.8. The carved festoons on this early sixteenth-century fireplace in the Castel San Giorgio, Mantua conjure up the scents of plants thrown into the fire to perfume the room (M. A.-W.).

warns that women, in particular, not satisfied with just using foot-warmers to warm their feet, have taken to filling '*caldani* and other vases' with embers 'which they enclose under their clothing so that the heat, finding no barrier, penetrates the skin burning it, inflaming the blood, giving rise to vapours which go to the head, even giving rise to toxic and impure flames'.[120] However, foot-warmers (see Fig. 3.9) were evidently in use much earlier than this, judging from their appearance in just under 10 per cent of our inventories—three of which are owned by former prostitutes in 1607.

Foot-warmers probably belonged to the larger category of braziers (*caldani*), another utilitarian and multifunctional object familiar to the Renaissance household, which could be used to burn scented substances whilst supplementing the heating. Braziers could most simply be obtained by filling generic metal bowls with hot coals, as in Fig. 3.10, hence the difficulty of using inventorial records for any quantitative analysis of this type of object. They could also be purpose-made, in

---

[120] Frediano, *Arca novella*, 52: 'è vero che l'uso delle cassettine assai introdotto la si cangia in abuso perchè non si contentato particolarmente le donne adoperarle in maniera che conservino calde le piante dei piedi ma servendosi alcuni di caldani e altri vasi con molta bragia rinserrano con l'ambito de' panneggiamenti il calore e quello penetrando senza alcun impedimento la pelle l'imbrostulisce, infiamma il sangue, solleva vapori alla testa e ha forza di destare fiamme nocive e impure'.

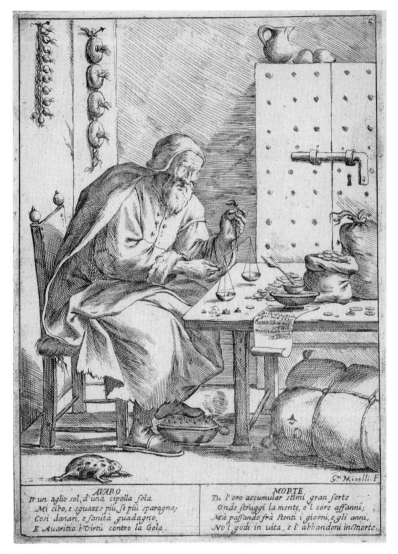

AVARO
Tr un aglio sol, d'una cipolla sola
Mi cibo, e sguazzo piu se piu sparagno;
Cosi danari, e sanità guadagno,
E Auaritia è Virtù contro la Gola.

MORTE
Tu l'oro accumular stimi gran sorte
Onde struggi la mente, e'l core affanni;
Mà passando frà stenti i giorni, e gli anni,
No'l godi in uita, e l'abbandoni in morte.

Fig. 3.9. This seventeenth-century print of a miser alludes to the fact that a foot-warmer was a comparatively cheap way of keeping warm.

many designs, sizes, and from less or more expensive metals (see Fig. 3.11). The handles meant that they could be also easily moved, allowing for scents to quickly reach all the rooms of the house (see Plate 7).

As noted earlier, scents had traditionally been understood as counteracting unhealthy air in various ways, but whilst late medieval authors had simply recommended fumigating the rooms without explaining how, sixteenth-century regimens go into far more detail, listing the ingredients and the techniques to be used

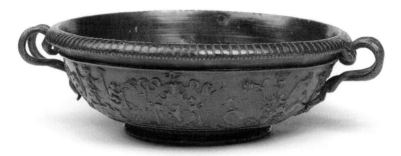

Fig. 3.10. This late sixteenth-century bronze bowl (h. 8.6 cm, d. 25.7 cm, w. 40.1 cm), decorated with swags and equipped with handles, could have been used as a portable brazier (M. A.-W.).

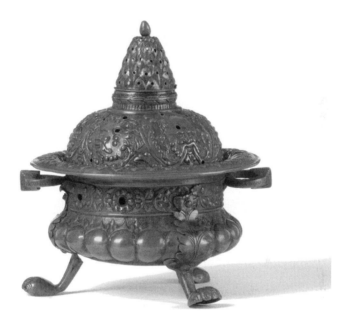

Fig. 3.11. This embossed and pierced copper brazier from the second half of the fifteenth century would have been a relatively cheap item. It could also easily be carried around from room to room (h. 21.9 cm, w. 20.5 cm) (M. A.-W.).

in producing domestic perfumes for the ambient air.[121] *Profumieri*, or *profumatoi*, were luxury objects designed specifically for the purpose of burning scented substances, so as to maintain healthy air within the home. Often originating in the Middle East, their gilt filigree perforations, fine enamel work, complex technology,

---

[121] In the 14th century for example, Maino de Maineri generically talks of 'fumigating with hot or cold aromatic things'; [Maineri], *Opera utilissima*, 104.

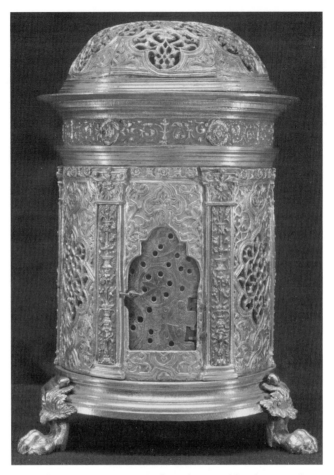

Fig. 3.12. Sixteenth-century Venetian perfume burners like this one (h. 23 cm, diam. 14 cm) were modelled on Islamic prototypes. Made of pierced gilt bronze and enamel, they could be moved about the house and placed on any surface to infuse the room with their scented vapours (M. A.-W.).

and exotic associations made them objects of distinction, suitable for use and display in a refined space (see Fig. 3.12).[122]

Smaller, spherical perfume-burners as shown in Fig. 3.13, documented in Italy from the late fourteenth century, also originated in Egypt or Syria. These objects grew in popularity and by the early sixteenth century they were perfectly replicated by local imitations made by Italian craftsmen, thus making them more easily available. The 'profumego di bronzo a la damaschina' ('in the fashion of Damascus'), recorded in 1513 in the inventory of the Venetian noblewoman Elena Capello,

---

[122] Aga-Oglu, 'About', 28–45.

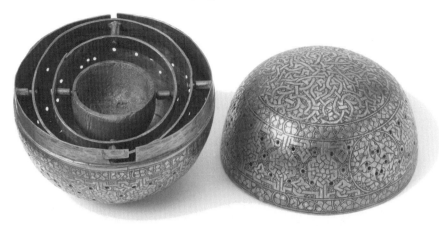

Fig. 3.13. This elaborate brass perfume burner (diam. 13.4 cm) was made in Syria or Egypt in the late fifteenth or early sixteenth century. It has a series of rings one inside another, which were attached to one half to ensure that the central saucer remained upright. This technology enabled the incense burner to be rolled around to purify the air while in motion (M. A.-W.).

may have been locally produced.[123] Generally made of brass which was pierced and inlaid with gold and silver, the *profumatoio* opened out into two half-spheres and in its centre was a small cup for burning perfumed essences with coal.

Surviving examples of spherical perfume burners, dated between the late sixteenth and the early eighteenth century, which are made entirely of cheaper metals—such as copper and brass—and display a much lower level of craftsmanship, support the hypothesis of a process of social dissemination (see Fig. 3.14).

There were also simpler and cheaper methods of perfuming the home. Amongst randomly picked Roman inventories from across the seventeenth century 10 per cent possessed objects for perfuming, three of which were spherical and were probably scented paste balls, of a kind mentioned in recipe books.[124] The author of a mid-seventeenth-century regimen likewise shows a pragmatic, artisanal approach to the manufacturing of perfume burners, instructing the reader on how one can produce a home-made one: 'By having a small pan on a slow fire covered with parchment with a small hole pierced in it.'[125] Ceramic hand-warmers, usually filled with hot water, would have also assisted in the daily battle against the cold, believed, as we have seen, to particularly affect the body's extremities (see Plate 8).

Doctors had long recommended using leaves, herbs, and flowers to counteract bad air by perfuming it. The petals of roses, violets, and myrtle for example corrected hot air, whilst spring flowers and the leaves of citrus trees were 'supremely'

---

[123] Contadini, 'Middle Eastern Objects', 315.
[124] For the 'palle di profumi' (scented balls): ASR, TNC, Uff. 2, vol. 218, 258ʳ–259ᵛ and 268ʳ–ᵛ, 4.8.1660, Maddalena Bartoloccia; and vol. 199, 422ʳ–425ᵛ and 430ʳ–431ʳ, 20.11.1655, Pietro Antonio Ricci.
[125] Panaroli, *Aerologia*, 86–7.

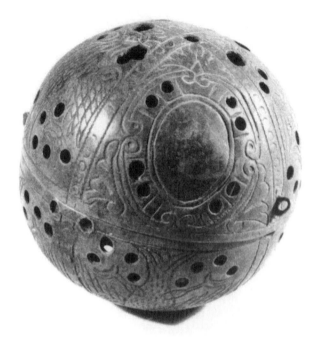

Fig. 3.14. Made in late sixteenth-century Italy this unsophisticated brass perfume burner could have doubled up as a hand-warmer (M. A.-W.).

useful against cold air.[126] Petals and leaves could be scattered on beds, tables, and on the ground whilst flowers and boughs could be hung or arranged in vases, something which the English apparently excelled at.[127] We also find that recommendations about perfuming the body to protect it from the noxious effects of dangerous air become more common and specific in the sixteenth century. One regimen mentions specific objects which can be carried and emit the required scents for summer use, such as a sponge bathed in rose water and rose vinegar or a scented ball (*palla odorata*) or a *pomo di ambra*—popular versions of the metal or ceramic pomanders discussed earlier.[128] Another way of ensuring that the air closest to the body would promote good health was by impregnating clothing and bedlinen with the preferred scents, thereby allowing the wearer to be enveloped in a cloud of appropriate scents.[129] Evelyn Welch has argued that although widely available by 1500, there was in fact a surge in the popularity of scented accessories (gloves, buttons, etc.) in the second half of the sixteenth century although she also notes that this was accompanied by criticism from numerous quarters, whether on the grounds of effeminacy, 'Spanishness', excessive luxury, or the danger of poison.

---

[126] 'Di sopremo giovamento.' Ficino, *De le tre vite*, 14ᵛ; Pictorius, *Dialogi*, 23; Panaroli, *Aerologia*, 86–7; Durante, *Il tesoro*, 4.

[127] See Lennio's praise for English use of flowers and boughs, *Della complessione*, 33.

[128] Durante, *Il tesoro*, 9.   [129] Durante, *Il tesoro*, 8–10.

There may also have been a 'schism' within the medical world as to the appropriateness of using exotic perfumes.[130]

The popularity of these domestic perfuming practices is confirmed by the many sets of instructions in cheap, popular printed booklets known as 'Books of Secrets' or 'Books of Recipes' which contained instructions for making a huge variety of perfumes, scented objects, and scented medicinal and cosmetic compounds, mostly using very simple ingredients which could be grown, or purchased from the apothecary or herbalist.[131] They included instructions for making little bags of herbs and flowers to carry around or to sweeten stored linen and clothes, or to make the perfumed pastes used in the domestic production of necklaces, earrings, buttons, and even paternosters (rosary beads). The need to protect the brain, in particular, from the impact of putrid air rising through the body was also at the heart of those recipes aiming to improve the breath, which ranged from sweetmeats (*moscardini*) to scented mouthwashes. Another solution was a scented unguent like that described in 1538, presumably to be applied around the neck and head—'which opens the pores of the brain...chases away windiness...gives good breath'.[132] Presumably, similar fears lay behind the many deodorant remedies circulating in the period; since as well as being unpleasant, the bad odour released by those who stink when they sweat or those who have stinking feet and armpits was perceived as a threat to health.[133]

FROM PERFUMES TO CLOTHING

Judging from the early regimens, such as one written just after the 1348 plague but printed in the 1540s, or Benzi's late fifteenth-century tract, it would appear that rectifying the air was initially only recommended in cases of pestilence.[134] But by the beginning of the sixteenth century the recommended uses of perfumes have shifted and perfuming is seen as an activity to be performed regularly to purge the air of all dangerous vapours. In reality, the evidence from both regimens and non-medical sources points to debates over perfuming, and a gradual decline in the use of perfume aimed at modifying the health quality of the air. For example, by the mid-sixteenth century using 'simples' such as local herbs, flowers, and available woods was both cheaper and more 'natural' whilst using products such as incense, myrrh, and similar expensive, imported 'odours' was seen as more extravagant.[135] Towards the end of the century some writers even started to reject the extensive use of perfuming to alter the air. Two strands of thought coexisted in the medical literature, with some regimens advocating perfuming (Lennio, Durante, Anguillara, and Fonseca) whilst others

---

[130] Welch, 'Perfumed Buttons'.   [131] See Ch. 1.

[132] *'Che apre i serrami del cervello [...] scaccia ventosità e fa buon fiato.'* Manente, *Col nome di Dio*, 15; also Lennio, *Della complessione*, 100.

[133] Piemontese, *Secreti*, IV. 417 and II. 56.

[134] 'Suffumigando e odorando cose aromatiche caldo o fredde'; [Maineri], *Opera utilissima*, 104 and Benzi, *Tractato utilissimo*, 4ʳ. Aldrobrandino da Siena is another medieval author who associates the need to purify the air only with pestilence; *Le Régime du corps*, 59–61.

[135] Gropretio, *Un breue*, 370; Pictorius, *Dialogi*, 23; Lennio, *Della complessione*, 33.

appear to ignore it almost completely. These latter, such as Rangoni, Petronio, Paschetti, and Pietragrassa are, not coincidentally, those authors who were most emphatically in favour of ensuring that the air, wind, and temperature in and around the home were healthy in the first place, and presumably if this was achieved, there was no need to correct the ambient internal air (although, interestingly, they do not attack it either). Panaroli was the only exception to this trend, combining both approaches. Indeed, an element in this declining emphasis on the possibility of changing the composition of the air through perfumes might have been linked to the growing environmentalism deriving from readings of texts such as *Airs, Waters, Places* and a corresponding attempt to purge medical knowledge of the taint of Arab influence.[136]

There was undoubtedly a link between the use of aromatics, expensive perfumes, and rectifying the air and the Arab medical tradition, and this link may have also contributed ultimately to a demise of the medical use of perfumes.[137] That the Arab influence existed in the minds of sixteenth-century authors we see in a passage from Rangoni's regimen. The text mentions in passing that one should 'allow the sun to enter the house, rectifying the air, as we have learned from the Arabs for the preparation of places in which to live'.[138] Whether or not there was a conscious rejection of perfuming and fumigating as an outdated practice tainted with Arabism remains to be studied.[139]

Also in those texts that mention perfuming the connection established between scenting and health seems gradually to have been lost—or at least, to have been regarded with some ambivalence. Writing in 1565 one physician merely concludes that scents 'please and comfort, so long as they are hot and dry' and in non-medical sources we find, from an even earlier date, evidence of ignorance about the medicinal power of smells.[140] In the introduction to a perfumery manual printed in 1555 the author explains that his book will teach the readers to 'govern' their stomachs, breath, and teeth amongst other areas. However, he has to remind his readers that this knowledge of the health properties of scented products is based on 'the rules of medicine', which physicians would defend, before explaining that his recipe for a product for washing the hair will 'benefit and comfort the brain and defend it from pernicious humours'.[141] So it would seem that even by this date amongst the

---

[136] In Petronio there is an attack on the dominance of Arab thought: 'Come se fossero padroni e che commandassero alla natura'; Petronio, *Del viver*, 324. On the ambivalent attitude to Arab authors see also Siraisi, 'The Changing Fortunes'.
[137] The extensive use of aromatics in medicine is generally attributed to the influence of the Arab medical tradition, transmitted into the Latin West between the 11th and 13th centuries with the translation of Arab medical texts. On the expansion of technical knowledge and availability of products see Morris, *A History of Aromatics*, 127–34.
[138] 'Acciochè il sole possa entrare in casa, retificando l'aere come s'ha dagli Arabi della preparazione de' luoghi habitabili.' Rangoni, *Consiglio*, 27.
[139] Scholars have shown that despite controversy over the place of Arabic texts Avicenna remained very popular until the 17th century. See Jacquart and Micheau (eds.), *La Médecine*, 96 and 200; and Siraisi, 'The Changing Fortunes'.
[140] Traffichetti, *L'arte di conservar*, 178.
[141] 'Governarsi il stomaco' and 'Che danno giovamento e conforta il cerebro e lo difende da humori perniciosi.' Rosetti, *Notandissimi secreti*, 3^{r–v}.

laity perfumes were regarded as something pleasurable rather than something used for health.

This declining appreciation of the health benefits of perfuming appears to be supported by the evidence from our analysis of Roman inventories. This suggests that by 1600 elaborate containers for perfume were not common household objects even in the houses of the most privileged. In the early seventeenth century, nobleman Vincenzo Giustiniani owned only two such objects; an engraved silver one 'with a lion's foot' and a cover, decorated with women's heads, and a smaller, plainer iron one.[142] About seventy years later Cardinal Virgilio Spada possessed only two *profumieri*, both silver.[143] This suggests that the practice was falling out of fashion in the seventeenth century, and their use confined to ceremonial or festive occasions, such as banquets, as indicated by Romoli in his advice book.[144]

A hundred years later we find an even clearer example of the way in which the belief in the ability of perfumes to counteract malignant air had been lost for the layperson, although it was still supported by the public health authorities. This transpires from the annoyance with which Eugenia Maldachini née Spada, confined in Viterbo, and her mother Maria Veralli Spada in Rome react to the public health measures adopted by authorities during the plague epidemic that hits the region in 1656–7: the letters that Eugenia and Maria write to each other are perfumed and fumigated by public health officers, or soaked with vinegar, but the two women's comments only betray impatience for these practices, which often erase the writing so that the letters become illegible and look 'almost burnt'.[145] They are more preoccupied by the breech of privacy that the opening of letters in order to scent them involved than by the danger posed by contact with goods from an infected area: 'You say you have no idea why there is a need to open the letters in order to perfume them, and nor do I.'[146] There seems to be little understanding of and support for these measures, as if all knowledge of the medical reasons behind perfuming had been lost, while it was still a practice required by the medical ordinances of the day. Yet, if the practice of perfuming as a preventive measure had declined, perfumes continued to be used widely both for the pleasure they gave as well as for the positive effects scents were supposed to have on the mind and spirits.

Although by the late sixteenth century preventive practices were shifting away from a reliance on perfuming, something else had stepped in to replace it. We see a new kind of attention paid to clothing used as a protective barrier against the elements in the late sixteenth century as authors provide instructions regarding how to 'arm' the body by donning clothing made of textiles appropriate to both season and air quality. Durante's *Tesoro di sanità*, published in 1586, is one of the

---

[142] Danesi Squarzina, *La collezione Giustiniani*, 36.

[143] ASR, FSV, vol. 269, 195, 21.5.1663, 220ʳ.

[144] Romoli, *La singolare dottrina*, 9ᵛ.

[145] 'Le lettere si profumano e quasi si abrasciano' and 'Sue lettere mi arrivano tutte bagnate di aceto.' ASR, FSV, B.410, 2.7.1656, 29.8.1656, and 13.9.1656.

[146] 'Vlll. dice che non sa che bisogno c'è di aprir le lettere per profumarle e manco io lo so.' ASR, FSV, B.410, 29.8.1656.

first sixteenth-century regimens to elaborate on the use of clothing, although some of his medieval precursors had briefly mentioned the clothing and textiles appropriate for each season.[147] Durante seizes on clothing firstly for the inherent properties of the materials to protect the body from the air, naming the qualities of various furs and skins particularly. He also focuses on specific body parts. For example, the chest and stomach ('mother of afflictions') should be 'defended' either with pieces of scented sheepskin or hare skin or a feather pillow or pieces of cloth.[148] This is echoed some years later by a doctor who recommends that those with weak chests 'should arm themselves by covering the whole chest with a leather skin, like a corset, and wear leather clothing'.[149] The feet, hands, and head, rarely considered in medieval regimens, also came in for particular attention. One author mentioned that 'The feet should be cared for because if they chill down the whole body is offended, leading to tiredness, stomach aches, and pains in the sides and colics.'[150] Another advises wearing gloves all year round as a way of protecting one's health with Durante specifying that one should wear fox skin gloves in winter, and hare, kid, or lamb skin gloves in summer.[151] And as we noted earlier, hats, caps, and berets were considered crucial elements of clothing.

Frediano, writing seventy years after Durante, takes the case for the protective powers of clothing to its most extreme, spreading his arguments over fifty pages.[152] He was particularly concerned in winter to prevent closure of the pores though the cold, and applauds the Spanish and Orientals for their tendency to dress heavily during the summer which 'allows the body to transpire and keep it free from superfluities, and fresh everywhere thanks to the continual ventilation and deflation caused by the opening of the pores'.[153] However, it is possible that by the time Frediano was writing, in 1656, even these ideas about the protective value of clothes were losing their hold, if we are to believe him. He claimed that in his youth everybody had heeded Durante's advice to protect the chest and particularly the stomach by wearing such heavily padded jackets and trousers that 'they could have been used as mattresses or pillows'. He also commented that different kinds of fur and skin gloves had been so popular that 'there were whole shops filled with them'. Alas, he laments, 'that was when most men sought to conserve their health and defend themselves', whilst now such careful advice is ignored.[154]

---

[147] Arnau de Villanova, Aldobrandino da Siena, and Maino de Maineri had all suggested the different materials which should be worn in each season to best maintain body temperature: Arnaldi, *Regimen sanitatis*, 424; Aldobrandino, *Le Régime du corps*, 62–5; [Maineri], *Opera utilissima*, 90–4.

[148] Durante, *Il tesoro*, 8, 10.

[149] Fonseca, *Del conservare*, 123.

[150] 'I piedi si custodiscano per lo cui tutto il corpo viene offeso. Temonsi strachezze, dolori di stomaco, di fianchi, colici e somiglianti.' Rangoni, *Consiglio*, 11.

[151] Lombardelli, *De gli vfizii*, 163; Durante, *Il tesoro*, 10.

[152] Frediano, *Arca novella*, 26–73.

[153] Frediano, *Arca novella*, 57: 'Gli Orientali e Spagnoli vestono molti panni anco d'estate acciò non restino le membra offese dal sole e rendano il corpo traspirabile e libero dalle superfluità e rinfrescato in tutte le parti per la continua ventilazione e deflazione causata dall'apertura dei pori e meati.'

[154] 'Imbottiti di tanto cotone che potevano servire di matarazzo o per coscino. . . . Ai tempi nostri ne eran fornite le botteghe intiere allora quando la maggior parte degli uomini aveva il fine di conservarsi e difendersi.' Frediano, *Arca novella*, 50–1.

'AND TAKE CARE OF YOURSELF, BECAUSE THE
WEATHER IS EXTREMELY CHANGEABLE, FIRST
COOL AND THEN HOT'[155]

We have seen that concerns about the quality of the air pervaded the vocabulary used by architects as well as that of doctors and informed their professional activity but how did the lay elite perceive the air and the dangers it posed to their health? Were these concerns also a part of the lay culture of prevention against illness and to what extent did they shape the precautions taken in daily life to keep in good health? To explore these questions we turn now to the private letters exchanged between members of the aristocratic Roman Spada-Veralli family in the first three quarters of the seventeenth century.[156] With residences in Viterbo, Castel Viscardo, Tivoli, and just outside Rome on the Salaria (see Plate 6, Figs. 3.4 and 3.15), as well as the Roman palace, Palazzo Spada, they had a wide choice of places in which to stay or visit and in their letters we certainly find confirmation that the attention paid by the regimens to the air quality and temperature also informed the daily lives of the elite.

Firstly we find the letters give considerable importance to the quality of the air in any given locality, both recommending stays in particular locations on that basis, or discouraging sudden moves between localities with different air. In 1678 a letter from Maria Veralli in Rome to her husband in Castel Viscardo betrays the awareness not only that certain types of air were good or bad, but that the individual body adapted with difficulty to sudden changes in the air and needed time to acclimatize: 'Many are of the opinion that Bartolomeo [their son, aged 21 and currently in Castel Viscardo] should not go to Viterbo so soon because its air is similar to that of Rome, all the more so since he is coming from places with perfect airs, such as Perugia and Castello. He could first go to Giove and then carry on to Viterbo . . . and the Duchess says that . . . the airs of Perugia and Castello are too perfect.'[157] The letter also suggests that numerous people have been consulted on the question of whether or not their son should travel directly to Viterbo from Castel Viscardo, given the change in airs this involves, as if it is a matter of considerable importance. This anxiety about changing place and air, so characteristic of the post-1540 regimens, was evidently widespread and still a matter of concern in the second half of the seventeenth century. For the same reason a change of air and a sojourn in a locality renowned for its air such as the hills and lakes around Bolsena, Frascati, or Albano is frequently recommended or undertaken after illness, as the air in Rome is judged to be quite poor. Thus when her husband has taken refuge at Bolsena for Christmas, she writes that she 'hears' what he writes about 'the many benefits' it brings for his health, and that anyone would happily do as

---

[155] 'E si abbia cura, che sono tempi stravaganti che quando e fresco e quando e caldo, e credo, l'istesso sia costi.' ASR, FSV, B.1115, 21.7.1660.
[156] See Ch. 2 for a discussion of this body of letters.
[157] ASR, FSV, B.618, 21.9.1678.

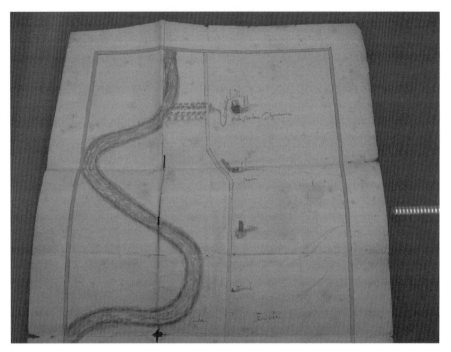

Fig. 3.15. This seventeenth-century watercolour map gives an impression of the seclusion of the Villa Spada (known as La Serpentara), on the Via Salaria leaving Rome.

he has done 'if they were effectively being damaged by the air in Rome'.[158] Likewise in an account of the health of the late Cardinal Bernardino Spada the writer notes that he paid the barest attention to medical advice: 'in the last three years the most he would do was use the villa at Tivoli continuously throughout the summer'.[159] The strictly medical benefits of good air also emerge in a letter from Orazio Spada writing from the countryside to his wife Maria dated April 1658, where he explains that he is recovering well, 'and I am already feeling the effects of this good air which serves to purge me without resorting to medicines and syrups which make me nauseous'.[160]

So, as stressed in ancient regimens, there is a given air for each place. But this also changes with the season. Hence the air of Tivoli, beneficial from late spring to early autumn, the long period that the Spada family spent there in *villeggiatura*, turns nasty in late October when, Maria writes, 'it no longer does my head any

---

[158] 'Sento le raggioni che VS mi apporta dello stare costì e trovare tanti beneficij per la sua salute,...ogn'uno ci starebbe volontieri quanto fa VS, e se dall'aria di Roma effettivamente riceve pregiuditio.' ASR, FSV, B.618, 31.12.1678.

[159] 'Della infermità e morte Cap. XXXII': 'La maggior che usasse fu negli ultimi tre anni di usare tutta l'estate la villa.' ASR, FSV, B.463.

[160] 'e già provo gli effetti di questa buon'aria. Che mi serve di purga senza nausearmi con medicine e siroppi.' ASR, FSV, B.607, 23.4.1658.

good' and 'my eyes have started to get worse'.[161] Hence she begs Cardinal Bernardino, the head of the family, to give her permission to return to Rome earlier than expected. Similarly sea air, normally beneficial, is not so in winter and a sojourn there needs to be postponed. In a letter dated December 1678 Maria informs her husband that Cardinal Rocci is getting better and 'they advise him to go to Albano [Laziale, on lake Albano] until he is able to freely take the sea air'.[162] Likewise, in the already-mentioned account of the health of Cardinal Bernardino Spada in the period leading up to his death in 1661, the correspondent notes that on one occasion the cardinal was urged by his doctor to return to Rome because the season was 'mature' enough for him to do so. He then comments that unfortunately 'that year a large proportion of those who changed location, even for the better, died', but that the cardinal himself was spared—though he then died as a result of his disorderly eating.[163] Even so, it was also deemed possible to have too much of a good thing. Thus, after the birth of her first child, Eugenia writes to her mother that 'today I was thinking of going out for the first time, but Signora Olimpia [Doria Pamphilj, her maternal great-aunt, also based in Viterbo] has said that on my first time out…is too early for me to take so much air'.[164] Many letters also express fears about the wind and the need to avoid exposure to it, in tune with the concerns of the early modern regimen. Thus severe winds, particularly the sirocco and the tramontana, are described by correspondents as extremely dangerous to the body, something one needs to shield oneself from which makes travelling or visits outside the palace or castle difficult. In September 1678 Maria cannot bring herself to leave Rome for Castel Viscardo: 'I would like to see the weather stabilize and this sirocco turn away, because it makes people ill.'[165] 'Too much wind' prevents Eugenia from going out on several occasions, as when there is a 'north wind [*tramontana*] so cold today that it was necessary to stay in the house'.[166]

There are also many recommendations regarding the cold, and a sense of great anxiety about the danger it poses to health. Travelling, for example, takes place in spring, summer, and early autumn rather than in winter. When, on the 28th December, Maria receives some visitors she is amazed they journey in such weather.[167] Cold is an ordeal from which even the most prosperous cannot successfully protect themselves, even with their great fireplaces. In December 1656 Eugenia warns her

[161] 'l'aria non fa più bene alla sua testa' and 'gli occhi hanno cominciato a star peggio.' ASR, FSV, B.619, 26.10.1659.

[162] 'Lo consegliano d'andare ad Albano sino a tanto che si possi pratticare liberamente l'aria della marina.' ASR, FSV, B.618, 31.12.1678.

[163] 'Della infermità e morte Cap. XXXII': 'Il caso portò che quell'anno gran parte di quelli che mutarono luogo, anche in meglio, vi lasciarono la vita.' ASR, FSV, B.618, 31.12.1678.

[164] 'Oggi avevo pensiere di uscire per la prima volta ma la Sig. Olimpia ha detto che sicome alla prima uscita…è troppo presto per prendere tanta aria.' ASR, FSV, B.410, 15.7.1657.

[165] 'Vorrei in tanto vedere il tempo fermo e voltar questo scirocco, che causa degli amalati'. ASR, FSV, B.618, 28.11.1678.

[166] 'Troppo gran vento' and 'Una tramontana assai fredda che oggi ci è bisognato stare in casa'. ASR, FSV, B.1115, 2.4.1662 and 14.11.1660.

[167] ASR, FSV, B.618, 28.12.1678.

mother that 'it is so cold my hands freeze when I write so don't be surprised if I don't write very much'.[168] And even in April, Maria's husband writes from Castel Viscardo: 'It is so cold I have to stay by the fire and I can't hold the pen in my hand.'[169] Getting ill because of the intense cold is very common. Hence warnings about 'avoiding the cold and wrapping up warm' abound. Indeed, when winter approaches servants are provided by their mistress with breeches and under-sleeves so as to increase the number of layers they wear. In the winter of 1678 Maria Veralli sends her husband, who is touring their country estates, a 'cassettina per i piedi', a small metal container with hot coals inside to keep the feet warm (see Fig. 3.8). Although, as we already know, the use of this object had been well established in the urban environment for several decades, the fact that she also sends instructions on how to use it suggests that this was perhaps a novelty in the countryside. 'I have sent the foot-warmer so that your lordship can use it whilst he is sitting writing at a desk, but they have to put the fire inside and then cover it with hot ash, so the heat is constant and the tin lid won't burn.'[170] A week later she writes to him that she has had a cap with ear flaps and a pair of woollen socks made especially for him in Turin which we learn he was very pleased with.[171] These precautions echo those found in regimens which, as we have seen, in this period place increased emphasis on the importance of protecting the body's extremities, 'avoiding any chill in the hands and feet, which often can be crippled and painfully afflicted with tumours and sores'.[172] Another health concern shared by letters and regimens alike is the change of season, the dangerous period when temperatures have not yet settled into a pattern. Special attention needs to be paid to these transitions and caution has to be exercised particularly in discarding any winter clothes: 'It's not the time for any haste in casting off thick clothes because the season hasn't settled yet, and in the same day it's hot one minute and cold the next.'[173]

Letters however also depart in some ways from the advice found in regimens. For example, exposure to the sun is seen as a major source of harm and repeatedly discouraged in letters, especially in those addressed to relatives in the countryside. In April 1658, for example, Orazio Spada, writing from Castel Viscardo, reassures his wife: 'Keep in good heart because there is no danger that I will catch the sun whilst the weather carries on like this.'[174] Long journeys in an open coach are

---

[168] 'Tanto è il gran freddo che mi gelo le mani a scrivere e non si meravigli se scrivo poco.' ASR, FSV, B.410, 3.12.1656.

[169] 'E' così freddo che bisogna star al fuoco e non posso tener la penna in mano.' ASR, FSV, B.607, 30.4. 1658.

[170] 'La cassettina da piedi l'ho mandato perche VS se ne serva quando lei stà al tavolino à scrivere, ma ci devono mettere il foco e poi coprirlo con la cenere calda, e così si mantiene e non si abrugi la latta di sopra.' ASR, FSV, B.618, 7.12.1678.

[171] 'Mando a V.S il berrettino dall'orecchie, et un paro di calzette di lana, fatte venire da Torino.' ASR, FSV, B.618, 14 and 21.12.1678.

[172] Frediano, *Arca novella*, 51: 'Fuggir la frigidità di mani e piedi, quali restano molte volte tormentati da tumori, piaghe, doglie e stroppiature.'

[173] ASR, FSV, B.618, 15.3.1679.

[174] 'Stia di buon animo perchè non è pericolo ch'io pigli sole mentre seguita così il tempo.' ASR, FSV, B.607, 23.4.1658. For an earlier example of a similar warning see the letter of Giulia Benzoni to her husband Giovan Battista Veralli; ASR, FSV, B.449, 11.8.1597.

expressly discouraged in summer heat for they expose the vulnerable head to too much sun.[175] Even the workers employed in the restructuring of the Spada palace in 1642 are protected from the sun when they work on the roof; Maria makes sure that awnings are put in place to shield them from the sun.[176] By contrast, the dangerous effects of the sun upon the head and the skin are only rarely mentioned in health-advice literature; in medical thought the sun's benefits to the air and therefore, indirectly, to the body, seem to largely surpass its negative potential.

Another remarkable feature of lay correspondence is the absence of any reference to the dangers posed by bad smells and the putrid or miasmatic air. Stench (*puzza*) from cesspits or infected bodies and animal waste is sometimes mentioned and remarked upon as disgusting and nauseous but not as posing a danger to health. In March 1601 Giulia Benzoni Veralli reports from Castel Viscardo to her husband in Rome about the health conditions of the cowman, who is seriously ill and infested with *rogna* (scabies)—a skin disease that, in tune with other contemporary accounts, she describes as repellent.[177] In another letter she explains how the unbearable, even 'pestilential', stench at the cowman's dwelling, makes her sick, preventing her from visiting him often. Interestingly, she justifies this with the delicacy of her stomach not by any infectious quality of the smelly air: 'Nobody but Smiralla has the stomach to look after him...and I really can't go up there because there is a pestilential stink and you know how my stomach is, the most I go there is every two or three days, I simply cannot go more often.'[178] Likewise, in a letter to her husband dated May 1678, Maria Spada worries about the stink emanating from the cellars of their Roman palace, which permeates the bedrooms and gallery. The cesspit needs cleaning out because it is full and Maria urges her husband to provide instructions, warning him that it is an expense which cannot be spared, 'because it is a necessity'.[179] In this letter, too, there is no mention of the infectious nature of stench. Smells are not feared but avoided because they are unpleasant and revolting.

CONCLUSION

All the sources examined in this chapter—from letters to architectural plans, from medical and lay advice literature to the objects used in ordinary homes to preserve one's health—concur in indicating that the quality of the air which one breathed was a major cause for concern, not just amongst physicians, but also amongst the

---

[175] See e.g. the letter of Maria to Bernardino Spada; ASR, FSV, B.619, 15.9.1642.

[176] ASR, FSV, B.619, 6.7.1660.

[177] We will return to this condition and attitudes towards it in Ch. 7.

[178] 'Et li è venuta talmente la rogna che l'ha insino sul mostaccio et credo che sia altro che rogna, che non c'è altri che la Smiralla che habia stomaco de governarlo et manegiarlo...et io la sù non ce posso andare, perché c'è una puzza che s'appesta et V. S. sa che stomaco io me ritrovo et ogni volta ch'io ci vado è ogni doi o tre gior/ni, più spesso non ce posso andare.' ASR, FSV, B.449, 27.3.1601. See also, a week earlier; ASR, FSV, B.449, 20.3.1601.

[179] 'Per essere cosa necessaria.' ASR, FSV, B.618, 4.5.1678 and B.1115, 21.9.1678.

educated non-medical elites and even the population at large, throughout the sixteenth and seventeenth centuries. The issues discussed at such length by the authors of healthy living guides were also those which worried noblemen and women and cardinals as they went about their daily lives; and some of them at least did their best to follow the advice which was handed out in the latest regimen, which they or perhaps their doctors had read. They built and restructured their homes so as to minimize damage to their health from the cold, damp, and winds; they organized their travel plans around the weather; they knew which towns and cities had good or bad air, and moved between them accordingly. Furthermore, it appears that early modern people deployed a whole range of strategies and objects to deflect, minimize, correct, and avoid bad air.

What these sources also make very clear is that there was no single concept of 'bad' or 'miasmatic' air, not even of 'mal-aria'; rather, there were multiple definitions of bad and good airs which could be inhaled through mouth and nose, or emitted by the body whether in the home or in the streets, in courtyard gardens or country villas. It also appears that over the 200-year period considered here ideas about air changed considerably. In the late fifteenth century concerns were particularly focused on putrid air, often connected to the danger of pestilence, and corrective perfuming was offered as the mainstay of health prevention. Yet starting in the last decades of the sixteenth century, the concept of 'putrid' or 'corrupt' air seems largely to have been replaced by that of 'good' and 'bad' air, and the main threat was that of cold, damp air, particularly when carried by strong winds. Lay practices seem to have mirrored this evolution, as early modern people implemented new measures to avoid the cold and the wind, adopting and experimenting with the new objects on the market. In this period we also find a shift away from fearing putrid air as a source of pestilence, to mere distaste for its unpleasantness, accompanied by a loss of awareness of the medicinal uses of perfumes. Indeed, this focus on wind, place, and temperature from the mid-sixteenth century may also have contributed to the declining emphasis placed on the medical agency of perfume, as the sensuous, exotic, and pleasant aspects of smell eclipsed their role as preventive medicines.

4
A Good Night's Sleep

The regulation of *sonno e vigilia* (sleep and wakefulness), is given considerable attention in the late Renaissance literature on healthy living; moreover, the definition of what constitutes a healthy environment for sleep increasingly becomes a matter of concern. The main principles that govern healthy sleep had already been outlined in the medieval regimens. These references were, however, relatively sketchy, consisting of practical advice on when, for how long, and how one should sleep rather than providing explanations of why certain ways of sleeping were healthy or otherwise. Even when the recommendations were more comprehensive, as in the case of Arnau's regimen, the approach remained prescriptive rather than explanatory.[1] In late fifteenth-century regimens, however, the physiological processes induced by different ways of sleeping and their impact upon health began to be expounded in greater detail.[2] These accounts become even more thorough in the second half of the sixteenth century. Just as in the discussions of air, traditional recommendations were now justified at length; furthermore, texts now include frequent references to ancient authorities scattered through them. This expansion of the space occupied by advice concerning sleep is evident, if we compare, for example, Savonarola's regimen (written in 1464) with the re-edition of this text issued by Boldo in 1575: the number of pages devoted to sleep in the revised text is at least three times that in the original edition.[3] In general sleep seems to have attracted increased attention and works devoted entirely to this Non-Natural were published around mid-century also by humanist scholars.[4]

At a superficial glance it may seem that old and new texts present substantial continuity in terms of the advice offered; even the examples and figurative images provided are similar. In reality sixteenth-century guides to healthy living include significant new approaches by comparison with their medieval predecessors. First, there is a shift in emphasis regarding the organs deemed to be affected by bad sleeping habits. The stomach remains the central preoccupation, due to the strong

---

[1] Alderotti, *Libello*, 16; Aldobrandino, *Le Régime du corps*, 21–2; and Arnaldi, *Regimen sanitatis*, 433–5.

[2] See Savonarola, *Libreto*, 50ᵛ–52ᵛ, 60ʳ–61ʳ, and even more Benzi, *Tractato utilissimo*, IVᵛ–VIᵛ.

[3] While Savonarola devotes two and a half pages to the matter in his chapter on the five non-naturals and returns only briefly to the theme in the two subsequent chapters, Boldo includes six pages on sleep and wakefulness as well as more specific sections later. Boldo, *Libro della natura*, 221–7, 260–1, 282, and 293–4.

[4] Tartaglini, *Opera nuova*; and Ugoni, *Dialogo*. The work authored by Tartaglini, a surgeon and herbalist, in reality deals also with exercise and includes recipes for remedies for various ailments.

association between sleep and digestion, but the impact of sleeping practices on the brain also becomes key. This is partly the consequence of the increased role this organ came to occupy in Renaissance physiology: initially, and in keeping with Aristotelian views, the brain had been judged important simply because it was seen as the site of memory—a position still reflected in Arnau's regimen.[5] In the Renaissance, however, the Galenic view prevailed. This sees the brain also as the site of what we would define as the nervous system, and hence as the source of motion and sensation, making the head the focus of health concerns, as already noted in Chapter 3.[6] Moreover, there is an increased emphasis on the dangers that cold and damp air represent for the sleeping, inactive, and therefore vulnerable body, in keeping with the growing preoccupation with the impact of environmental factors on health that replaces the previous emphasis on putrid, corrupted air. Finally, medical advice becomes more flexible, less prescriptive than in medieval regimens; there is no attempt to create universal rules but greater room for exceptions. Amplifying elements of caution already present in the late fifteenth-century texts, the recommendations about healthy sleep become less prescriptive from the late sixteenth century, allowing much more room for exceptions on grounds of age, season, or in view of what the complexions of particular groups might require. The power of custom and the potential dangers to health arising from deviation from ingrained sleeping habits is also increasingly underlined. This may be seen as a consequence of the enhanced emphasis on the specificity of place that we have already encountered in Chapter 3. Particular ways of life were seen to have developed in different regions, being forged by specific environmental conditions that had become part of the cultural make-up of the local population.[7] Originally used to explain ethnic and cultural differences between nations or continents, this approach was extended in the second half of the sixteenth century to make sense of regional diversity and even of micro-local variation in custom within the Italian peninsula. Ideas of healthy and unhealthy sleep were profoundly affected by this new sensitivity to the power of place.

It can be argued that this new interest, in the healthy-living literature, in the complexions of certain groups and the Hippocratic emphasis on the custom of place gave doctors considerable leeway vis-à-vis sleeping habits that did not conform to the traditional principles of healthy living in terms of time, duration, and manners. By taking to the extreme the precept that what is good for one body is bad for another, doctors managed to legitimize unorthodox sleeping practices that, as contemporary testimonies suggest, were becoming common in society, at least among the most privileged. Indeed, sleeping patterns were changing fast in the sixteenth century and the sleeping environment was being redesigned.

---

[5] Arnaldi, *Regimen sanitatis*, 434.
[6] There are however some exceptions: Viviani (*Trattato*, 195–6) seems to side with Aristotle in seeing the heart as the origin of all sensations, and Tassoni (*Pensieri*, 271) adopts an intermediate position, seeing some of the senses as originating in the brain and others, such as touch, in the heart. Traffichetti (*L'arte*, 113) summarizes the dispute but does not take sides. On the Galenic–Aristotelian controversy regarding the role of the brain and the heart, see Jacquart, 'Cœur'.
[7] Wear, 'Place'.

Sleep is therefore a particularly useful instance for exploring the thorny question of the relationship between medical authority and lay practice. Did precepts for healthy sleep simply adapt to changing habits or did doctors manage to maintain some influence over the changing culture of sleep? Were the innovations introduced into the sleeping environment affected by health anxieties? Household inventories and family letters, together with the evidence from surviving exemplars of the material culture of sleep and their visual representations, will help us address these questions. Though ideas of privacy, comfort, and fashion have been seen as the main driving force presiding over the transformation of beds, bedding, and bedrooms, health concerns might also have played a powerful, though neglected, role.

SLEEP AND DIGESTION

'Sleep comes from the vapours which rise from foods [which have been eaten] to the brain and, once in touch with the frigid brain, they freeze and in falling obstruct the sensitive passages, just as rain is formed in the midst of the air through rising vapours.'[8] In his customary clear and vivid language Durante explains the basic process whereby, according to the physiology of the time, sleep came about; the link with digestion is immediately clear: it is after the main meal of the day, the evening meal, that the so-called animal faculties, that is the five senses, enter into a state of quiet due to the drop in temperature caused by the vapours rising to the brain from the full stomach, and are subsequently frozen by this cold organ. As a consequence of this 'binding of the senses' ('ligamento dei sensi'), as some authors put it, 'when we sleep we are more like the dead than the living'.[9]

Due to the inactivity of the senses, sleep is considered a state of vulnerability of the body, but it is also a necessary and beneficial state since it restores physical strength, while simultaneously comforting the mental faculties. As a result sleep was seen both as 'a refuge from labours [and] repose for the soul' ('rifugio delle fatiche, riposo dell'anima').[10] An equally important function of sleep however, is that it promotes digestion: during rest the 'natural heat', without distraction from the exercise of the senses and intellectual faculties, can concentrate on the inner parts of the body—the stomach and the intestines—and process food, transforming it into nourishment. It is paramount therefore that any interruption or disruption of sleep be avoided lest it upset the digestive process.

Indeed most of the recommendations concerning sleep proceed from its role in digestion. This preoccupation dictates the time when sleep should occur: after the evening meal but only once the food has descended to the lower part of the stomach

---

[8] 'Si fa il sonno elevandosi da cibi i vapori, che arrivati al cervello, e ritrovandolo fridigo, e denso, si congelano, e fatti gravi, e discendendo, opilano i meati sensitivi de i membri, in quella maniera, che si genera la pioggia nella meza regione dell'aria, per l'ascenso de i vapori.' Durante, *Il tesoro*, 24–5.

[9] 'quando dormiamo siamo più simili a morti che a vivi.' Durante, *Il tesoro*, 24–5; Petronio, *Del viver*, 324. The expression 'ligamento dei sensi' is found in the *Commentarii*, 112.

[10] Paschetti, *Del conservare*, 205. Durante, *Il tesoro*, 24.

and the first absorption of food has been completed; hence sleep immediately after supper is to be avoided since, among other things, it would cause tossing and turning in bed, impeding profound sleep and blocking digestion. Some authors recommend that a precise interval of time, ranging from one and a half to four hours, should elapse between eating and going to bed.[11] To facilitate the descent of the food many recommend gentle walking during this interval.[12] Others discourage any activity and simply suggest resting and remaining seated after supper, with the head and upper body not bent but erect, listening to pleasant and not overly demanding conversation so that the intellect is not too engaged and natural heat is not diverted to the brain.[13]

These principles are repeated again and again in the health-advice literature, but there are also dissenting voices: Petronio, writing in 1592, denies the need to avoid sleeping immediately after the evening meal, 'as the Arabs suggest' ('come gli Arabi vogliono'). He defines as 'most peculiar diligence' ('diligentia troppo curiosa') the recommendation to wait until food descends to the bottom of the stomach before going to bed, and he uses the example of infants who alternate eating and sleeping in a continuous cycle without suffering ill effects.[14] In his view it all depends on how the individual reacts to different sleeping patterns, so a general rule cannot be established. Interestingly, the fashionable anti-Arab stance of the day provides the ideological justification for this increased flexibility. Petronio's attack on a rigid timing for sleep seems to be one of the first manifestations of a general rejection of universal rules about sleep that is also articulated in other regimens at the turn of the century. Paschetti, for example, likewise seems unconvinced by the obligation to space food and sleep and restricts the recommendation to those who drink a great deal while eating little: the latter should wait one or two hours before sleeping or else the food will float in their stomach.[15]

If the damage of sleeping on a full stomach is slightly controversial there is general consensus about the negative effects of the opposite circumstance. Sleeping on an empty stomach is very bad since the natural heat, which moves to the internal parts during sleep, finds no food to digest and hence turns upon flesh and blood and even upon radical moisture which is the very source of natural heat.[16] This shortens life, dries up and thins the body, makes man weak and sad, and also thinner, so that Petronio can suggest, with his usual irreverence, that one can go to bed hungry on purpose as an expedient to lose weight.[17] The dangers of sleeping on an

---

[11] e.g. Fonseca, *Del conservare*, 79; Durante, *Il tesoro*, 27–8; and Traffichetti, *L'arte*, 115.

[12] Benzi, *Tractato utilissimo*, Vᵛ; [Maineri], *Opera utilissima*, 45; and Camaffi, *Reggimento*, 135.

[13] Camaffi, *Regimento*, 138.

[14] Petronio, *Del viver*, 326–7.

[15] Petronio, *Del viver*, 328; and Paschetti, *Del conservare*, 209. The orthodox rule is embraced however in bk. I of Paschetti's regimen, which sets the scene in which the framing dialogue between gentlemen is taking place: each evening after their meal, they sit and talk about their health, precisely because they have to while away two hours before going to bed. *Del conservare*, 11.

[16] Benzi, *Tractato utilissimo*, Vᵛ; similarly, Camaffi, *Reggimento*, 135. On radical moisture (*humidum radicale*) see Pomata, 'Editor's Introduction', 46–52 and 81.

[17] Petronio, *Del viver*, 324.

empty stomach are also part and parcel of folkloric wisdom; Camaffi recalls a popular saying which warns: 'Go to bed without supper and be left cold all night.'[18]

Sleeping positions also attracted considerable attention and were defined by the dual need to promote digestion and protect the brain. Sleeping on the back was to be avoided, because the superfluities that ascend to the head in the form of vapours and are normally expelled through the nose and the mouth do not follow the natural routes but are drawn back to the brain, causing damage that creates even greater concern as we proceed into the early modern period. While Arnau, writing in the thirteenth century, was mainly preoccupied with the effects on memory, later authors talk of paralysis, apoplexy, phantoms, *incubi*, or lethargy as possible consequences of sleeping in this unorthodox position.[19] This growing concern for the effects upon the nervous system testifies to the increasing acceptance of a conceptualization of the brain as the source of motion and pathway of the nerves. To prevent superfluities from following the wrong pathways during sleep it was also important to keep the head and all the upper parts of the back 'proportionally elevated'. This was seen as a key principle of healthy sleep, one that also prevented food from being regurgitated; the use of sufficiently thick pillows (*guanciali convenevoli*) was therefore explicitly recommended.[20]

The issue of whether one should sleep on the stomach or not appears to be more controversial in the health-advice literature. In some cases this position is praised because it keeps the stomach warm, thus facilitating digestion, and is recommended especially for those with a cold stomach or when foods that are difficult to digest have been eaten; but it is bad in other cases, for example for those with discharge from the eyes.[21] A long tradition, dating back at least to the thirteenth century, recommends sleeping with a small feather pillow pressed upon the stomach, such that it can be hugged or else tied around the waist. Durante suggests this can be replaced by a plump boy or a fat little dog ('fanciullo carnoso o un cagnolo grasso').[22]

Lying on one's side is regarded as by far the healthiest way of sleeping. One should go to sleep lying on the right side for a couple of hours, then turn to the left for a longer stretch of time, then move back to the right side, at the end of the digestive process, for the rest of the time asleep. Extremely clear and graphic explanations of the benefits of this sequence of positions are offered by Tartaglini and Durante. Since the stomach tends towards the left while the mouth of the stomach tends toward the right, lying on the right side allows the stomach to straighten out so that food can descend more easily; moreover, by resting upon the liver, the stomach comforts natural heat and eases the digestive process. Then, turning to the

---

[18] 'chi la sera non cena tutta la notte dal freddo si rimena'; Camaffi, *Reggimento*, 134.

[19] Arnaldi, *Regimen sanitatis*, 435; Savonarola, *Libreto*, 51ᵛ, 60ᵛ; Tartaglini, *Opera nuova*, 24; and Durante, *Il tesoro*, 268. Durante however introduces an exception to the general rule: sleeping on the back is preferable for those affected by *renella* (kidney stones); *Il tesoro*, 268.

[20] Rangoni, *Consiglio*, 26.

[21] Benzi, *Tractato utilissimo*, Vʳ; Savonarola, *Libreto*, 60ᵛ; and Durante, *Il tesoro*, 29.

[22] Durante, *Il tesoro*, 28–9; Arnaldi, *Regimen sanitatis*, 435; and Benzi, *Tractato utilissimo*, Vʳ–VIʳ.

left has the effect of speeding up digestion, since the liver is wrapped around the food that has descended into the stomach, like the fingers of a hand or a hen enfolding its chicks. This again comforts natural heat by warming the stomach like the fire below a pan of water; moreover, the liver is in this way closer to the bowels from which it draws in the chylous humidity generated by the process of digestion and more easily absorbs it. Finally, with a shift to the right side at the end of the process, the mouth of the stomach opens wide, hence allowing the remaining superfluities produced by digestion to be expelled.[23] An additional expedient recommended by some authors is to sleep with the legs bent in order to keep one's precious natural heat focused on the stomach, thereby favouring digestion.[24]

Though these general principles are indicated by most authors as the universal rules presiding over healthy sleep, many exceptions are then introduced to adapt them to the specific needs of individuals and their differing complexions. Hence the order of sleeping positions can be inverted by those who have a cold stomach and a hot liver, and for those ill with diarrhoea sleeping on the left side is more advisable.[25] While these recommendations are usually presented as exceptions to a universal paradigm, Petronio is the only author who goes a step further and attacks head-on the view that sleeping modes can in any way be regulated by general guidelines. As we have already mentioned, he rejects the assumption that sleep should be delayed until food has descended to the bottom of the stomach, but he also criticizes the advice to sleep on different sides at different times. In his view both recommendations lack foundation, for there is no way of knowing whether the first concoction has been completed and the food has fallen on the side to which the sleeper turns. He accuses those who give this advice of talking 'as if they were the masters of nature and could rule over its operations'. Only individual experience, he argues, should dictate the best sleeping position for the individual:

> Each one of us can dispense with this pointless precaution and having eaten may at once or shortly after go to sleep on either right side or left as it suits provided that we can then wake up in cheerful spirits, with agile bodies and happy faces, without either damp eyes or mouths full of saliva, because otherwise if we arise from our beds sad, weary, and slothful, with damp eyes and much saliva in our mouths, it is best for us to change such habits and be at ease in the time, the place and in those things that we know make us feel better.[26]

Petronio is not unique in exposing elements of the traditional paradigm to criticism: the *Commentaries* attributed to Arnau and published in the vernacular in

---

[23] Durante, *Il tesoro*, 28–9; and Tartaglini, *Opera nuova*, 22–3.

[24] Savonarola, *Libreto*, 61ʳ; Rangoni, *Consiglio*, 26; and Tartaglini, *Opera nuova*, 25.

[25] e.g. Tartaglini, *Opera nuova*, 23; and Durante, *Il tesoro*, 31.

[26] 'Potrà ognuno, lassando questa vana diligenza da canto, subito o poco dopo preso il cibo coricarsi sul lato destro o sinistro come gli pare purchè però si svegli con l'animo allegro, il corpo agile, la faccia lieta, non avrà gli occhi humidi nè la bocca piena di sputi, perchè altrimenti, se si leverà tristo, lasso e pigro, con gli occhi humidi e molti sputi in bocca gli converrà mutare quest'usanza e accomodarsi nel sito, nel tempo e a quelle cose nelle quali conoscerà sentirsi meglio.' Petronio, *Del viver*, 327.

1587, and, ten years later, Paschetti's regimen, also describe the prescription of adopting different positions at different stages of sleep as a waste of time.[27] This stance represents a fundamental challenge to the traditional rules. As suggested by the quotation from Petronio, these authors go well beyond the classification of bodies in types with specific characteristics and requirements. By taking the idea that each body is different to the extreme they reach the conclusion that only individuals themselves, on the basis of personal reactions, can identify the pattern of sleep most suitable to the specific make-up of their bodies.

As we shall see further on, this call for a more radical deregulation of advice regarding sleep is evident in many passages of Petronio's text. However, challenges to the traditional body of knowledge coexist with a more cautious and conventional approach. Hence, limiting somehow the scope of their previous criticism, both Petronio and Paschetti note that it will be safe to lie on the side that one finds more convenient especially when considerable time has elapsed between the evening meal and going to bed, for by then the food, tending to liquefy while one is awake, will occupy very little space in the stomach. As is often the case in regimens, change emerges gradually and in an apparently contradictory fashion. Innovative ideas are certainly present but stand side by side with the reiteration of traditional principles.

SLEEPING DURING THE DAY: OLD AND NEW VIEWS

In terms of the best time for sleep this should come at night and not during the day because the silence, cool temperature, and darkness of the night are ideal for rest; moreover, mind and body are tranquil at night because all occupations come to a standstill.[28] The idea that night is destined for rest and day for wakefulness and activity is presented by some authors as 'part of the order of nature'.[29] Others suggest it is a habit (*consuetudine*) but so ingrained that we no longer desire to sleep during the day.[30] There are also serious physiological reasons why daytime sleep is not advisable: it would be impossible to sleep long enough to complete digestion, hence this will be interrupted, causing great damage to health. Incomplete digestion would generate 'oxiremia', acid disturbances, overmuch wind, and various infirmities ranging from fevers to catarrh, from headaches to hoarseness. Sleeping during the day also induces laziness, forgetfulness, dazed states, and lack of appetite, and causes sadness and anxiety.[31] For all these reasons daytime sleep is strongly condemned by most authors, especially as we move into the late fifteenth century;

[27] *Commentarii*, 114; and Paschetti, *Del conservare*, 209.
[28] Arnaldi, *Regimen sanitatis*, 439; Benzi, *Tractato utilissimo*, Vʳ; Lennio, *Della complessione*, 42; Durante, *Il tesoro*, 26; and Traffichetti, *L'arte*, 115.
[29] Fonseca, *Del conservare*, 79.
[30] Viviani, *Trattato*, 200.
[31] Camaffi, *Reggimento*, 136; Frediano, *Arca novella*, 178; Boldo, *Libro della natura*, 223; *Scuola Salernitana*, 2, 112; and Pictorius, *Dialogi*, 59.

earlier regimens mention the issue only in passing or not at all, or sometimes they simply point to necessary precautions without completing forbidding naps. Thus Arnau recommends that daytime sleep should occur in a fresh and dry place, with the feet bare but covered and he lists the ill effects of sleeping with socks. Similar admonitions are reiterated in the late fifteenth century in the regimen attributed to Benzi, but by now the prohibition on sleeping during the day seems to have become more severe.[32]

Some exceptions to the general rule are however conceded: daytime sleep can be allowed if one has not slept at night, especially if it is so hot that sleep is difficult, or the body and stomach are particularly weak.[33] In addition, age, complexion, and above all custom are increasingly taken into account as factors that temper the universality of the prohibition: if day sleep is customary it will not be harmful, provided that it is short.[34] Even in these circumstances however, day rest should be limited only to the summer season and be separated from food and digestion, hence take place before lunch; moreover, it should not last longer than an hour.

The potential for deviating from even this body of precepts becomes, however, increasingly significant towards the end of the sixteenth century. Progressively, both the seasonal restrictions and the daytime injunction to sleep only at midday are dropped, while custom and complexion come to be seen as more powerful determinants of healthy sleeping practices. Sleeping after lunch is initially allowed in men with hot and dry complexions, scholars, and those who are thin, but in Camaffi's regimen this habit is tolerated simply to 'please the young' ('compiacere la gioventú')—an acknowledgement perhaps that this practice was becoming common among the younger generation.[35] And although the limitation of daytime sleep to the summer is still upheld, it is stressed that ingrained habits cannot be dislodged without causing serious damage. Hence, as argued by Camaffi in 1610, 'there are those so accustomed that even in winter and other seasons they wish to take a little nap every day and are so fond of it that if they wanted to do without it for a few days it would be to their detriment because the habit and the disposition introduced have become second nature to the limbs and the whole body and spirit'.[36] For them it is preferable therefore to stick to bad old habits. Petronio stresses instead the variety of individual reactions, in order to argue once more against the value of universal guidelines also in matters of daytime sleep: 'if however a person who for some personal reason sleeps in daytime should wake more agile in body, lively in spirits and cheerful in expression, he may also sleep after the

---

[32] Arnaldi, *Regimen sanitatis*, 434; and Benzi, *Tractato utilissimo*, V^r.

[33] Lennio, *Della complessione*, 44; Paschetti, *Del conservare*, 206; Fonseca, *Del conservare*, 79; and Zacchia, *De mali*, 102.

[34] Benzi, *Tractato utilissimo*, V^r; Savonarola, *Libreto*, 52^v; Durante, *Il tesoro*, 26; Boldo, *Libro della natura*, 224; *Commentarii*, 113; Traffichetti, *L'arte*, 115; and Pictorius, *Dialogi*, 60.

[35] Fonseca, *Del conservare*, 136; and Camaffi, *Reggimento*, 136.

[36] 'Si trovano alcuni tanto assuefatti che anche d'inverno e altre stagioni vogliono fare un sonnetto ogni giorno e vi sono inclinati talmente che se per qualche giorno se ne volessero astenere ne sentirebbero non mediocre detrimento per la consuetudine, natura e disposizione introdotta e habituata nei membri e in tutto il corpo e nell'animo.' Camaffi, *Reggimento*, 137. On a similar note Boldo, *Libro della natura*, 224.

midday meal'.[37] Though the justifications provided are slightly different in each author, the overall trend is towards an increasing legitimization of the daytime nap. This tendency reaches the apex in Viviani's regimen (1626), which praises post-prandial sleep without reservations and, entirely reversing the old paradigm, describes it as a healthy practice that favours digestion rather than impeding it: 'the habit of that rest taken by men after the midday meal is a very suitable one for ensuring that the digestion of food should have greater calorific value'.[38]

Another limitation that is gradually lifted concerns the position of the body during daytime sleep. From the second half of the sixteenth century health-advice literature recommends that, when unavoidable, daytime sleep should at least not occur in bed but in a sitting position, with the head leaning against the wall, a *spalliera*, or against the back of a chair.[39] Durante even specifies this should be a leather chair, indicating a precise type of armchair with a back high enough to support the head, a type becoming common in the second half of the sixteenth century (see Fig. 4.1) and which was evidently also used for this purpose.[40]

A few decades later, however, sleeping in a horizontal position during the day has become acceptable also among health advisers. Fonseca recommends: 'and be seated or else lie on hard mattresses with leather pillows under the head' (see Plates 9, 10).[41] Here he is echoing the preoccupation expressed also by earlier authors that day sleep should not be too comfortable, so that it does not last too long; his concern is in any case more for the quality of the couch than for the reclining position adopted.[42] On a similar note Camaffi warns against 'relaxing too much, instead keeping the head higher and sleeping on the right side', clearly taking it for granted that one could lie down when taking a daytime nap.[43] By the first decades of the seventeenth century day sleep appears to be widely authorized, the only restriction still in place in health-advice literature being that it should not exceed one hour.

THE CULTURE OF DAYTIME REST

The development of advice regarding daytime sleep in the healthy-living texts seems to indicate the growing acceptance of a practice that, as revealed by other sources, had become common, at least among the better-off. Indeed the appearance

[37] 'se invece chi dorme di giorno per qualche proprietà si sveglia più agile di corpo, l'animo pronto e la cera allegra, potrà dormire anche dopo pranzo.' Petronio, *Del viver*, 327.
[38] 'la consuetudine di quel riposo che gli uomini prendono dopo pranzo è di molto comodo acciò che la cottura del cibo abbia più valido calore.' Viviani, *Trattato*, 200.
[39] Paschetti, *Del conservare*, 209; Petronio, *Del viver*, 325; and *Commentarii*, 113.
[40] Durante, *Il tesoro*, 27.
[41] 'e stiasi a sedere overo a giacere sopra duri materassi con guanciali di cuoio sotto la testa.' Fonseca, *Del conservare*, 79. For surviving leather pillows see the examples in Rosignoli, *Cuoi d'oro*, 115–23.
[42] Benzi, *Tractato utilissimo*, V[r]; and Durante, *Il tesoro*, 27. Similar recommendations are found in tracts for the education of children. See e.g. Antoniano, *Dell'educazione*, 354.
[43] 'di non si adagiare troppo ma stare con la testa elevata e porsi a dormire sopra il destro lato.' Camaffi, *Reggimento*, 137.

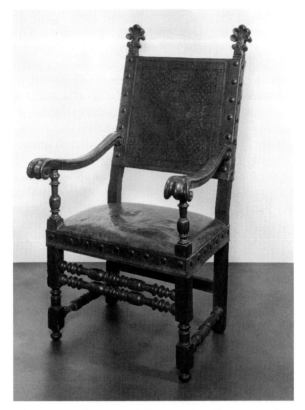

Fig. 4.1. This early seventeenth-century Italian armchair (h. 129.5 cm) exemplifies a type that became popular among the elites in Italy after 1600. Made of walnut—a prestigious wood—the frame is designed for comfort as the flowing arms provide excellent support and the upholstered seat and back are made of smooth leather. This is an object of some distinction, as shown by the ornamental gilding on the leather, and the gilded coat of arms of the Chiaramonti family of Verona. The high, slightly sloping back is a novel design aimed at supporting the head and would have made this chair well suited for naps. This design links it to more customized reclining chairs, made for the elderly and for periods of ill health, as we can see in Plate 11 (M. A.-W.).

of objects specifically designated for daytime naps suggests that by the early decades of the seventeenth century sleeping during the day was regarded as a regular component of genteel life.

In this period Roman household inventories show the presence of *sedie da riposo* (see Plate 11) and *lettiere da riposo* (resting chairs and frames for daybeds) in cardinals' palaces, suggesting that specialized objects had been created for this purpose.[44]

---

[44] The first examples in our sample of inventories are the 'gilded daybed' ('lettiera indorata da reposo') in the wardrobe of Cardinal Belmonti (ASR, TCG, Notai degli Uffici della Curia Romana, vol. 177, 19.12.1618, 116) and the 'painted daybed with little mattresses and two red and yellow

These furnishings differ in many respects from the *lettuccio* that is a feature of the Tuscan patrician house of the fifteenth and early sixteenth centuries. This imposing object, invariably placed in the bedchamber, often forms a set with the nearby adjacent night bed, chests, and hat rack, and sometimes it is part of the same inbuilt wooden panel (as in Plate 12).[45]

Normally positioned close to the bed, the *lettuccio* provided seating for visitors at a time when the bedroom still represented a focus for sociability and chairs were rare, as well as a couch for convalescents and those afflicted by minor ailments.[46] By contrast, the *letto da riposo* (daybed) that our evidence highlights as a feature of the late sixteenth and the early decades of the seventeenth centuries is a self-standing object, and one that does not necessarily belong to the bedroom but can be moved to different rooms, to the outdoor space, and from the palace to the villa. Moreover, it is designed exclusively for individual use and for daytime rest. The terminology also reflects this shift in function: in the seventeenth century the word *lettuccio* is hardly used but has given way to the word *letto da riposo* or *lettiera da riposo*.[47]

Doctor Paolo Zacchia, writing in 1639, acknowledges this development in the material culture of sleep: 'in order to avoid sleeping too long, many use the practice of not sleeping in bed, nor removing any of their clothes, but rather sleeping on chairs *that are made for this purpose, or on little day beds also fashioned for this*' (our emphasis).[48] The injunction that daytime sleep should not be too comfortable in order to be brief, a leitmotif in health-advice literature since the fifteenth century, was therefore taken seriously in everyday practice and was reflected in the characteristics of furniture serving the ritual of resting during the day. Indeed a letter written in October 1643 by Maria Spada in Rome to accompany the dispatch of a daybed with a gilded headrest to Uncle Bernardino (in one of the Spada villas) shows that a clear difference was made between 'mattresses only for daytime rest' and 'mattresses for ordinary sleep'. The fact that the daybed was equipped also with 'two leather pillows' completes the picture, echoing closely the recommendation in Fonseca's regimen that day sleep should take place either on a chair or lying on 'hard mattresses with leather pillows under the head' so that one would not sink into them and run the risk of falling into a too pleasurable and long sleep.[49]

Venetian satin pillows' ('lettuccio dipinto con materazzini e due cuscini di rasetto di Venetia rossi e gialli') in the villa of Cardinal Benedetto Giustiniani outside Porta del Popolo in 1621. In 1638 the same object is found in the inventory of Benedetto's brother Vincenzo; Danesi Squarzina, *La collezione Giustiniani*, vol. i. *Inventari I*, 200 and 497.

[45] Thornton, *The Italian*, 149–51 and 381.

[46] Musacchio, *Art, Marriage, and Family*, 107.

[47] It is unfortunate that no examples seem to have survived for this object. However, both Giulio Romano and Lambert Sustris provide idealized representations of the self-standing daybed described in our sources. See Ch. 2 n. 77.

[48] 'Molti per fuggir di dormire piu lungamente di quello che converrebbe usano di non dormire ne' letti, ne' per alcun modo spogliarsi de' panni, ma piu' tosto sopra alcune segge a questo fine fabricate, o su alcuni letticciuoli per il medesimo fine fatti.' Zacchia, *De mali*, 102.

[49] See n. 41.

We are sending the daybed with the gilded headrest in accordance with Your Excellency's orders, along with two leather pillows. The mattresses and the palliasses have never been here; when Your Excellency slept in it we would put out those used ordinarily by Your Excellency. Just now the satin ones were on, the ones left by Monsignor Matalino, which are only mattresses for resting during the day and not for ordinary sleeping, but we shall not send them; mattresses can be put on from one of those beds that are upstairs, where I think there are some large beds.[50]

Interestingly Maria's letter also suggests that these bed frames could be used interchangeably for night and day sleep, by just altering the type of mattress used, pointing to the importance that daybeds had acquired as prestigious objects in household furniture, not second in appearance to the night bed. The comment about the possible use of large mattresses in a *lettiera* previously used for daytime sleep also suggests that these objects could be quite imposing in size. Indeed by mid-century daybeds have become the focus of creative design, existing in aristocratic households in a variety of shapes and materials with different kinds of ornamentation. In 1655, for example, an elaborate 'daybed of *fico d'India*, embellished with gilded brasses: knobs, studs, bed heads and their fittings, each of them with 12 screws' is listed among the goods belonging to Cardinal Virgilio Spada.[51] A few years later, a plainer walnut daybed is also present in the Spada palace together with the already-mentioned daybed with a gilded headrest.[52]

The Spada villas also appear to be equipped with several items devoted to daytime sleep: 'una sedia di vachetta di riposo con scabilletto da piedi simili' (a reclining chair of cowhide with a footstool of the same kind) is found among the furnishings of the Serpentara villa in 1664. A 'lettiera di riposo alla napolitana' (a Neapolitan-style daybed) is listed in another chamber and another old daybed of walnut in the *tinello*, the space where the household staff normally took their meals, suggesting that by now postprandial rest was also practised by domestic servants.[53]

The letters exchanged between members of the Spada family in the seventeenth century provide some evidence about the circumstances when day rest was desirable. A period of generous rest was a regular occurrence after travelling. On their arrival at Tivoli from Rome (a journey of only two hours), Maria and the family

---

[50] 'Si manda la lettiera de la testiera dorata conforme l'ordine di VEcc, assieme con due cuscini di corame; li matarazzi e i pagliericci non ci sono mai stati, quando VEcc ci ha dormito ce se metteva quelli che adopra di ordinario VEcc. Hora stavano sopra quelli de' Rasetti [di rasetto, a type of fabric] che furono lasciati da Mons. Matalino, quali non sono materazzi se non per riposo il giorno e non da dormire ordinariamente, che però non si mandano, si potranno mettere li matarazzi di uno di quelli letti che sono di sopra che me pare ci siano alcuni letti grandi.' ASR, FSV, B.619, 9.10.1643.

[51] 'lettiera da riposo di fico d'India guarnita di ottoni dorati con pomi, colonnette, testiera e suoi finimenti, tutti con dodici vite.' ASR, FSV, B.481, 190. It is difficult to say what is meant by *fico d'India*, literally prickly pear. It may be a wood of Asian origin such as ebony, as we know that this precious wood started to be used in the manufacture of beds towards the end of the 16th century. Thornton, *The Italian*, 154 and 382.

[52] These are among the goods found in Virgilio's inventory at his death. ASR, FSV, vol. 269, 21.5.1663, 217, 234, and 245.

[53] ASR, FSV, vol. 359, fasc. 471, 'Inventario dei mobili esistenti nella villa della Serpentara nel Tempo del Sig. Marchese Orazio Spada, 1664'.

had a meal and then rested for three and a half hours before starting to organize the house for their stay.[54] A period of rest was also requested after activities seen as medicinal, such as going to the spas. As Bernardino reports, with some annoyance, from the thermal baths of San Casciano in September 1642, one was expected to take the waters for one hour and then rest for another hour in a 'small structure made of boards for this purpose and in a good little daybed'.[55] A much longer period of rest, varying from half a day to several days in the case of an old person, was required when one submitted to bloodletting.[56] Day sleep was also practised as a remedy against debilitating conditions such as *fiacchezza* and stomach pain, a recurrent source of suffering for Maria.[57]

Though letters do not make clear where day rest took place, whether on a chair or *lettiera da riposo* or on the bed itself, the phrasing in some of these accounts suggests that even if the bed was used for this purpose the sleeper rested 'on the bed' rather than 'in bed'. In keeping with contemporary advice concerning healthy sleep therefore, day rest did not involve getting undressed and sleeping under the covers. So, although medical authors had gradually accepted the surging tide of day rest and progressively adapted their advice to the new habits of their clients they certainly made their voice heard: they stipulated that day sleep, if unavoidable, should take place according to different criteria from those of night sleep and this was largely complied with. And in fact, unlike ordinary beds, daybeds in household inventories never appear to be furnished with blankets and quilts. 'At 18 hours [2.30 p.m.] on the 6th I sent a courier to Rome and I settled down to some much-needed rest, lying *on the bed* until at least 20 hours [4.30 p.m.]' (our emphasis).[58] The letter, written in May from Tor de' Buonacorsi when Bernardino is 42 years old and in good health, also suggests that day rest was often simply used as an enjoyable and restorative activity and not only as a response to ill health or exhaustion. That day rest was increasingly conceptualized as a form of comfort to which the elite might resort also several times in a day seems to be confirmed by a letter dated 7 July 1655 in which Bernardino gives Maria an exceptionally detailed account of his first day in Tivoli:

> When I reached home it was already 14 hours [11 a.m.],...[and] I at once lay down on my bed to rest and after three-quarters of an hour I got up and said the office. We could not dine until after midday...After dining I rested until 18 hours [3 p.m.], but before it became dark I returned to my bed three or four times, which accounted for some two hours more, which I passed partly in reading and partly in sleeping.[59]

---

[54] ASR, FSV. B.619, 7.5.1652. For another example, ASR, FSV, B.491, 26.5.1636.

[55] 'camerino di tavole fatto fare a posta e in buon letticciolo.' ASR, FSV, B.619, 9.9.1642 and 10.9.1642.

[56] See e.g. the letters in ASR, FSV, B.619, 9.9.1642 and 11.7.1655.

[57] See her letters to uncle Bernardino in ASR, FSV, B.619, 10.9.1642 and 6.7.1660.

[58] 'Alle 18 del 6 mandai un corriere a Roma e mi misi a riposare che ne avevo bisogno, e me ne stetti sul letto fino a ore 20 e oltre.' ASR, FSV, B.491, 9.5.1638.

[59] 'Arrivai a casa a hore 14 sonate,... mi posi subito sul letto a riposare e dopo tre quarti d'ora ne scesi e dissi l'uffizio. Non si poté pranzare se non dopo il mezzogiorno...Dopo pranzo riposai fino alle 18 ore, ma inanzi che si facesse notte tornai sul letto 3 o 4 volte, che portarono via circa un paio di altre ore, delle quali ne passai parte leggiucchiando e parte dormendo.' ASR, FSV, B.481, 7.7.1655.

Day rest is presented as a source of pleasure and well-being, in spite of taking place after lunch, in a reclining position, and also for longer than an hour—all practices that a few decades earlier were energetically discouraged in health-advice literature.

It would seem however that the elite indulged in these forms of pleasure especially in the summer and during their stays at the villa—a period of licence from many of the strictures associated with the winter and with city life. All the accounts about this practice found in letters refer in fact to the summer months and we should not forget that the regimens had traditionally tolerated day sleep in the heat of the summer. Indeed, day sleep seems to be particularly conversant with the lifestyle of *villeggiatura* and the pursuit of classical *otium* that was seen to characterize the villa stay; it is no accident that the first furnishings designed for this activity seem to have been introduced in the villa environment. By the late sixteenth century the garden of the Cardinal of Ferrara's villa in Tivoli is equipped with 'outside summer beds for daytime rest'. These are positioned next to the rooms that had been created within a grotto and, embellished with columns, a fountain, and a combination of ancient statues, paintings, and marble tables with various sorts of stones, were 'all designed to voluptuous pleasure' ('dedicata al piacer voluttuoso').[60]

It is interesting to compare Bernardino's relaxed and self-satisfied account of his afternoon napping in Tivoli with the fears about the negative effects of sleeping during the day experienced a century earlier by the painter Pontormo. As he recorded in his autobiography on 31 March 1554, 'on Monday morning I found it painful to move; I got up and because it was cold and windy I went back to bed and stayed there until the 18th hour [1.30 p.m.] and for the whole day I felt unwell…I think that going back to bed was altogether bad for me.'[61] Tainted with a sense of guilt for the strain inflicted to his own body, Pontormo's testimony suggests that in the mid-sixteenth century disapproval of lying in bed during the day was deeply ingrained and shared also by the artisan class. A century later, the rise of the culture of *villeggiatura* and the increased value attributed to custom in medical thinking have transformed the perception of daytime sleep. No longer regarded as damaging for health if limited in duration, this is now universally seen as a treat in the summer months and a form of regeneration for those who have experienced infirmities, debilitation, or fatigue.

NIGHT SLEEP: A NEW ROLE FOR THE BED

How long should night sleep last? The general indication is that sleep should range from seven to nine or ten hours, but the possibility of establishing a fixed rule is denied by most authors: some argue that the length of sleep depends on how long

---

[60] 'letti esterni d'estate per risposarvisi di giorno.' 'Descrittione di Tivoli, et del giardino dell'Ill/mo Cardinal di Ferrara' in Coffin, *The Villa d'Este*, 144.

[61] 'lunedí mattina mi si smosse il corpo con dolore: lévami e poi per esser fredo e vento ritornai nel letto e stettivi insino a hore 18 e in tuttodí poi non mi sentii bene…penso che mi nuocesse assai quello ritornare nel leto.' Pontormo, *Diario*, 24.

one was awake for: 'let sleep be proportional to waking'; others that sleep should cease on the completion of digestion—signalled by the color of urine—and when energies (the spirits) have returned.[62] Moreover it is impossible to regulate the duration of a night's sleep because this varies according to age, habit, exercise, and strength of the body.[63] The type of complexion is also an element to consider: those with a hot body, especially if young, digest quickly and six hours' sleep are sufficient for them, while others, like children and the elderly, take longer and need longer sleeps. After 22 years of age, however, sleeping longer than nine hours goes beyond the bounds of good health.[64] The season of the year is another relevant factor: sleep should be longer in winter and spring, when more solid food is consumed. There is particular encouragement for sleeping generously in springtime, when nights are short and morning sleep is particularly pleasant, as reflected in the popular saying: 'nel mese di aprile dolce è il dormire' ('April is a month when sleep is sweet').[65]

While advice on the duration of sleep has therefore become highly flexible there are exceptions. Excessive sleeping is regarded as particularly damaging and as a sign of moral decay. Although authors list the unhealthy effects of lack of sleep or limited sleep, it is especially with the risks of immoderate sleep that early modern texts are concerned.[66] It would seem that there is an increased dislike for superfluous sleep, which is discussed more at length by late sixteenth-century authors than by earlier ones. Those who sleep too much are depicted in disparaging terms and as undignified: he yawns, stretches his body, is weak and lazy, he is sad and tends to be taciturn. His senses will be dumb, the mind dulled (*balorda*), the head heavy, and the sleeper will experience memory loss; his body will be cold, filled with phlegm, and with a bad colour.[67] Hence 'he who sleeps too much is like half a man and almost a dead one', for the protracted paralysis of sensation and functions (not seeing, not hearing, and not speaking) are like death.[68] Superfluous sleep also predisposes towards sundry infirmities—including asthma, apoplexy, epilepsy, paralysis, stupor, fever, and constipation—and it prevents the elimination of superfluities since, with the exception of sweating, all evacuations come to a standstill.[69]

The offensive against superfluous sleep is carried out in similar tones by a group of doctors who unanimously depict immoderate sleep as a form of anti-civic behaviour and a barrier to the public role the elite is called on to perform. The idea is conveyed through the presentation of a number of exemplary figures who sacrificed sleep to the requirements of an active life. Hence in his annotations to Benzi's

---

[62] Rangoni, *Consiglio*, 26; Pictorius, *Dialogi*, 59–60; 'sia il sonno proporzionato alle vigilie'; Benzi, *Tractato utilissimo*, Vᵛ; Bertaldi, *Regole della sanità*, 31; and Durante, *Il tesoro*, 29.

[63] Savonarola, *Libreto*, 52ᵛ.

[64] Durante, *Il tesoro*, 29; Paschetti, *Del conservare*, 207; Pictorius, *Dialogi*, 59–60; and Petronio, *Del viver*, 325.

[65] Petronio, *Del viver*, 352.

[66] Savonarola, *Libreto*, 52ᵛ; Benzi, *Tractato utilissimo*, Vᵛ; Durante, *Il tesoro*, 24 and 29–30; Paschetti, *Del conservare*, 210; Rangoni, *Consiglio*, 22; and *Commentarii*, 115.

[67] Durante, *Il tesoro*, 30.

[68] 'chi dorme troppo è simile a un mezzo uomo e quasi morto.' Durante, *Il tesoro*, 24.

[69] *Commentarii*, 115; Camaffi, *Reggimento*, 131; Frediano, *Arca novella*, 174 and 176; and Bertaldi, *Regole della sanità*, 31.

regimen (1618) Bertaldi declares that 'wakefulness was estimed by great princes and celebrated by philosophers'.[70] He then refers to Celio's suggestion that one should to get up at night to attend to public affairs and businesses of consequence and mentions the case of Diogenes who, to avoid sleepiness, held a ball in his hand above a copper vase so that he would be awakened by the noise of the ball hitting the vase if he fell asleep. He also praises Carlo Emanuele XI, Duke of Savoy, who spends entire nights dealing with state and military affairs and studying history and moral philosophy, cultivating therefore the kind of moral education expected in leaders. He rarely sleeps longer than five hours and never eats unless he feels his stomach is empty.

Moderate sleep is thus presented as a sign of virtue and, together with frugality in eating habits, is associated with alertness and industriousness, with clear minds and active engagement in activities of public interest. In a similar vein, a dialogue between sleep and wakefulness, published in 1562 by Ugoni da Brescia, condemns the habit of sleeping without need and the sophisticated expedients introduced to conjure sleep and make the experience particularly gratifying:

> drinking poppyseed, eating cooked lettuce, hearing the murmur of a brook or gently falling rain, a thorough soak in a sweet-smelling evening bath, to say nothing of soft silk bedding and delicate and fragrantly laundered sheets, along with other entice-ments in cool well-appointed bedrooms scattered with as many varieties of flowers as can be found in the season.[71]

Such a hedonistic culture of sleep is depicted as contrary to the divine order and to nature and a comparison is made with the excessive eating in which the wealthy indulge: 'the sumptuous dishes and the many kinds of food with which man indis-criminately fills himself, setting out tables for banquets which are like spectacles of every cruelty both against himself, his overindulgence leading to so many illnesses, and in devouring the needs of the poor, who would live off his leftovers'.[72]

Recent studies have suggested that the way in which societies in Western Europe understood and used the night changed dramatically in the early modern period. Elite entertainments spread to the hours of darkness, the time of dining and going to bed moved progressively later. The fact that from the last decades of the six-teenth century the discourse on sleep, especially in its relation to time, is imbued with moralistic overtones might be related to these developments.[73] Interestingly,

---

[70] Bertaldi, *Regole della sanità*, 31.

[71] 'il bere del seme di papavero, il mangiare della lattuca cotta, il sentire il mormorio di qualche fiumicello o pioggia che soavemente cada, il lavarsi la sera bene bene in qualche bagno di buon odore, per non dire dei morbidissimi letti di seta con le lenzuola di bucato sottilissime e profumate e degli altri dolci inviti delle camere fresche et ornate e sparse di tante varietà di fiori quante secondo le sta-gioni è possibile ritrovarne.' Ugoni, *Dialogo*, 73.

[72] 'le sontuose vivande e i tanti cibi di che l'huomo si empie indiscriminatamente mettendo tavole e facendo conviti i quali sono come spettacoli d'ogni crudeltà sì contra di sè medesimo, in prendere dalla incontinenza sua le tante infermità che poi perciò gli sopravengono, come in divorare le necessità dei poveri, i quali degli avanzi suoi vivrebbero.' Ugoni, *Dialogo*, 73. A similar analogy between overeat-ing and oversleeping is drawn by Pictorius (*Dialogi*, 59), who defines these habits as bestial and diabolical.

[73] Cabantous, *Histoire de la nuit*; and Koslofsky, *Evening's Empire*.

while regimens have grown increasingly indulgent towards daytime naps, they strongly disapprove not just of exceedingly long sleeps but of the habit of turning the day into night and vice versa. The involvement of doctors in the pleasures of the *villeggiatura*, in which they were often invited to participate by their patrons, was perhaps a factor differentiating the attitudes they display towards these unorthodox sleeping practices. While resting at the villa, far from equalling idleness, maintained the classical connotation of a period devoted to study and intellectual pursuits, meant to uplift the spirit oppressed by civil duties, oversleeping in the morning was simply a sign of laziness. In 1603 Fonseca thunders: 'Sleeping must be by night, because by day we must be awake, as required by the order of nature and lest we wish to live in the guise of the bat or the owl as is the custom of pirates or wretched courtiers.'[74] Doctors clearly identify disorderly sleep with certain sections of the nobility. A few years later this kind of social critique is developed even more overtly by Camaffi:

> as we seek to know when that hour is we say that the hour for sleep is not as the nobles would have it, for they do all the things the opposite way, since when we speak of eating they never have a time for sitting down at table and once they are there they do not seem to remember having to rise from it, and when we speak of rest they never consider the time for going to bed and when they are in bed in the morning nor do they think likewise of getting up, for to them it is odious, and I have observed in many of them that when one should have slept they have not yet dined, whether it be summer or winter...and by dint of these things they make night day and day night...

Camaffi, a university teacher in the town of Perugia, then goes on to identify two figures who on the contrary stand out for their positive behaviour and set an example that all those with public responsibilities should follow: the late Pope Paul III, an assiduous visitor to Perugia, and the late Cardinal della Corgna.[75] A few decades later Bartolomeo Pietragrassa, another provincial doctor, a university lecturer in Pavia, more broadly chastises the general corruption of the present century in which, 'with no little prejudice to his health, he is wont to go to sleep at dawn, and almost at midday, and he stays up all night, indulging in gluttony for most of it'.[76] It is perhaps significant that the authors most overtly critical of aristocratic extravagance are provincial doctors, while court doctors like Petronio favour physiological explanations of excess sleep rather than a moralistic one. In his view this tendency

---

[74] 'Dormir deve esser di notte perchè di giorno dobbiamo vegliare, così richiede l'ordine della natura se pure non vogliamo vivere a guisa di pipistrello o di civetta come hanno in usanza i corsari e i miseri cortigiani.' Fonseca, *Del conservare*, 79.

[75] 'cercando noi di sapere quale sia quell'ora disciamo che l'ora di dormire non è secondo l'uso dei nobili, i quali fanno tutte le loro cose al rovescio imperochè se parliamo di mangiare mai trovano l'ora di andare a tavola e quando vi sono non par che si ricordano di haversene a levare, se poi parliamo del riposo non pensano mai l'ora di andare a dormire e essendo in letto la mattina poco meno che all'ora di mangiare gli è odioso levarsi e io ho osservato in molti che quando bisognerebbe aver dormito non hanno ancor cenato tanto d'estate che d'inverno...a tal che gli è forza della notte far giorno e del giorno far notte'; Camaffi, *Reggimento*, 132.

[76] 'con pregiuditio non leggier della salute, si dedica al sonno l'aurora, e quasi il mezzodi, e si consacra alle vigilie, e alle crapole gran parte della notte.' Pietragrassa, *Politica medica*, 413.

to sleep excessively is caused by lack of good exercise through which superfluities are normally burned up; as a consequence humours build up, creating many and strange vapours which in turn provoke lethargy. The best remedy for this kind of affliction is not discipline but a change in diet that would prevent sleepiness.[77]

How can we explain this increasing preoccupation with the effects of excessive sleep? It is likely that doctors were targeting new sleeping habits among their readers, especially the younger generations. As the studies on the history of the night have demonstrated, the hours of darkness were increasingly colonized by the elites in the seventeenth century, and these transformations were generationally driven.[78] It is interesting to observe how, in the last decades of the sixteenth century, similar concerns were raised by authors of educational treatises. While what is expected of the young noble, destined to a career in the Church, at court, or in public office, is an active life, increasingly devoted to studying a range of academic subjects as well as to practical training in drawing, playing music, singing, and dancing, it would also seem that there was a growing distance between generations. Hence Lombardelli rails against the bad habits of the young, whose families kindly allow them 'to sleep from nightfall until the second hour of the day as well as some hours after the midday meal, issuing orders that no one in the house should disturb them'. He prescribes a rigid routine that includes 'getting out of bed two or three hours before daylight according to their calling or profession' and 'staying up two or three hours at most after dinner, both summer and winter, and then going to sleep'.[79] The motivations for these rules are spelled out in his 1594 treatise:

> in every season you will rise from bed as the day breaks rather than as the sun shines, because were you to do otherwise you would yourself become subject to many bad habits of temper, because sleeping too much generates many superfluities and it never rouses the spirits to any honourable enterprise. When it is time to go to sleep it is only a matter of doing so at a somewhat early hour so as not to spoil the morning with the fault of late nights.[80]

The moral value of getting up early in the morning seems to have been recognized by noblemen of mature age and well established in their duties, like Cardinal Bernardino Spada. Bernardino often gets up remarkably early to begin work and makes a point of mentioning this in his letters—though, as we know, long periods of rest are also embedded in his day, at least in the summer.[81] Getting up at five or six in the morning is also common for his nephew Orazio (married to Maria and

---

[77] Petronio, *Del viver*, 241.   [78] See n. 73.

[79] 'dormir dal principio della notte fino a due ore di giorno e anche alcune ore dopo il pranzo per gentilezza, con espresse commissioni per la casa che nessuno li interrompa. Levarsi dal letto due o tre ore inanzi giorno secondo la loro arte o professione [and]...dopo cena veglieranno due o tre ore al piú, tanto il verno che l'estate e poi andranno a dormire.' Lombardelli, *De gli vfizii*, 217.

[80] 'ad ogni stagione vi leverete piuttosto all'apparir del giorno che a un'ora di sole perche' se altrimenti faceste la persona verrebbe a farsi soggetto a molte cattive disposizioni perche' il troppo dormire ingenera molte superfluitá e non lascia mai levare l'animo ad alcuna impresa onorata. Quando sia l'ora di andare a dormire basta che si faccia un poco a buon'ora per non marcire poi la mattina col darne al tardi della sera la colpa.' Lombardelli, *Il giovane studente*, 23.

[81] ASR, FSV, B.491, 9.5.1638 and 7.7.1655.

father of a large cohort of offspring), a very active man, constantly engaged in the running of the large landholdings of the family and in the management of the Roman properties.[82] Letters represent these men as incessantly at work and often on the move, stressing their industriousness and scorn for inactivity. Nor are there instances of them going to bed at impossible hours at night; even when the family entertains, it is just for a few hours after supper.[83] Even during their stays at the villa adult members of the family get up very early, at 5 or 6 a.m., to take advantage of the cooler air.[84] Young nephews and children are on the contrary described with some anxiety as being feebler than their parents, easily tired, and unable to get up at dawn. Bernardino Spada, for example, is depicted by his father as being made of 'ricotta, so soft and delicate is he, that the smallest movement tires him out and robs him of his appetite, though not for sleep, and yet he is my son, and still today I can walk much more than him, I feel robust, I have a good appetite and I get up at dawn'.[85] It is likely that a generation gap was appearing in attitudes to idling about and sleeping in. For this reason, the departure of sons from the home to be educated in another city is regarded positively by fathers, in the hope that the new environment will make 'men' of them and perhaps remedy the damage done by the overindulgent education received at home.[86]

In spite of Spartan sleeping habits among nobles like the Spadas, the bed had undoubtedly come to play a new role in the life of the well-to-do, increasingly becoming a focus for leisure. As Ugoni had claimed in the second half of the sixteenth century, it had also grown more comfortable.

Household inventories, as well as visual evidence, reveal that several mattresses would be piled one upon the other on the beds of the most privileged (see Plate 13). In the Spada palace the adult members of the family sleep on three mattresses, high-ranking servants have two, and only the lower staff sleep on one mattress, sometimes with a mattress set atop a base of straw.[87] Moreover, according to Doctor Fonseca, writing in 1603, mattresses were to be made of different materials in winter and summer; silk wadding was to be used in summer and wool in winter—to make sleep cooler or warmer according to the seasons.[88] Outside the noble palace the distance between the sleeping conditions of the rich and the poor was widening: inventories show that the lower classes slept on just one mattress, often stuffed with hair. The difference between *letti civili* (civilized beds) and *letti incivili* (uncivilized beds) is made in letters: those defined *civili* have a bed frame (*lettiera*)—not resting simply on benches and boards—but presumably are also made *civili* by

---

[82] See e.g. the letter dated 21.7.1661 in ASR, FSV, B.607.

[83] A dancing 'veglia' that lingers on until 1a.m. is considered exceptional; ASR, FSV, B.410, 11.2.1657.

[84] ASR, FSV, B.410, 5.8.1657.

[85] ASR, FSV, B.607, 31.5.1661. On the feeble complexion of the Spada children; B.607, 6.4.1678.

[86] See e.g. the case of Alviano Spada, 'che qui non fa molto' ('who does very little here'), sent to the grand ducal court in Florence at age 13; ASR, FSV, B.607, 21.5.1658.

[87] ASR, Notai AC, vol. 5933, 'Inventario bonorum Cardinal Bernardino Spada', 23.11.1661.

[88] Fonseca, *Del conservare*, 80. Both Fonseca and Zacchia regard the use of feather mattresses as unhealthy, seeing this as a German custom alien to Italian ways. Zacchia, *De mali*, 69.

the thickness of the mattress and by the bedding.[89] In fact inventories also distinguish between matresses and bedsheets *da patrone* ('for the masters') and those in use *per la famiglia* ('for the household', that is to say the servants). Made more comfortable by the number of mattresses and pillows and their filling, by the quality of bedlinen, blankets, and quilts, and rendered more luxurious and attractive by the ornament of *trabacche*, valances, and canopies, beds have become the focus for pleasurable activities other than a night's sleep.

As we have seen, extended daytime rest is common among the nobility after travelling, bloodletting, and also in response to minor ailments, but the bed is also a place for retreat, for spending time alone. Reading in bed, for example during the day or before sleeping at night, seems to have been common for Cardinal Bernardino, who even had a rudimentary bedside table made out of 'a smooth board resting on the arms of his chair near the bed, where he would set the light and some books'.[90] The habit of reading in bed is also praised by Lombardelli, who instructs young people to do so for half an hour after the evening prayers and before going to sleep.[91]

Eating in bed was another common practice that would have been anathema to doctors, since it flies in the face of the golden rule that sleep should never occur immediately after a meal. Cardinal Bernardino often eats in bed, presumably on the 'tavolino da mangiare in letto' ('little table for eating in bed') found among his goods at his death.[92] It is the same item he wants to be sent to him when he is at San Casciano to take the waters, together with two other personal objects of comfort he keeps in his bedroom in Rome: his own *seggetta* (commode) and the board for placing the light and the books when he reads in bed which we have already mentioned.[93] His fondness for these items illustrates the enhanced role acquired by the bed and bedroom as a space for relaxing in peace and solitude during the day, as well as before going to sleep at night.

This fashion for what would have been considered unhealthy sleeping habits was something doctors had to come to terms with in the recommendations provided in advice books. Some articulate their dissatisfaction with the practices of their patients and readers by drawing on the long tradition of critical writing about the mores of the nobility that portrayed it as idle and socially useless, a tradition undergoing a revival in this period. Others, like Petronio, take to extremes the option of stressing individuality in the body's response to the strictures of healthy living, in an effort to accommodate varied sleeping habits within a paradigm by now perceived as too rigid. At the same time however, the influence of medical ideas about healthy sleep was far from irrelevant; as we shall see, these ideas also played

---

[89] ASR, FSV, B.491, 15.6.1655.

[90] 'quella tavoletta liscia che sta sui bracci della sua sedia, accanto al letto, su la quale soleva tenere il lume e qualche libro.' ASR, FSV, B.491, 4.9.1642. Twenty years later, at his death, the item is still listed among the goods present in his bedroom. ASR, Notai AC, vol. 5933, 'Inventario bonorum Cardinal Bernardino Spada', 23.11.1661: 'una sedia d'appoggio per il letto et una tavoletta'.

[91] Lombardelli, *Il giovane studente*, 29.

[92] ASR, FSV, B.491, 18.6.1656. Even when he does not eat in bed he seems to disregard the recommendation that dinner should be followed by a little walk or one or two hours of light conversation; B.491, 7.7.1655.

[93] ASR, FSV, B.491, 4.9.1642.

a role in the transformations that were affecting the look and use of bedrooms, beds, and bedding.

A HEALTHY ENVIRONMENT FOR SLEEP

Many elements converge in defining the material culture of sleep and the construction of the ideal sleeping environment in the early modern period. Among these, health concerns certainly occupy a significant place. The constant preoccupation with digestion inspires the recurring recommendation in regimens to sleep with the body well covered and not exposed to draughts from windows or doors. There is evidence that some of these prescriptions were taken seriously.

In the architectural drawings for the plans of villas and palaces in the sixteenth century, beds were no longer placed facing the centre of a room but in a corner, away from windows and doors and not too close to the fireplace either.[94] In this way they would be protected from sources of both cold and heat (see Fig. 4.2). Letters also confirm these preoccupations: having to sleep in a room without any door hanging while visiting his daughter in Viterbo, Orazio Spada was forced to spend the night with his head under the covers to shelter himself from 'the wind'.[95]

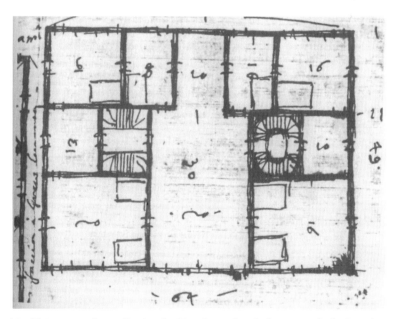

Fig. 4.2. This project for a villa, dated 1597, shows the ideal position for beds, in line with medical advice.

[94] Burns, 'Letti'.
[95] 'Dormisse...in una camera dove per non esservi portiera alcuna haveva l'entrata libra al vento per lo che tenne sempre il capo sotto le lenzuola.' ASR, FSV, B.607, 25.2.1659.

Regimens advise against opening the windows at night even in the suffocating heat of the summer. Windows were to be kept shut and the bedroom to be sealed everywhere so that the bed was not exposed to draughts.[96] As already highlighted in Chapter 3, cold and wind were increasingly seen as the principal threats to health; hence it was deemed better to suffer from excessive heat than from the cold.[97] Medieval authors consistently recommended that head and feet should also be covered in bed because natural heat moves away from the body extremities during sleep and digestion, causing these parts to cool down, with considerable ensuing damage for the brain.[98] The advice was reiterated by certain early modern authors, especially those writing in the second half of the sixteenth century. Durante adds the arms to the body parts that should not be exposed to night air.[99] In seventeenth-century texts, however, these recommendations have largely been dropped and they seem to have been disregarded also in daily practice. Writing in August from the villa, Eugenia remarks that the air is so cool in the evening that they cannot sleep with bare arms ('con le braccia scoperte'), implying that on hotter nights this was indeed common.[100] Moreover, the nightcap is an item rarely found in Roman inventories of this period. It is possible that the growing recourse to canopy beds, dressed with thick, heavy curtains hanging from the so-called *trabacca* or *padiglione*, now represented a more effective protection from the chill of the night.

In 1560 Rangoni prescribed in his regimen that 'the bed should never be without a canopy [*padiglione*]'.[101] The remark is interesting because it suggests that the increasing popularity of canopy beds in this period may have been partly determined by health concerns, as well as by the desire for greater privacy and by new aesthetic trends. The dissemination of the canopy bed is a phenomenon that develops in Italy precisely in the second half of the sixteenth century. It has thick curtains that envelop the bed on all sides, including the top, where it spreads out either from a cap (*cappello*), a round device hanging from the ceiling (see Plate 14), or from a flat or domed canopy sometimes defined as *cielo* (sky), supported by bedposts (see Plate 13).[102] On the basis of representations in paintings and household inventories of the ruling families Thornton has traced the emergence in Italy of these two typologies back to the end of the fifteenth century (for the pavilion bed) and to the first decades of the sixteenth century (for the four-poster bed).[103] Our study however, suggests that in this period *padiglioni* and *trabacche* are still elite objects, and they only begin to be listed in household inventories from Rome and Genoa, with increasing frequency, in the last decades of the sixteenth century. By the beginning of the seventeenth century they can be found right across the

---

[96] Rangoni, *Consiglio*, 11; and Fonseca, *Del conservare*, 80.

[97] Fonseca, *Del conservare*, 80.

[98] Arnaldi, *Regimen sanitatis*, 434; Alderotti, *Libello*, 15; and *Commentarii*, 113.

[99] Durante, *Il tesoro*, 27. This is repeated by Frediano, *Arca novella*, 177.

[100] ASR, FSV, B.410, 12.8.1657.

[101] Rangoni, *Consiglio*, 11.

[102] The evidence from Rome indicates that the former was called a '*padiglione*' and the latter a '*trabacca*'.

[103] Thornton, *The Italian*, 124–49.

social spectrum. For example, all the former prostitutes who chose to withdraw to the Roman house of the convertites in 1604 and 1605, have *padiglioni* among their goods.[104] Certainly, we still find beds without this structure in humble houses like that of fruit vendor Ghiringhelli in 1619 and among the household goods of the patients dictating their last will in the hospital of the Consolazione.[105] *Padiglioni* are also absent from the rooms destined for domestic staff in the palaces of the nobility; there, the bed, often *a credenza* (bunk bed), is equipped with a mattress, a pallet, and bolster, and with lighter or heavier blankets according to the season, but not with bed curtains.

With few exceptions therefore, bed curtains and the associated canopy have become very common elements of furniture by 1600 and have thus transformed the look of the bed. While the iconography suggests that bed curtains, though not integral to the bed, were often used also in previous centuries, it highlights differences in their physical characteristics and role (see Plate 15). The absence of a canopy left the bed exposed to cold temperatures; moreover, the curtains often seem to be made of light, thin fabric, and of less fabric (normally there are only one to three lengths) so that once pulled they would hang flat rather than be draped in multiple pleats; while they would create a partition of sorts that temporarily hid the bed from the rest of the room, this merely provided privacy rather than protection from the cold.[106] By the mid-sixteenth century, in contrast, they created a completely enclosed space, thanks to the introduction of the pavilion or canopy, the thickness of the fabrics deployed, and the increasing quantity and width of the hangings (we learn from inventories that in the seventeenth century these were sometimes made with as many as twenty-six lengths). The range of materials employed in the draping of the bed—silk, lawn, damask, twill, linen, ticking, wool and silk mixtures, net, figured silk, or taffeta—made it possible to adapt the structure to the season. Certainly, by mid-century, members of the Roman nobility possessed a large selection of *padiglioni* and *trabacche* of different colours and materials and suitable for all occasions and seasons. At the time of his death, in 1661, Cardinal Bernardino had twelve of these sets of bed hangings with matching canopies and coverlets; a year later, his brother Virgilio, who had also inherited Bernardino's assets, had twenty-one of them.[107]

These lavishly dressed beds also deployed a wide range of bright colours (green, turquoise, red, white, and yellow), creating a strong visual effect.[108] As well as proving the appeal of this new decorative item in the second half of the sixteenth

[104] ASVR, MCI, vol. 198, 1605–6.

[105] ASR, Ospedale della Consolazione, 244, 21.9.1619, 470, will of Navilia, wife of Gio' di Cocolla da Chieti; 22.4.1620, 484, will of Camilla, from Florence, wife of Lorenzo di Santo; 30.11.1619, 488, last will of Persia, daughter of Antonio Cappone da Valmontone.

[106] They were either hanging from hooks in the walls or sliding on rods protruding from the wall. Thornton, *The Italian*, 121.

[107] ASR, Notai AC, vol. 5933, 23.11.1661, 'Inventario bonorum Cardinal Bernardino Spada'; and ASR, FSV, vol. 269, 21.5.1663, 195, Inventory of Virgilio Spada.

[108] Their value also varies considerably, from 1 to 9 *scudo* just considering the *padiglioni* held by former courtesans at the beginning of the 17th century. ASVR, MCI, vol. 198, 20.4.1605 and 13.12.1605.

century, the rise in the use of the draped and canopied bed also offered an effective response to the growing preoccupation with climatic factors and their impact on sleep. In fact, besides protecting the body, and especially the head, from wind and cold, and in particular from the freezing air of the *bora*, the *padiglione* performed other important health functions: it shielded the sleeper from the first light of the morning and from noise, both factors that were described in regimens as disturbing, since they could prematurely awaken the sleeper, fatally interrupting the crucial process of digestion.[109] The other harmful agent from which shelter was needed during sleep was moonlight.[110] Traditionally classified as a cold planet, the moon was supposed to generate *rheuma* (catarrh of the brain) if it shone directly on the head; this encounter between the coldest planet and the coldest organ of the body was deemed to be particularly dangerous and more damaging than sleeping outside in the open, where the moon irradiates the whole body, another practice that was vigorously discouraged.[111]

The development and widespread use of the canopy bed thus took on a set of concerns related to healthy sleep, and it can be seen as an example of how preventive discourse went hand in hand with the emergence of new forms of display and decorative trends that redefined the furnishings of the home. Histories of the domestic interior have seen the quest for privacy as a key driving force behind many of the developments that transform the Renaissance palace, and the replacement of the 'open bed' with the enclosed one may be understood as an expression of this increased hunger for intimacy.[112] Certainly, the new bed structure also created an undisturbed, intimate space for sleepers and sexual partners. This concern for privacy, however, might have been felt strongly in the limited living spaces of the lower classes, but by now it was scarcely significant in the homes of the upper and middle strata, where the bedroom was becoming an increasingly secluded space, accessible only to the personal *cameriere* (chamber attendant) and separated from the rest of the house by a suite of small adjoining rooms (*salette*, *studioli*, and *camerini*) that acted as a kind of buffer.[113] Among the most prosperous, who already had the benefit of considerable private space at their disposal, the principal purpose of the canopy bed seems to have been that of creating a warm, dark, and noiseless environment around the sleeper, conducive to uninterrupted and quiet sleep and to a complete digestion.

The bed and its canopy functioned in conjunction with the fireplace, a regular feature of the bedroom even in the house of the artisanal classes.[114] The practice of warming the bed with bedpans before getting into it also seems to have been widespread.

---

[109] Benzi, *Tractato utilissimo*, Vʳ and Durante, *Il tesoro*, 26.
[110] Durante, *Il tesoro*, 26; Rangoni, *Consiglio*, 28; Fonseca, *Del conservare*, 80; and Traffichetti, *L'arte*, 116.
[111] Benzi, *Tractato utilissimo*, VIʳ.
[112] See e.g. Sarti, *Europe at Home*, ch. 4, esp. pp. 119–46; Roche, *History of Everyday Things*, chs. 5 and 7; Ranum, 'The Refuges'.
[113] Thornton, *The Italian*, 300–13; McIver, *Women*, 109–10.
[114] Cavallo, 'The Artisan's *Casa*', 74.

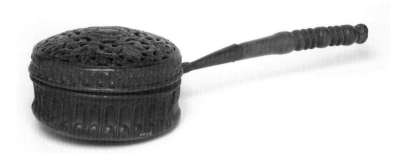

Fig. 4.3. In sixteenth-century Italy copper warming pans like this were commonly used across the social spectrum. Filled with coals and equipped with a long pole they were drawn through the sheets before going to bed.

Bed-warmers, commonly made of copper, but sometimes of wood and even silver, with an ebony handle, are listed among the household goods of all classes and from an early date (see Fig. 4.3).[115] Their use is also documented in family letters, which often mention the practice as a sign of cold, unseasonable weather.[116]

Regimens recommended warming the bed not just to take the edge off the cold, but to dry the sheets, since the other climatic threat to healthy sleeping was in fact the excessive humidity in the air. It was assumed that dampness, when not absorbed by the walls, was inhaled through breathing by the sleeper. This was particularly dangerous at a time when the body, being inactive, was incapable of dispersing dampness through its normal daily activities. As a result, the excess humidity caused the humours to become denser and to obstruct the pores, so that the trapped vapours filled the head, with serious consequences for health.[117] Elderly people, in particular, were therefore advised to take precautions against dampness at night. It was better for them to sleep in rooms with wooden ceilings rather than in vaulted rooms, or at least in rooms draped with woollen wall hangings which would absorb the dampness from the wet walls. Doctor Frediano recommended following his example and in winter sleeping only under the heaviest blankets from Romagna and in a tiny room, easier to keep warm and lined with leather wall hangings.[118] Leather was indeed regarded as a particularly efficient agent against dampness probably because of the impermeability of the material that was often employed in the making of waterproof vessels such as travelling flasks. The belief in the insulating properties of leather is confirmed, in daily practice, by the extensive employment of this material in the bedroom and its furnishings: here we find not only leather panels lining the walls but leather pillows (see Plates 9 and 10) on the bed

---

[115] For examples of different materials see the inventories of Francesco Ghiringhelli (ASR, Notai UG, vol. 177, 1618–23, 163), Jo Baptista Serlupi (ASR, TNC, Ufficio 4, vol. 77, *c.*246ʳ–266ᵛ) and the Spada inventories (see n. 107).

[116] e.g. ASR, FSV, B.491, 7.9.1642 and 3.7.1655; B.607, 7.5.1658; and n. 124.

[117] Petronio, *Del viver*, 295.   [118] Frediano, *Arca novella*, 70.

or daybed, leather throws to cover chests and the bed itself, and leather *cieli* and *tornaletti* (valances decorating the bed frame).[119]

The expansion in the use of textiles and leather in house furnishings that many have noted as a feature of the sixteenth and seventeenth centuries, was therefore justified by health considerations as well as by new models of home consumption and by aesthetic preoccupations. Similarly, the fireplace was broadly understood as a key agent in the battle against dampness as well as a source of heat, for, as stated by the scholar and chronicler Sansovino, it 'dries up the damp that gathers while one sleeps during the night'.[120]

HEALTHY SLEEP, GENDER, AND PRIVACY

As suggested by Frediano, the size of the room is also viewed as an element influencing the quality of sleep. The bedroom should be small in winter because it can be kept warm and dry more easily, but in other seasons it should be 'spacious and with the means, wherever air may flow freely, to promote its movement, for in small rooms it may more easily be corrupted'.[121] While travelling to Castel Viscardo in May 1653, Maria complains that she slept very little, having been a guest in a narrow house with small bedrooms, and hence unsuited to the great heat.[122] In other words the ideal size of the room changes with the season and this is also attested in practice. As already noted in Chapter 3, the well-off use different bedrooms in different periods of the year. In the Spada palace in Rome Cardinal Bernardino has rooms for the summer, overlooking the square and facing north, but in winter he lives and sleeps in his winter apartments, facing south. Initially he had partitioned a large *camerone* overlooking the garden into *camerini*, then, with the acquisition and incorporation into the palace of Casa dell'Arco in 1648, he was able to enjoy a more spacious winter apartment.[123]

For health reasons people also move from one room to another according to the temperature of the day. During a stay in Tivoli in June 1656, in order to cope with the unusually low temperature Bernardino decides to sleep in the side room below the loggia, which is clearly more sheltered from the cold.[124] Indeed, sleeping arrangements are even more flexible in the villa than in the palace. Having reached

---

[119] The practice is attested also in Genoa: the draper Simone de Amigdola has 16 leather pillows beside 12 feather pillows in his house (ASG, Notai Antichi, 1402, 18.5.1568) and Agostino Marchi, silk maker, has both a leather bed valance and a leather *cielo* in his bedroom (Notai Antichi, 2445, 5.3.1583). In Italy the use of leather furnishings in the home became frequent in the second half of the 16th century and reached its apex in the following century. Rosignoli, *Cuoi d'oro*, 23–42.

[120] Sansovino, *Venetia*, cited in Fortini-Brown, 'The Venetian *Casa*', 58.

[121] 'grande e capace, dove l'aria abbia libera uscita, acciò possa più speditamente muoversi perchè negli stanzini più facilmente si può corrompere.' Fonseca, *Del conservare*, 80.

[122] 'e dormí pochissimo per il gran caldo in quella casa angusta e con camere piccole'. ASR, FSV, B.619, 20.5.1653.

[123] Neppi, *Palazzo Spada*, 137 and 165.

[124] 'ieri sera mi scaldai il letto e dormii nella stanza che guarda per fianco sotto la loggia'. ASR, FSV, B.491, 18.6.1656.

Tivoli with some of her children and her brother-in-law, Maria lets Bernardino know which rooms she has assigned to whom; evidently there is no fixed sleeping space, but arrangements change at each stay according to the number of residents.[125] This fluidity was certainly nurtured by contemporary modes of travelling: not just individuals but large groups of people, sometimes families and their servants, stopped by in the course of their journeys, expecting to be accommodated by distant relatives, friends, and even acquaintances.[126] Hence homes had a large number of beds in store, which could rapidly be assembled to provide temporary hospitality. Casual visitors were numerous in particular during the months devoted to the *villeggiatura*, when the weather conditions made travelling easier. But long-standing guests were also a feature of villa life and this explains the large number of beds among the furnishings of summer residences.[127] The disproportionate number of bunk beds among these suggests that sleeping arrangements at the villa might have been much more informal and lax about status requirements than in urban residences.

Even in the palace, bedrooms were occasionally swapped, and also on health grounds. On 4 September 1642, Cardinal Bernardino, writing from San Casciano, offered his niece Maria his bedroom in Rome, so that she could recover from her illness by moving away from her own room, which was small and also polluted, in his view, by the concentration of many small children and the *donne* who look after them, in the adjacent rooms: 'No one has ever entered your ladyship's bedchamber and others nearby without being assailed most acutely by the foul odours of so many infants and their natural needs, and those looking after them, and it must give no pleasure to your good self.'[128] By now Maria already had five children, aged between 5 and 1, and the room 'delle donne e putti' (for the maids and children) is indeed in direct contact with her bedroom, constituting an integral part of her own apartment on the east side of the palace, facing vicolo del Polverone.[129] If, following the advice found in regimens, windows were normally kept shut at night, even in summer, we can imagine that the stench in this string of rooms must indeed have been remarkable.

In the end the swap did not take place, Maria politely rejected Bernardino's generous offer on the grounds that the weather was cooling down and the temperature in her room was falling. But other passages in her uncle's letter reveal how this concern with the salubriousness of the sleeping environment might clash with different imperatives governing the allocation of sleeping space. First with the gendered organization of space in the aristocratic palace: had Maria moved into Bernardino's area she would have had to be accompanied by her *donne* moving to

---

[125] ASR, FSV, B.619, 7.5.1652.
[126] Letters provide numerous instances of this practice.
[127] See e.g. the list of goods in the *casino* in Tivoli in the inventory of Bernardino Spada ASR, Notai AC, vol. 5933, 23.11.1661, 752–9.
[128] 'Non é mai venuto in camera di VS e altre vicine che non gli abbiano offeso la testa, tanto per esser piccolo, tanto per ritrovar sensibilissimo il tanfo di tante creature e lor bisogni e di chi le governa e crede che anco a VS non giovi molto.' ASR, FSV, B.491, 4.9.1642.
[129] Tabarrini, *Borromini e gli Spada*, 55.

the adjacent *saletta*, thereby creating a sort of buffer between female and male space so that the swap, as Bernardino was eager to underline, 'would not mean abandoning the female area'.[130] A second problem prompted by the suggested move was the breach in privacy it would have entailed, as Bernardino's *scritture* (papers) would have needed to be removed in his absence, a reminder of the way in which by the seventeenth century the male bedroom had become a secluded space, suited to prolonged periods of solitary retreat, rest, and work.[131]

Indeed the evolution in layout and furnishings of the bedroom testifies to its gradual transformation from a space for sleeping but also for family meals, musical performances, and social gatherings to a more private and individual space.[132] In the fifteenth century the monumental bed would be positioned at the centre of the wall and would rest on a protruding platform, with benches built in all around (see Plate 12) which facilitate storage and provided seating for visitors. During the sixteenth century, it has been noted, 'the projecting bases disappeared and beds acquired freestanding legs' losing in this way their function as a focus for sociability as well as a storage structure.[133]

Other aspects of the transformation of the bedroom into a space for individual use have however gone unnoticed. On the one hand the size of the bed diminished substantially: while in the fifteenth century it measured between 3 and 3.5 metres wide, surviving examples suggest that in the following century it became much narrower (Fig. 4.4) and close in size to the ideal measurement of what Doctor Fonseca in 1603 regarded as the standard bed: 'the bed must be 1.8 metres long [*tre braccia*] and 1.5 metres wide [*due braccia e mezzo*]', less than the width of a modern double bed.[134] On the other hand, as we have seen, bed curtains and the associated *padiglione* or *trabacca*, previously not an integral part of the structure, became a regular and permanent feature of the bed in this period, while the accompanying *lettuccio* (Plate 12), a bench providing additional seating, disappeared and was replaced by the daybed, suitable only for reclining.[135]

The reduction of the size of the bed might also be related to the consolidation of the already-mentioned segregation of genders in the noble palace. Husband and

---

[130] 'Questo non si chiamerá allontanarsi dalla camera femminile poi che dalla camera della signora Giulia a quello di lui non c'é che la saletta in mezzo e ne la saletta stessa si possono mettere dei letti e delle donne.' ASR, FSV, B.491, 4.9.1642.

[131] From other letters we know that Bernardino used to take the key to his rooms with him when away from Rome. ASR, FSV, B.491, 24.10.1638.

[132] Fortini-Bown, 'The Venetian *Casa*', 58 and 60–1; and Preyer, 'The Florentine *Casa*', 41 and 44–5.

[133] Preyer, 'The Florentine *Casa*', 40. Surely the privatization of the bedroom was a slow process and did not occur at the same time everywhere. According to Frommel (cited in Waddy, *Seventeenth-Century Roman Palaces*, 10), in early 16th-century Roman palaces the bedroom was still 'a small room to be used both for sleeping and for receiving guests' and in his *Quattro Libri di Architettura* (1570), Palladio described bedrooms as spaces where 'one sleeps, eats and receive foreigners'. Burns, 'Letti', 135.

[134] 'il letto sia di lunghezza tre braccia e due e mezzo di larghezza', Fonseca, *Del conservare*, 80. The measure of 1 *braccio* varied from 59 cm in Florence to 66 cm in Naples; Guidi, *Ragguaglio delle monete*, 24.

[135] The measures of the 15th-century bed are provided by Preyer, 'The Florentine *Casa*', 40. See also Thornton, *The Italian*, 288; and Musacchio, *Art, Marriage, and Family*, 106.

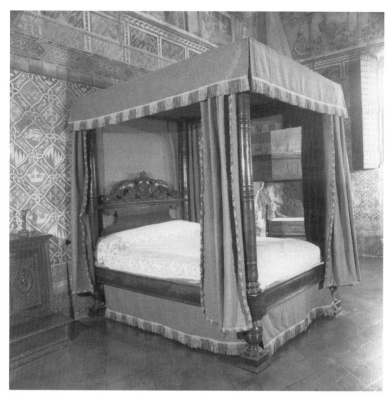

Fig. 4.4. Beds became free-standing and narrower in the second half of the sixteenth century and lost their multifunctional character. The width of this sixteenth-century bed frame from Palazzo Davanzati in Florence (163.5 m) is close to the ideal bed size indicated by Doctor Fonseca in his regimen. (The bed curtains and valances in this photo are modern additions and are not accurate for the period.)

wife now regularly slept apart in the residences of the nobility. Whilst instances of spouses sleeping separately already existed in the previous period, this seems less to have been a permanent arrangement than one related to childbirth and the resulting period of confinement.[136] By the beginning of the seventeenth century however, individual bedrooms and apartments had become the norm at least in the urban context.[137] We find a tangible example of this transformation if we compare the sleeping arrangements of two consecutive generations in the Spada-Veralli family. At the close of the sixteenth century, Maria Spada's father, Giovan Battista Veralli, apparently shared a bed with his first wife, Giulia Benzoni, at least in the

---

[136] Musacchio (*Art, Marriage, and Family*, 89, 46) suggests that a separate room might have been used by the wife only for the duration of her confinement. See also the observations in Preyer, 'The Florentine *Casa*', 40: in reducing its size the bed also lost its previous symbolic value as a 'monument to the very idea of procreation'.

[137] For Rome see the evidence in Waddy, *Seventeenth-Century Roman Palaces*, 26, 28–30, and 38.

short periods during which they lived under the same roof. This is suggested by a letter from Castel Viscardo dated 16 January 1596, in which Giulia complains, as she frequently does in her conjugal correspondence, about her husband's absence, which has now lasted thirty-four days. This time she protests that it is not appropriate in this period of the year and in 'this extreme cold', to sleep alone, even more so given that she 'has a cold'.[138] For some patrician spouses sleeping together seems therefore still to have been common in the late sixteenth century, at least in the rural environment. Forty years later, on entering the marital home, Giovan Battista's daughter, Maria, is allocated a separate bedroom from that of her husband Orazio, as part of the personal apartment.[139] As vividly described by Bernardino however, this space soon became suffocating and unhealthy, positioned as it was in close communication with the set of cramped rooms occupied by her children and her *donne*.[140] Yet it remained Maria's sleeping space for at least twenty years. Only in 1656, following her repeated complaints about the inconveniences caused by the uncomfortable accommodation of women and children (by now there were eight of them still living in the palace and ranging in age from 2 to 18), were works undertaken in that side of the palace. These substantially increased the space in the female quarters. Nevertheless, the living spaces allocated to mother, children, and female attendants still communicated through an internal *scala a chiocciola*.

The creation in noble residences of separate female and male bedrooms and quarters therefore had a different meaning for women and for men. The construction of an individualized, peaceful, and salubrious environment around the sleeper, conducive to healthy sleep and to digestion, related primarily to the aristocratic male. For nobelwomen on the other hand, maternal and household duties meant that their bedroom was rarely a healthy space to which they could withdraw for peace and quiet and a good night's sleep. Though the children normally slept with the *donne*, their mothers were constantly on call at night in case of problems, and when a sick child needed to be separated from its healthy siblings the mother was ready to take one of her offspring into her bed.[141] In any case, the proximity and the lack of significant sound barriers between the sleeping space of children and their mothers would make it hard for the latter to remain unaware of any disruption in the children's rooms. Similarly, the lady of the house was the first to be woken if any other member of the household was feeling unwell,

---

[138] 'ritrovandomi raffreddata nè mi pare tempo di havere a dormire sola, maxime per questi grandissimi freddi, sebene qua per ancora non habbiamo hauta neve...che di già sono trenta quattro giorni che partì di qua et mi pare siano trentaquattro anni che non l'ho visto'. ASR, FSV, B.449, 16.1.1596.

[139] A 'marriage bed' (*letto degli sposi*) to be placed in a room that until then has served as an antechamber, is also mentioned in the arrangement. It is likely however that this was a space of purely ceremonial value, to be exhibited during the wedding celebrations and perhaps during the visits to the lying-in mother at the birth of a child, or an extra bedroom reserved for the spouses' encounters throughout their marital life. Neppi, *Palazzo Spada*, 144; and Tamburrini, *Borromini e gli Spada*, 59–61.

[140] Tamburrini *Borromini e gli Spada*, 56–61; and Neppi, *Palazzo Spada*, 144 n. 81.

[141] ASR, FSV, B.1115, 16.7.1662.

for she was in charge of health care for the whole family, including the servants. This contrasts with the reverential attitude towards the sleep of the head of household: even when a distinguished guest was seriously ill during the night and not only the doctor but the confessor too was summoned, the master would not be disturbed until early morning.[142] While the male sleeping space was becoming increasingly secluded, and accessible only to the male attendants who acted as the master's personal valets, the privacy of the female bedroom could easily be violated.

Sleeping arrangements in the palace were not only gendered but class-related. Sleeping alone remained a social privilege. Grouped together according to their rank, male servants shared a bedroom often furnished with bunk beds; so did the *donne*, and if one of them lay awake sobbing her companion could not sleep.[143] Even in the privileged environment of the noble palace only the adult male aristocrat could enjoy the uninterrupted sleep advocated by regimens of health.

CONCLUSION

The last part of the sixteenth and the early decades of the seventeenth centuries were a highly dynamic period for the material culture and spatial aspects of sleep: a range of chairs and beds for daytime rest were to be found in villas and palaces, while individual free-standing beds, closed on all sides by bed curtains and covered on top by a canopy, replaced the monumental platformed open bed that was a feature of the fifteenth century. Bedrooms became more secluded in the aristocratic palace and male and female sleeping spaces were separated. The use of multiple mattresses increased the comfort of lying in bed for the most privileged, and the extensive deployment of bright varied textiles in bedrooms made the sleeping environment more attractive. Birds brought from remote parts of the globe and especially the New World, costly purchases for some, gave pleasure to the ears with their song, as did the portable fountains with their gentle sound of quietly gushing water, all pleasantly inducing sleep.[144]

These transformations went hand in hand with new sleeping habits, and more generally with the development of a new culture of rest. Resting during the day came to be seen as one of the pleasures of genteel life, especially in summer and during the *villeggiatura*, as well as a way of restoring strength after debilitating activities. Reading in bed became so common as to be recommended in manuals for the education of young men. To judge from contemporary complaints, times for getting up and going to bed became less strict, especially among the young and socially privileged, and the time-honoured principle that required a significant interval to elapse between a meal and sleep seems to have been often ignored when not completely overturned by the habit of eating in bed. Bedrooms were also losing

---

[142] ASR, FSV, B.491, 3.7.1638.   [143] ASR, FSV, B.410, 6.8.1656.
[144] Rangoni, *Consiglio*, 13; Petronio, *Del viver*, 222.

their social and display functions and were reconceptualized as the focus of solitary leisure time. Even in the court environment the Italian rulers perceived their bedroom as private rather than as a ceremonial space, used for example to give audience in the French fashion.[145]

Inevitably, medical advisers were forced to adapt time-honoured precepts for healthy sleep to these changing habits; they increasingly deregulated prescriptions stipulating bedtime, the length of sleep, and sleeping positions. It would be far too simple, however, to say that authors of regimens were merely driven by the desire to accommodate the new habits of their patients. Aspects of the sleep culture of the time were fiercely criticized in some of these works, the disorderly sleeping practices of the nobility and of young nobles specifically were particularly under attack. Unhealthy sleeping habits clearly abounded and while doctors came to terms with some of them, in other cases they clearly articulated their concern with these practices by drawing on the long tradition of critical writing about the mores of the nobility. At the same time however, they continued to exert a significant influence on the everyday culture of sleep. The increased space that regimens of health devote to rest, especially from the second half of the sixteenth century, demonstrates an awareness of the growing importance of the culture of sleep and the wish of medical professionals to play a role in directing and monitoring those changes. Various elements converge to inspire the transformations that were changing resting and sleeping practices and the sleeping environment: the ethos of privacy; the enhanced culture of the *villeggiatura*; the construction of a pattern of aristocratic life in which leisure occupies more time; the growth of a gendered division of space in the noble palace; and the increased investment in house furnishings characterized by the widespread use of textiles. Undoubtedly, however, many of the innovations in the material environment of sleep also had implications for health. They made for more salubrious sleep according to the principles of healthy life promoted in the advice literature: chairs for daytime rest guaranteed that this always took place with the head raised; daybeds fitted with leather pillows and hard mattresses ensured that daytime rest was short and not too comfortable, while woollen and leather wall hangings absorbed the night-time humidity that was so dangerous to the vulnerable sleeper. Finally, bed curtains and canopies protected the sleeper from cold draughts, as well as from light and noise and the dangerous rays of the moon. Even if the new culture of rest pushed the boundaries of medical definitions of healthy sleep, it did not disregard medical advice but was the result of a complex negotiation between new genteel lifestyles and medical preoccupations.

---

[145] This contrasts with the customs of the French court (Waddy, *Seventeenth-Century Roman Palaces*, 9). However, the *zampanaro*, a representational bed placed in a room next to the audience room but not in the actual sleeping room, was introduced in 17th-century Rome in cardinals' houses (*Seventeenth-Century Roman Palaces*, 13 and 28). The Spada cardinals had one *zampanaro* each. For their inventories, see n. 110.

5

Gentle Exercise and Genteel Living

In medical literature exercise was traditionally regarded as a key component of a healthy lifestyle. According to classical humoral theory its benefits were multifarious: exercise hardened the organs and limbs and improved their functions, increased intrinsic heat therefore promoting digestion and the distribution of nutrition around the body, and vigorous respiration opened the pores, allowing the expulsion of superfluous, dangerous wastes left in the body. Although the basic principles held over time, by 1600 we find significant shifts in emphasis in comparison with the ancient and medieval regimen. More specifically there are some departures from Galen's *De sanitade tuenda*, whilst Avicenna's *Canon*, understood to be a translation and reworking of Galenic medicine, appears to have provided the impetus for this new approach to exercise.[1] This chapter will trace how definitions of exercise gradually shifted in the medical advice literature, showing how they closely intertwined with the new views of the ideal male body and the new patterns of genteel life brought about by an emerging aristocratic culture. In Italy, the reasons for this early transformation of the physical qualities associated with being noble rested on two key pillars: the early development of court life, codified by Castiglione in his celebrated *Cortigiano*, and the demilitarization of the nobility and of urban society at large that had taken place in the states of northern and central Italy earlier than elsewhere in Europe. These are important contexts that need to be taken into account when considering changing ideas of what constituted a healthy forms of exercise. Useful sources for the study of these cultural shifts are the various strands of conduct literature written for the perfect gentleman (sometimes called 'civility treatises') that flourished in Italy in the sixteenth and early seventeenth century, as well as the various sport treatises compiled in this period. This large and varied body of didactic literature has been impressively analysed by literary scholars and their work has represented an important point of reference for our discussion. Imbued with medical notions of the impact of exercise upon the body these texts contributed a great deal towards adapting medical ideas to meet the requirements of the new aristocratic society that was taking shape at the time.

Another important though less obvious influence on medical thinking about exercise is to be found in the advice literature on the education of children directed

---

[1] Whilst the influence of Arabic medicine in the 16th century has been questioned by some, Nancy Siraisi has emphasized the importance of Avicenna in the Italian peninsula up until the early 17th century; *Avicenna in Renaissance Italy*, esp. 80–9, 105.

to their parents and tutors that flourished in Italy in the wake of the Counter-Reformation. Aimed at propagating Tridentine precepts, and disciplining the body as well as the mind and the soul in keeping with broader church policy, this literature was largely penned by ecclesiastics and directed to a wider social audience than civility treatises.

Though these two genres have tended to be discussed separately as part of different historiographical fields, they both contributed to disseminate the new values and practices associated with physical conduct, though with different nuances.[2] Yet important cross-fertilization also took place between them. For example both paid attention to class and the need to differentiate the body language of the privileged from that of plebeians and both participated in the definition of new forms of exercise for the well-off as well as types of exercise considered more appropriate to different sexes and age groups. In addition to exploring how medical ideas about exercise responded to these broader transformations in society and the refashioning of social identities, this chapter will investigate how medical definitions of what constituted healthy exercise were appropriated by the laity as reflected in contemporary letters and diaries and contributed to generate new social practices such as new sports, new ways of travelling, and the universal fashion for walking.

'WE MUST AVOID ANYTHING WHICH TIRES US EXCESSIVELY'[3]

Understandings of exercise in early modern regimens drew extensively on Galen and Avicenna for whom its aims included increasing and distributing body heat, consuming superfluities, helping to expel excrements through sweat, and hardening the limbs and internal organs—this last being a particularly important concern for Galen. In *De sanitate tuenda* Galen had stressed that not all movement was exercise, only that which was vigorous, swift, or a combination of both, and which caused an acceleration of one's breathing.[4] He included under this rubric a lengthy list of highly demanding physical activities, ranging from wrestling to racing, hunting, ball games, and agricultural and artisanal activities such as ploughing, reaping, and building ships and houses. In *The Canon*, Avicenna's definition of exercise resembled Galen's, but emphasized that it should be 'voluntary', and 'undertaken for its own sake' and the benefits accruing from it, thereby creating a sharp distinction between physical labour and recreational, athletic, or medical exercise—one which we will later see accentuated in the late Renaissance.[5] Avicenna also gave more specific consideration to a broader range of slower and gentler movements as exercise, including activities later termed 'gestational', whereby the body—like a

---

[2] While civility treatises have sparked the interest of historians of the body, women, and the family (see e.g. Herman Roodenburg, *The Eloquence of the Body*), educational tracts have been the territory of historians of the Church and education (Ottavia Niccoli, 'Creanza e disciplina').

[3] 'Dobbiamo lasciare tutte le fatiche superflue e troppo grandi.' Auda, *Breue compendio*, 249.

[4] Galen, *De sanitate tuenda*, 53.   [5] Avicenna, *The Canon*, 384.

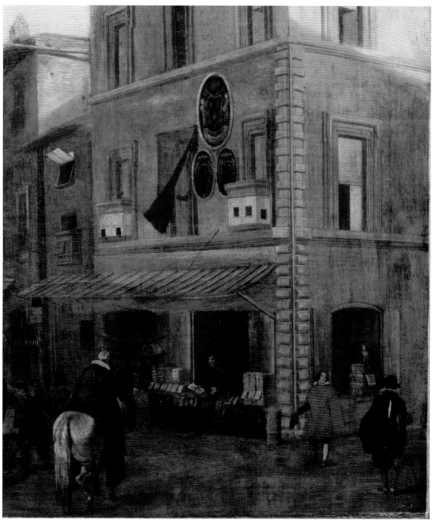

Plate 1 An early seventeenth-century bookshop in central Rome showing unbound books on display outside.

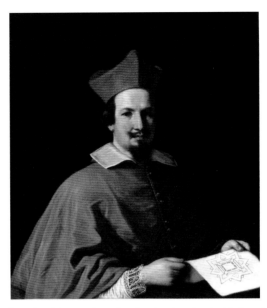

Plate 2 Portrait of Cardinal Bernardino Spada; the drawing in his hand may allude to his architectural interests.

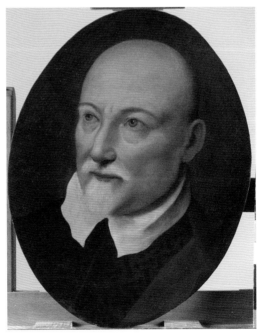

Plate 3 Portrait of Orazio Spada, 'adopted' nephew of Bernardino (Plate 2) and husband of Maria Veralli (Plate 5).

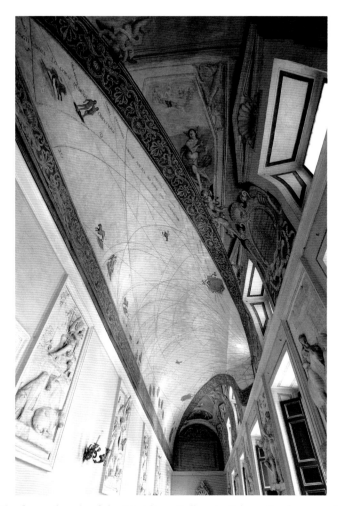

Plate 4 The frescoed vault of the Meridiana Gallery in Palazzo Spada, commissioned in 1644 and designed by the French mathematician Maignan, demonstrating Bernardino Spada's interests in astronomy and optics.

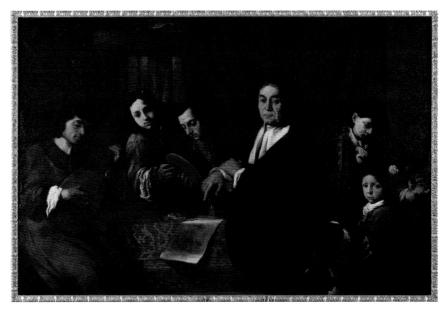

Plate 5 This portrait, said to be of Maria Veralli with her male children, reinforces the impression given by the letters of a robust and dominant figure at the centre of the family.

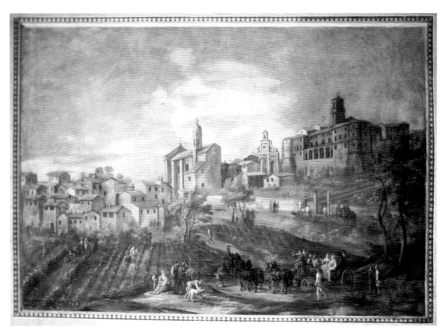

Plate 6 A fresco showing Castel Viscardo in the Room of the Fiefdoms in the Palazzo Spada. Originally frescoed in the mid-seventeenth century and retouched in the eighteenth century, the room celebrated the family properties in Romagna and around Orvieto. The Spadas had acquired the fief and mansion of Castel Viscardo as part of the dowry of the heiress Maria Veralli (see Plate 5), who married Orazio Spada (Plate 3) in 1636.

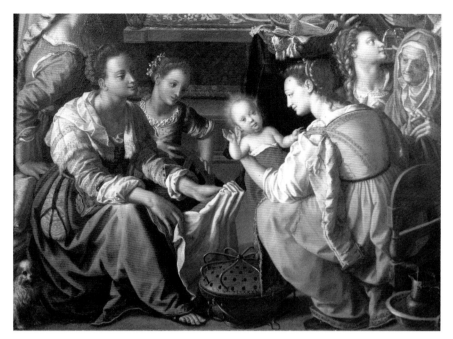

Plate 7 The elaborate brazier (also suitable for hanging) in this 1595 painting suggests that this apparently workaday object may also have been a fashionable one.

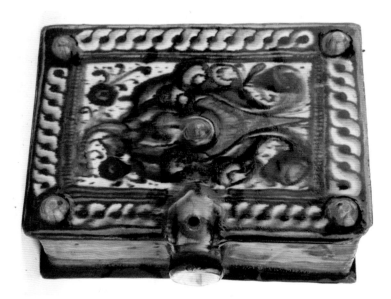

Plate 8 This ceramic hand-warmer shaped like a book was made in Pesaro in the late fifteenth or early sixteenth century. The four holes near the edge of the front and the back were probably designed for a string that would have enabled it to be carried or possibly worn. The tin-glazed earthenware and the simple design would have rendered it affordable to a wider cross-section of society than its metal equivalents (M. A.-W.).

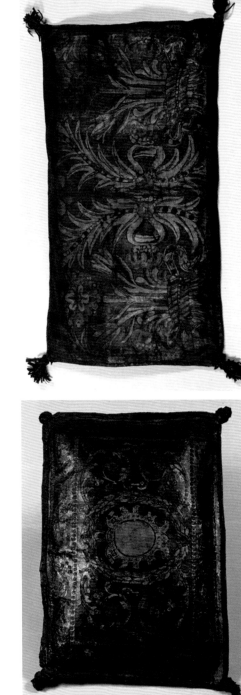

Plates 9–10 These small leather pillows, decorated in silver and red and stuffed with horsehair, were made in Italy during the late sixteenth and seventeenth centuries. Whilst the smaller one (33 × 47.5 cm) (Plate 9) was more likely to have been used for devotional practices, the longer one (35.5 × 68 cm) (Plate 10) might have been used for day sleep.

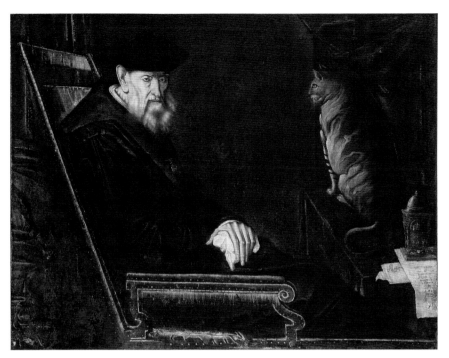

Plate 11 In the 1550s, when this portrait of Prince Andrea Doria was presumably painted (he died in 1560), reclining chairs must have been the preserve of the highest echelons of society. The example still preserved at the Victoria and Albert Museum, London (Fig. 4.1) shows the penetration of this typology amongst the provincial nobility fifty years later.

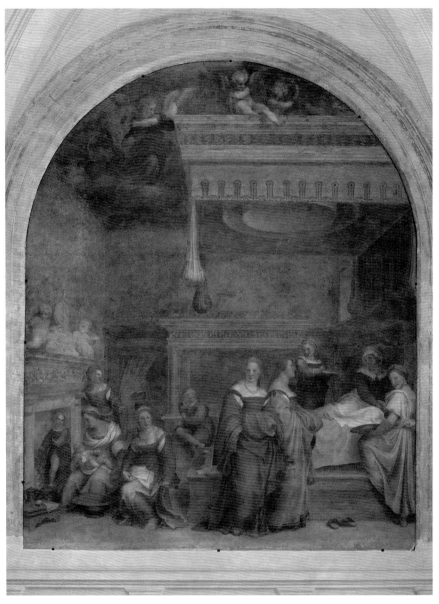

Plate 12 This 1513 fresco shows a man in the background sitting on an inbuilt *lettuccio*. These structures were a feature of Tuscan patrician bedrooms in the fifteenth and early sixteenth century and were used as extra seating and not simply for resting.

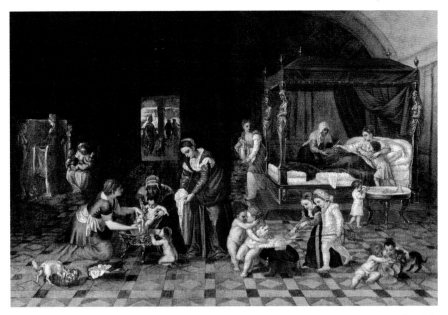

Plate 13 In late sixteenth-century paintings like this one we often notice how comfortable the beds look, with several mattresses laid on top of one another and large pillows and bolsters to lean back on.

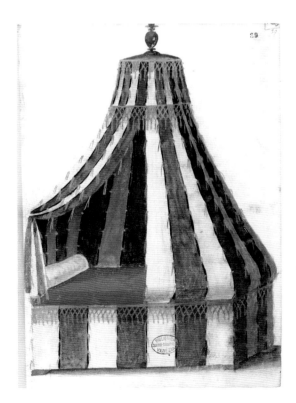

Plate 14 This drawing of a bed with a pavilion and *cappello* hanging from a rope fixed on the ceiling was commissioned by the Milan court in the mid-sixteenth century (Thornton, *The Italian*, 127). While at this time the *padiglione* was still an elite object, its use spread in the decades that followed.

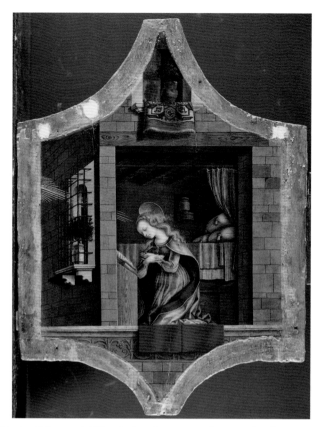

Plate 15 This detail from a 1482 painting shows an early example of a curtained bed. The light curtain (not part of the bed structure) and lack of any form of canopy make it far less enclosing and protective than its sixteenth-century counterparts.

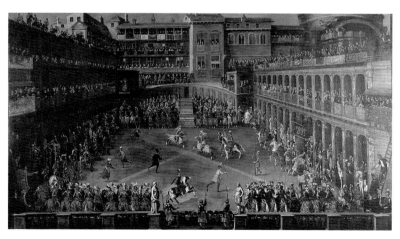

Plate 16 This painting depicts a tournament which took place in Rome in 1565. By this time such events were more a sumptuous display of elegant horsemanship and outdated military techniques such as jousting than of physical prowess and force.

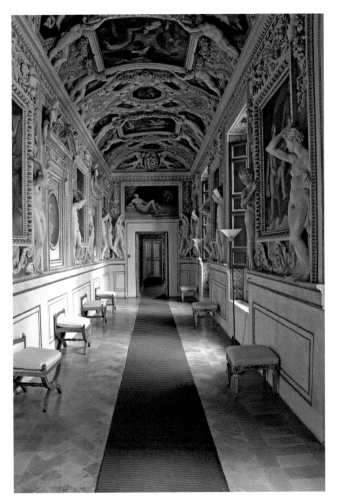

Plate 17 Galleries like this, built *c*.1548 for Palazzo Capodiferro (later Palazzo Spada) (measuring 3.4 × 11.75 m), were dotted with large windows normally oriented towards the garden, as well as with paintings and antiquities. All these elements were meant to cheer the spirits of those who took their exercise indoors by strolling up and down the long corridor.

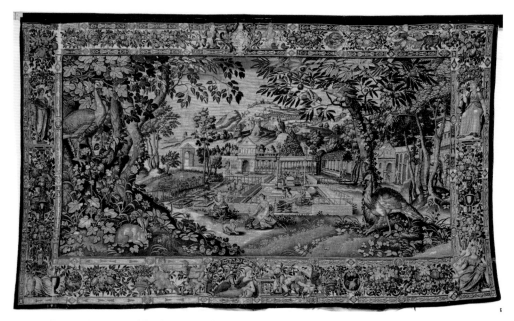

Plate 18 Tapestries like this one with the arms of the Contarini Family in Venice (h. 233.7 cm, w. 402.8 cm), were used to absorb dampness from the air whilst the imagery was deemed to comfort the animal spirits and thereby promote health. The intricacy of the scene stimulates the intellect; the sight of greenery and water pleases the eyes; flowers and plants allude to their invigorating perfumes; and the activities—such as fishing and boating around the pool—remind the viewer of the healthy pleasures to be enjoyed at the villa.

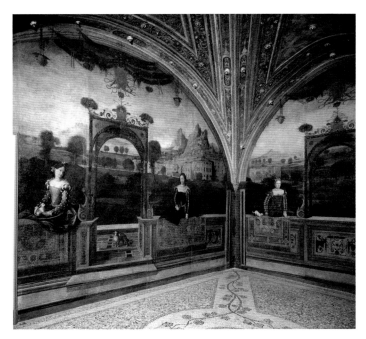

Plate 19 The frescos around the walls in this room in a palace in Brescia were intended (like the tapestry in Plate 18) to imitate the effects of actually gazing at a rural view. It is thought that music may often have been played in this room (Norris, 'Women on the Edge', 128–31), in which case listening to music whilst looking at the painted verdant countryside would have been beneficial to all the spirits.

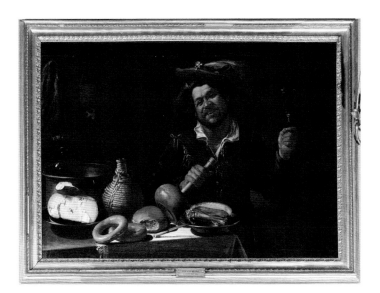

Plate 20 This early seventeenth-century painting of a man dining shows various objects associated with cold drinking. The long-necked vessel—perhaps a 'snow flask'—has presumably been removed from the wine cooler on the left. The rounded glass flask already cooling may have been another kind of snow flask.

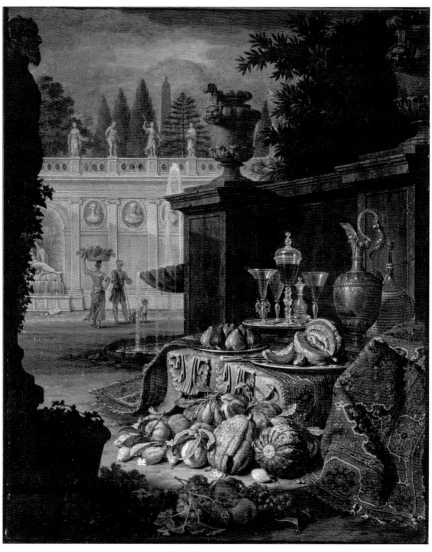

Plate 21 This still life painted in Rome at the turn of the eighteenth century shows the preparations for elegant refreshments and includes a fine set of glasses, one of which has a lid, resembling the goblets in Figs. 7.9 and 7.10.

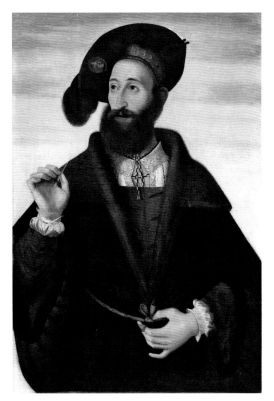

Plate 22 This portrait of a well-off man proudly exhibiting his ear- or tooth-cleaner (painted around 1530) suggests that hygienic care was embraced by the upper classes as a sign of distinction in the first decades of the sixteenth century.

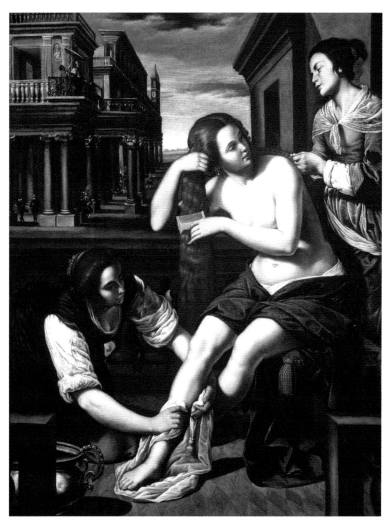

Plate 23 As illustrated in this early seventeenth-century painting by Artemesia Gentileschi chamber personnel were increasingly involved in the routine hygienic rituals of their masters and mistresses, reflecting growing attention to the appearance and health of the body.

foetus—was moved by another force, as when a baby is carried or rocked, or when one travels in a litter, boat, or carriage. Although Galen had described such movements in the context of his discussion of babies and young children, and mentions them in passing as a form of passive exercise, it is Avicenna who explains in detail how they can replace other exercise forms for the frail, the ill, and convalescents. He also elaborates on a scheme of so-called 'particular' exercises suitable for individual organs and limbs, mentioned only in passing in Galen's *De sanitate tuenda*, such as breathing, singing, and 'vociferation' exercises which benefited the chest, voice, throat, and neck, or looking at tiny objects specifically to exercise the eyes, or listening alternately to loud and quiet sounds to exercise the ears.[6]

Definitions of exercise in late medieval regimens varied. Maino adopted the Galenic emphasis on vigour, claiming that 'Unless exercise provokes many frequent and rapid breaths it does not merit being called by this name.'[7] He also opined that it should be voluntary. Benzi took the opposite view, arguing that one should avoid exercise 'which induces heavy breathing and overheating' and observe 'moderation' whether walking, hunting, or riding.[8] Otherwise there were broad similarities, as authors provided lengthy instructions on when and how one should exercise according to one's constitution, the season, and the proximity of mealtimes, along with detailed advice on different kinds of what were described as 'frictions' or massages and baths.[9] The massages were drawn from models found in both Galen and Avicenna and were used to prepare the body for exercise, thin waste products, and dilate the pores, thus enabling the rapid evacuation of superfluities from within. These formed part of a complicated series of obligatory phases which included the anointment of the body before and after exercise, a period of rest, and immersion in waters of different temperatures afterwards. Other than this, discussions of specific activities were virtually absent from late medieval accounts—in contrast to Galen's lengthy accounts of gymnastics and ball games—with the exception of brief references to walking, running, small ball, and riding.[10]

From the mid-sixteenth century, regimens differed from their late medieval predecessors in three main ways. Firstly, the aim of making the body stronger became secondary when not completely absent from discussions of the advantages of exercising. Secondly, and this was linked to the first change to some extent, these changed priorities meant that the cycle of frictions, exercise, further massage, rest, and bath was broken, whilst anointment disappears as does the subsequent bath, in all but one or two regimens.[11] Frictions, if still mentioned at all, are no longer

---

[6] Avicenna, *The Canon*, 386–7.

[7] '*L'esercitio* non merita il nome se non quando provoca la moltitudine del spirare e la frequenza.' Maineri, *Opera utilissima*, 33.

[8] 'Si deve ancora contenere da gl'essercitij, per quali l'annelito e respiratione siano troppo frequentati.' Benzi, *Tractato utilissimo*, iiiiᵛ.

[9] e.g. Maineri, *Opera utilissima*, 33–6. Benzi discusses baths as part of exercise in some detail; *Tractato utilissimo*, iiiiᵛ.

[10] See Nutton, 'Les Exercices', 298. Also Ulmann, *De la gymnastique*, 85; and Sotres, 'The Regimens of Health', 306.

[11] Traffichetti, for example in *L'arte*, does discuss frictions and baths in each of his sections on exercise.

understood as lengthy massages and tend to be passed over very briefly, a difference which some authors comment on themselves.[12] Furthermore, since they were understood as performing the same functions as movement but in a more gentle way (comforting the heart, helping to increase the limbs, and aiding the expulsion of superfluities), frictions were more likely to be recommended purely in their capacity to replace exercise if required for the weak, the sick, the very old, and the very young.[13] Gropretio for example simply observes that whoever cannot take vigorous exercise can use bathing, or 'have himself rubbed' (*stroppiciare*), and 'fare le fricationi' in the morning, 'and this will almost have the same benefits as exercise'.[14] Fonseca saw frictions as not only redundant, but 'very tiring', which was a good reason for abandoning them.[15] With the loss of these elaborate procedures and guidelines, early modern exercise was gradually depicted as more of an everyday activity, a simple part of one's daily routine. Petronio for example gives the impression that it can be slotted in just before breakfast: 'In the morning on waking,... before eating... go somewhere open, and quickly do whatever exercise he can.'[16] On returning home he just needs to wait until his breathing has returned to normal, then he may eat. However, if actually performing exercise became simpler, the discussions about it became ever more complicated, as physicians showed increasing concern for the potentially detrimental effects of strenuous and tiring movement on the body. The dangers of exercise were reviewed with great clarity by Paschetti. These included the belief that anything in continual movement consumes vital heat, therefore accelerating old age; that it leads to overheating, which is accompanied by poor 'concoction' (or what we would describe as digestion); and that it exhausts and weakens the body.[17] To this the popular seventeenth-century author Auda added the danger of losing too much weight, loss of sleep, and fevers.[18] This is not to say that vigorous exercise was dropped altogether from discussions in the regimen, but that physicians tended to recommend it only for particular categories; essentially healthy males between the ages of 14 or 21 (depending on their views) and 35 or 40. Furthermore, almost without exception, they interpolated continuously the words 'moderate' and 'temperate' in these discussions.

The most well-known representative of moderate exercise today is considered to be Girolamo Mercuriale, the author not of a regimen, but of an antiquarian reconstruction of exercise in ancient Greek and Rome, *De arte gymnastica*, which was published in Latin in 1569. Although famed for his attention to Galen's work on exercise, Mercuriale's definition of exercise owes much to Avicenna's. Firstly he accentuates the division between labour and exercise, by maintaining that 'true'

---

[12] See Fonseca, *Del conservare*, 15.

[13] Petronio, *Del viver*, 282–3.

[14] 'E quasi conseguirá l'utilità dell'esercizio'; Gropretio, *Un breue et notabile trattato*, 359. See also Petronio, *Del viver*, 283; and Viviani, *Trattato*, 190.

[15] 'di gran fatica'; Fonseca, *Del conservare*, 16. Boldo's re-edition of Savonarola, which claims that massages are still practised in Italy, seems to be the exception to this trend; *Libro della natura*, 214.

[16] 'deve la mattina quando sarà levato... prima che pranzi... partendosi dal luogo dove è stato a seder un pezzo, andar in uno aperto, e ivi presto, e in poco tempo far quell'essercitio, che potrà'. Petronio, *Del viver*, 255.

[17] Paschetti, *Del conservare*, 166–7.   [18] Auda, *Breue compendio*, 249.

exercise is vigorous but is undertaken voluntarily with a view to maintaining one's health. Secondly he legitimizes milder exercise by asserting the validity of 'exercise in the common sense of the word', which broadly includes any daily movements, the most important of which he considers to be walking.[19] In addition, throughout the text he reiterates 'incessantly', as noted by Vivien Nutton, that excessive and violent exercises are bad and must be replaced with moderation.[20] Mercuriale's contribution to this debate should not be overemphasized however, for it was not made in isolation and formed part of a broader approach to exercise which was coalescing around several issues: the dangers of vigorous exercise, the status of light and gestational movement for the healthy, and, as a way of accommodating these new views, the appropriateness of different exercise forms to different age groups.

The status of light exercise had already shifted by the mid-sixteenth century, as we can see in Pictorius' praise for those who have a garden by their house, because it provides them with a place where 'instead of exercise' after work they can 'wander with a book in hand or accompanied by children'. He also recommends 'light exercise' such as standing or strolling both before and after meals to aid digestion.[21] This was echoed fifty years later when the benefits of 'the kind of walking one does in the day around the house' were noted by one physician, whilst by the mid-seventeenth century Auda's only suggestion for exercise is that one should take a gentle stroll after meals, or on getting up in the morning one should go for a walk and stretch the arms and legs.[22] In Paschetti's definition of healthy exercise we also see the blurring of distinctions between vigorous, moderate, and light exercise. For him, exercise is 'not a swift or violent movement' but 'a mediocre' one.[23] He adds that by this he means 'every slightest movement, every minimal agitation of the body', so that when a man is standing, moving, and walking, 'then he is exercising and tiring himself'.[24] He was not the only nor the first physician to advocate such extremely light exercise—but only eighty years earlier that level of movement had been considered appropriate for elderly convalescent nuns![25]

Recommendations that individual organs, limbs, and muscles—particularly those related to the voice and chest—needed to be exercised in addition to one's need for overall physical movement had been largely neglected in late medieval regimens but gained popularity in the second half of the sixteenth century. Lennio notes the health benefits of declaiming to music. Rangoni suggests that one 'wanders here and there singing psalms, verses and other things in a loud voice, and speaking to one's domestic servants' for the same reason. Romoli explains one should exercise the chest, tongue,

---

[19] Mercuriale, *De arte gymnastica*, 211–13. Walking is discussed at pp. 323–9 and 587–602.

[20] Nutton, 'Les Exercices', 303.

[21] 'In esso horto in luogo d'esercitio dopo le fatiche publiche o vero private *spasseggiare con libretti in mano*, o vero accompagnati da fanciulli' (our emphasis). Pictorius, *Dialoghi*, 52.

[22] Paschetti, *Del conservare*, 164–5 and Auda, *Breue compendio*, 251, 254.

[23] 'Non é movimento gagliardo, ne violento, ma moderato e fatto ad opportuno tempo.' Paschetti, *Del conservare*, 150.

[24] 'Per essercitio intendiamo ogni lieve movimento, ogni minima agitatione di corpo.' Paschetti, *Del conservare*, 155. 'Ma quando sta in piedi stendendo I muscoli delle gambe, quando si muove, e camina, all'hora si essercita, e fatica.' *Del conservare*, 166.

[25] Magagni, *Compendio de la sanità*, ch. 6.

mouth, and breath by increasing the volume gradually when reading aloud or just vociferating. Exercising the eyes is also mentioned however, by looking at tiny objects, and the ears by listening to very faint sounds then loud ones.[26] One explanation for this renewed emphasis may be the revived interest in Avicenna in mid-sixteenth-century Italy which coincided with the fact that in their subtlety and lack of vigour, such exercises were extremely compatible with this new medical ethos which feared sweat and exhaustion.[27] It also lent itself particularly to regimens addressed to men with more sedentary, scholarly, intellectual pursuits.

It was not just that many physicians were veering towards far more gentle exercise forms, but around the mid-sixteenth century some also collapsed the traditional distinction which had reserved gestational exercise as something recommended just for the young, ill, and frail, turning it into an acceptable practice also for healthy adult males. Petronio suggests carriages as a form of light 'after-dinner' exercise, recommending it on the grounds that 'it can never be harmful to walk a little, ride, or go in a litter moderately, pleasantly, and slowly'.[28] Lennio advocates it as an alternative to other exercise, dismissing vigorous exercise as suitable only for robust men 'like soldiers' and suggesting that for 'others . . . there are other kinds of bodily exercise which are less demanding and disagreeable such as being carried, which can be in a coach or boat, many kinds of massage, and walking'.[29] By the 1560s the topic of gestational exercise had evidently polarized medical writers, with some arguing that its uses had been taken too far. Rosaccio argued that it is not 'as good as those kinds of exercise which one does through one's own effort'.[30] Even Paschetti, fervent advocate of gentle exercise, takes pains to clarify that by exercise he means movement which men have initiated themselves, so that 'if he is carried in a chair [*carega*] or litter, or boat, and does nothing, properly speaking he is not exercising, even if he appears to be'.[31]

'THERE CANNOT BE JUST ONE KIND OF EXERCISE FOR ALL NATURES, TIMES, AGES, AND PLACES'[32]

Driven by this increasing anxiety about the dangers of exercise new attention was paid by physicians to the appropriateness of specific activities for different bodies,

[26] Lennio, *Della complessione*, 37; Romoli, *La singolare dottrina*, 264; and Rangoni, *Consiglio*, 38–9. Gropretio (*Un breue e notabile trattato*, 359ᵛ) mentions exercising the tongue, ears, and nose by talking, listening, and smelling. For a detailed discussion of such exercise see Gage, 'Exercise'.

[27] On Avicenna, see n. 1.

[28] 'Dopo pranzo poi, e dopo cena, non noce mai passeggiar al quanto, overo cavalcar, overo andar in lettica, moderatamente, piacevolmente, e lentamente.' Petronio, *Del viver*, 310.

[29] 'Ma vi sono altri generi d'esercitare il corpo, meno operosi e manco molesti, cioè l'essere condotto, il quale si fa o in c arro o vero con barche, molte differenze di fricazioni, passeggiare, il quale si fa o con lento o con più presto passo.' Lennio, *Della complessione*, 37.

[30] 'Il cavalcare, l'andare in carrozza o in nave o altri eserciti non son cosí giovevoli come quelli che si fanno da sè'; Rosaccio, *Avvertimenti*, unnumbered. See also Durante, *Il tesoro*, 11.

[31] 'Percioché se cavalca, se viene portato in carega, in lettica, o in barca nulla operando propriamente non si essercita, benche' gli paia essercitarsi.' Paschetti, *Del conservar*, 166.

[32] 'Che non puol essere un sol' moto d'esercizio a tutte le nature, all'età, à i tempi, à i luoghi, e à diverse maniere di vivere proporzionato'; Fonseca, *Del conservare*, 12.

in effect resolving some of the more conflictual aspects of these debates by following the dictum that what suited one body type would not be likely to suit another. Physicians therefore started to categorize bodies by age, broadly following the scheme adopted in Galen's *De sanitate tuenda*, but also by gender, and as we will see later, by social class. Only the gentlest form of gestational exercise was permitted for babies, such as being rocked or carried, as well as gentle massage and washing. Until the age of 4 riding or travelling in carriages, litters, or boats were all considered too vigorous, and once permitted, must be done very gently. After age 7, both Fonseca and Traffichetti allow 'moderate, not vigorous' games and activities, such as walking, 'measured running', and playing some ball games and riding placid horses.[33] From the age of 14 to 21 doctors agreed that the levels of vigour could be increased, though the majority were still far from comfortable about very active games and activities, and diverged considerably in their opinions. An exception was Petronio who described children and youths under 21 as 'like young goats', consuming superfluities constantly in order to grow, so that they have no need for 'artful' exercises.[34] Traffichetti also allows running, jumping, and wrestling and he and three other authors now mention dancing, hitherto not discussed in regimens.[35] One of them, Fonseca, specifically suggested that from this age young men might dance the lively galliards which were popular at the time, although he later contradicts himself when he expresses the view that the only safe form of exercise for all is *pallamaglio*, an early form of golf, or hunting with a crossbow—generally used for hunting birds.[36]

It is only when men are in their twenties or thirties that medical authors finally consider the body to be sufficiently well formed, robust, and in need of exercise so that it can withstand vigorous activity. The two authors who followed Galen most slavishly were, not surprisingly, most permissive, allowing them to jump, throw the discus, joust, and engage in the military arts.[37] Bertaldi notes that 'nowadays the kind of exercise praised by doctors' is walking, riding, playing small ball, hunting, and *giocar d'armi*.[38] Petronio announces that now exercise should be 'as strenuous as possible'.[39]

Youth was considered to end after the age of 35 or 40, and there was some disagreement about how robust men were after then.[40] Some encouraged them to

---

[33] Fonseca, *Del conservare*, 15–16. Traffichetti, *L'arte*, 154–5.

[34] Petronio, *Del viver*, 272; to some extent echoed by Paschetti, *Del conservare*, 167.

[35] Traffichetti, *L'arte*, 156 and 161; Boldo, *Libro della natura*, 213; Bertaldi, *Regole della sanità*, 22–3; and Fonseca, *Del conservare*, 17. Alessandro Arcangeli also finds that dancing appears in French regimens around this time; 'Dance and Health', 13–16.

[36] He calls it 'Caccia con balestra', Fonseca, *Del conservare*, 17. For the definition see Accademia della Crusca, *Vocabolario degli Accademici della Crusca*, 31.

[37] Traffichetti, *L'arte*, 161; Boldo, *Libro della natura*, 213.

[38] 'Ma adesso l'esercitio lodato da medici e l'andare a piedi, cavalcare, il giuocare alla palla piccola overo andar a caccia d'animali, giuocar d'armi.' Bertaldi, *Regole della sanità*, 22. Petronio advised similar activities; *Del viver*, 305–6.

[39] 'Bisogna far essercitio piú vehemente.' Petronio, *Del viver*, 274.

[40] Scipione Mercurio says for example that youth ends at 35 and after this one is 'verde-vecchio', or a 'green old man'. *De gli errori*, 451. On definitions of the stages of life see Sears, *The Ages of Man*.

continue with whatever exercise they had done when youths, but gently reminded them that, particularly towards their fifties, although they might feel young, they should recognize their physical limitations and exercise caution and moderation.[41] The same advice pertained for the 'old', variously described as over 49, 63, and 65 although the main activities mentioned now are running, walking, riding, and going by carriage, litter, and boats.[42] The feeble, delicate, thin, and very old should guard against overexertion and in such cases doctors only recommend 'weak' forms of exercise; advising that gentle walking, just pottering about the house, 'frictions', or even 'putting on one's socks' could be sufficient.[43]

Overall then, doctors were exceedingly cautious in their advice: they feared damaging the body of the pre-adolescent child through overexertion, which might dry them up, weaken them, and stop growth; they were also concerned about the consequences of pushing the adolescent body to extremes too early, hence really vigorous exercise was only recommended after the age of 21. The duration of the phase in which the adult male was at the peak of his strength was however relatively brief—as after 35 he had already entered the long decline towards old age and from then onwards must once again guard against excessive exertion.

Within these elaborate discussions on exercise even the female body makes a rare appearance. According to Petronio up to age 12 girls could be treated much like boys, though after puberty his comments are restricted to that which pertains to pregnancy.[44] Paschetti is more forthcoming, explaining that because women's bodies tended to be excessively humid, the healthiest, longest-lived women are those 'who exercise most and tire themselves out', since they 'consume' this inner plethora. It appears however that such advice may have contrasted with what was considered appropriate exercise for women given the requirements of decorum, since he omits to give specific advice on what women's exercise should consist of. He mentions only that when they go out to visit friends and family, or to church, they are carried in sedan chairs rather than walking or riding horses or mules as was once customary (see Fig. 5.1).

This, he implies, was an opportunity for women to exercise—one which has been lost, as a consequence of which he warns that their inactivity will undoubtedly damage their health.[45] Likewise, his contemporary, Doctor Fonseca, alludes to women's relative confinement within the home, explaining that since women are unable to exercise as they should, they can make the most of going up and down stairs, sweeping, and decorating the house, and should not overdo activities like sewing, which are too inactive.[46]

The only other comments about women regarded the dangers of excessively violent or strenuous movements and the lifting of heavy objects when pregnant. Doctors advised them to rest at the start of pregnancy, exercise gently from the

---

[41] Traffichetti, *L'arte*, 164–5 and Petronio, *Del viver*, 276 and 279.

[42] See also Fonseca, *Del conservare*, 18.

[43] 'Mettersi da solo i calzetti e le vesti senza aiuto di servitori che così si esercita mediocremente il corpo.' Durante, *Il tesoro*, 14. Paschetti, *Del conservare*, 155; and Petronio, *Del viver*, 282.

[44] Petronio, *Del viver*, 272.   [45] Paschetti, *Del conservar*, 172.

[46] Fonseca, *Del conservare*, 21.

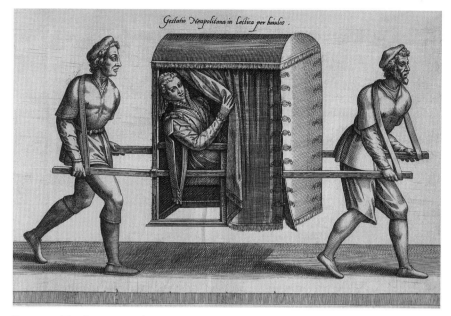

Gestatio Neapolitana in Lectica per baiulos.

Fig. 5.1. This late sixteenth-century Italian engraving illustrates the kind of sedan chair which became popular for women towards the end of the sixteenth century, attracting opprobrium from physicians who felt women would benefit from walking rather than being carried.

fourth to the seventh month, with good breaks, rest in the eighth month so as not to break the waters, and in the ninth start to do light daily exercise again so the baby is prepared for leaving the body. And, although riding in carriages was often recommended for women, when in this delicate condition they were to avoid it or any other vigorous or swift movements which might shake up the seed.[47]

There was however one form of exercise which everybody agreed was universally beneficial for all bodies according to how it was practised, and that was walking. This enjoyed a surge of popularity in medical advice literature, which after the mid-sixteenth century tended to include more detailed instructions on how to do it. This represented a considerable departure from earlier regimens in which it had been mentioned, but as something which should be made more demanding, for example by stopping to pick up stones, turning around and stretching out the arms, holding the breath to strengthen the lungs and stomach, or by climbing hills and 'tiring oneself in other ways'.[48] However, starting in the 1560s with Lennio's comment that walking may be done at different speeds, and later on Boldo's explanation of the ideal modes according to the seasons, the advice starts becoming

---

[47] Fonseca, *Del conservare*, 14; and Petronio, *Del viver*, 259–63.

[48] 'Chi non fa mestiere di esercizio alle mani debon camminare e passeggiare e piegare spesso la schiena e drizzarsi, montare in luoghi alti e fare altre fatiche.' *Libro di Arnaldo di Villa Nuova*, 115ʳ. There is a very similar passage in Maineri, *Opera utilissima*, 36.

more complex and evidently walking has begun to matter.[49] Soon afterwards, Petronio takes into consideration the terrain—whether stony or soft, whether in sun or shade—and even whether that shade is given by trees or walls. Also discussed are the ideal time of day for walking according to the seasons and weather conditions, and whether one should walk up or down hill, in straight lines or circles, according to one's constitution and the required health benefits![50] All these topics had already been aired in the *De arte gymnastica* by Mercuriale, and both he and Petronio were probably drawing on two key classical texts whose advice they were following: the *Problems* of Aristotle and the *De dieta* from the Hippocratic corpus.[51]

One consequence of the extremely detailed instructions regarding walking was that it could now be presented as a safe yet effective form of exercise, suitable for almost everyone, combining versatility with practicality. Paschetti, when distinguishing between different kinds of exercise, describes the most gentle as being any movement used inside the house, such as 'that kind of walking that we do in the house during the day'.[52] It was presumably the practicality and safety of walking as an exercise for all which contributed to the other development in the regimens, which was for the term 'exercise' to become almost synonymous with 'walking'. For example, Petronio makes few references to specific exercise forms, the single most common example given being walking (*passeggiare*), as when for example he refers to those whose exercise is to 'go around the city' ('andar in volta per la città'), whilst his key discussion of movement and rest hinges on an analysis of walking which covers several pages.[53] One after another authors tend to conflate the two, whether mentioning walking after dinner, or morning strolls on the Caelian Hill in Rome, or even just gently pottering about the house, when seeking to illustrate the value and ideal modes of exercise.[54]

EXERCISE FOR THE ELITES

In Traffichetti's regimen movement is divided into three distinct forms of exercise: movement for the sake of exercise alone; movement for exercise and labour or other such outcomes, like hunting and fishing; and movement for 'meditation and speaking'. For this last category he gives as examples the study of philosophy or

---

[49] Lennio, *Della complessione*, 37; and Boldo, *Libro della natura*, 217. See also Gropretio, *Un breue e nobile trattato*, 359; Romoli, *La singolare dottrina*, 261; and Rangoni, *Consiglio*, 40.

[50] Petronio, *Del viver*, 300–6. Paschetti (citing Aristotle, Hippocrates, and Galen), *Del conservar*, 168–70.

[51] Aristotle's *Problems* discuss the muscles involved in different types of walking, and the effects of terrain and temperatures. Hippocrates, *De dieta* discusses walking for different body types, as part of therapy, and with different speeds. Arcangeli points out that five complete editions of *De Dieta* appeared in either Greek or Latin in the 100 years after 1512; 'Una controversia veronese', 167.

[52] 'Quel passeggiar che alla giornata usiamo in casa.' Paschetti, *Del conservar*, 164.

[53] Petronio, *Del viver*, 255, 306–9.

[54] For examples see Paschetti, *Del conservar*, 130–1, 165; Auda, *Breue compendio*, 251, 254; Panaroli, *Aerologia*, 15–16; and Salando, *Trattato sopra la regola del vivere*, 7–9.

medicine, or speaking about an art, which he notes is 'often mistakenly called exercise of the body but is actually, of the soul'.[55] With this comment Traffichetti was underscoring the connection between body and soul, since the animal spirits governing sensation, thought, and the 'passions' were renewed and invigorated by the intake of pure air during exercise. Indeed, pleasant exercise in pleasing surroundings also 'delighted' the spirits, which resulted in that most positive state of well-being, *allegrezza*, of great benefit to one's health. It was therefore a short step from this to the argument that movement cannot merely be 'unpleasant exhaustion', and is only properly exercise if 'it delights the soul and makes man happy and cheerful'.[56] We see here how by establishing enjoyment as one of the criteria of valid exercise, Avicenna's view that exercise must be voluntarily undertaken was reinforced, enabling physicians not only to legitimize weaker and more pleasurable exercise forms for their elite readers, but to appropriate exercise and specific exercise forms in particular as an elite activity.

Other authors were not as subtle. Bertaldi noted simply that there were three types of exercise: 'violent' which was performed by 'people of low status', moderate 'used by nobles', and mild 'for the weak, ill and convalescent'.[57] This enhancing of the divisions and distinctions between exercise appropriate for the body of the patrician and gentleman and that suited to the body of the labourer was another important departure from antique literature. That is not to say that Galen had not also made the distinction between those who were free from labour and labourers: but in Galen these groups were not attributed different complexions but were simply associated with different levels of care of their bodies.[58] What changes is that around the turn of the seventeenth century we find lifestyle transformed into an innate, natural inclination, and ancient ideas being manipulated to fit the new social distinctions now embedded in forms of exercise. The first stage in this process was surely the emphasis on Avicenna's formulation of exercise as only that movement which is voluntarily undertaken, not physical labour, a distinction which we find taken up in many authors from the late Middle Ages onwards. A second step lay in the deployment of the Hippocratic notion whereby one should avoid deviating from conditions and habits which a body was already used to. These concepts could both be carefully stretched to fit the new exercise styles of patrician readers and patients.

Paschetti manages to use these two dictums to create his distinctions between the exercise needs of the leisured classes (those who live quietly and restfully, even 'lazily'), and of those whose bodies are used to fatigue such as hoeing and

---

[55] Traffichetti, *L'arte*, 110.

[56] 'Che diletti l'animo e renda l'huomo allegro e giocondo.' Traffichetti, *L'arte*, 110. He cites Galen as having advised that motions of the soul should be regarded as more important than motions of the body.

[57] 'Cioé violento, usato da gente di bassa conditione, mediocre, usato da nobili, e debole, usato da deboli, valetudinarij, e convalescenti.' Bertaldi, *Regole della sanità*, 24.

[58] Galen simply suggested that those devoted to a life of leisure were free to dedicate themselves entirely to the care of their body and were therefore bound to be healthier than those who performed time-consuming and harmful occupations.

threshing.[59] Part of his argument rests on the idea that each of these groups of people is used to particular forms and levels of exercise, and therefore can survive, if not actually thrive on it, whilst change could be very dangerous. The other part of the argument rests on ideas of nobility. Since Paschetti has already established that taking care of one's health is both prudent and virtuous, even a duty for those weighed down with affairs of state, it is also therefore synonymous with class, a point emphasized when he adds that it is necessary for the health of everyone 'who lives civilly and delicately'.[60] Thus physical labour, for a member of the elite, would not be 'appropriate for anyone who esteems his life'.[61] And the most swift and vigorous exercise he will allow his 'robust' patricians, if they are used to it, is the game of small ball, or *pillota*, and the like. When it comes to noblewomen however, as noted earlier, he is even more extreme in his application of class-based distinctions. For, having admonished Genoese gentlewomen for their laziness, he goes on to make an exemption for nobly born women, whose bodies can be differentiated from those of lower status women through their noble birth and their 'delicate' nourishment which (implicitly) result in their having less 'plethora' to evacuate and greater sensitivity to the heat produced by agitation. Hence in order to avoid the dangers of excessive or fast walking after meals he concedes that they may be carried in litters.[62]

Fonseca, writing at the same time, takes these arguments further, distinguishing between bodies that do not have to work, and bodies subject to servitude.[63] The latter are then divided into those who perform sedentary activities and those who are engaged in manual work, with different types of exercise being naturally associated with these categories. Only moderate exercise suits those 'used to a restful life' and vigorous movement would be damaging to them. Playing with the small ball, hunting with the bow and the crossbow but not with the arquebus (a heavy kind of primitive gun), walking, riding a mule, being carried in a litter or in a coach, and dancing are considered exercises fit for a gentleman (*esercizi da gentiluomo*), although age restrictions also apply to some of these activities. Moderate or even light exercise is also suited to the first category of those in servitude, by which he means scholars and politicians, but this should mainly consist of walking, since ball games, hunting, and dancing would be unbecoming in those who are expected to behave in a demure and austere way.

Fifty years later this view of vigorous exercise as unsuitable for gentleman was evidently so well established as to become the target of anti-noble stances. A provincial doctor named Frediano, writing in Lucca in 1656, vehemently criticizes the laziness of the nobility by contesting what had clearly become a prevailing assumption,

---

[59] 'In ozio'; Paschetti, *Del conservar*, 161, 167. He rehearses the arguments related to this over some 16 pages: pp. 150–66.

[60] 'Che civilmente e delicatamente vive per conservar la sanità sua.' Paschetti, *Del conservar*, 160 and 5–6 on the link between caring for one's health, prudence, virtue, and duty.

[61] 'Onde l'essercitio, che fanno i zapatori, i metitori, e altri lavoratori a niuno che stimi la vita sua si conviene.' Paschetti, *Del conservar*, 167.

[62] Paschetti, *Del conservar*, 173.

[63] '*Corpi liberi*, non soggetti ad alcuna occupazione e corpi soggetti alla condizione servile.' Fonseca, *Del conservare*, 23.

that 'exercise has been given as a punishment to the poor'. Drawing on classical sources he urges his readers to ignore those authors who fear sweating and vigorous physical labour, hinting that such concerns are not manly, and pointing to the example set by Galen who recounts splitting wood in winter, cutting and threshing barley, and performing other activities which countrymen did as their work. 'It is far from true that the nobility is not suited to fatigue,' he thunders; 'it was common among the ancients that all sorts of people exercised.'[64]

THE BODY OF THE GENTLEMAN, THE BODY OF THE DEVOUT CHRISTIAN

These changes in medical definitions of exercise need to be considered in the context of the wider transformations of codes of gesture and posture that started to affect the elites from the early sixteenth century. The flourishing genre of conduct literature for gentlemen acquired added vigour after the 1550s and was largely centred upon the body. Attention has focused on Castiglione's *The Courtier* and Guazzo's *Civil Conversation*, but in reality there is a much larger production of treatises directed to the aspiring gentleman that aim to regulate his occupations and time and advise him on how he should behave in all sorts of specific circumstances.[65] These texts support the creation of a new paradigm of the noble body that stresses grace and harmony and artlessly expresses elegance and refinement in all its manifestations. This is in stark contrast not only with the robust body of the peasant but also with the physique of the soldier, who in the new military treatises of the second half of the sixteenth century, is represented as vigorous, strong, and showing the marks of training and discipline.[66]

As the sixteenth century advanced, the ideals expressed in conduct literature for gentlemen meshed ever more tightly with the new models of behaviour and demeanour expected from a good Christian which were articulated through manuals for the education of children and youths. These texts, penned by ecclesiastical authors in the sixteenth century, were profoundly influenced by the values of the Counter-Reformation and their contribution to the establishment of new models of corporeality cannot be ignored. They played a significant part in the dissemination of ideals of posture, demeanour, and gestuality that were characterized by stricter notions of decorum and sobriety of movement. These then acted as a corrector to the emphasis on gracefulness, elegance, and proportion advocated by manuals of civility. Their message would inevitably have had an impact on both medical and lay ideas about exercise, even more so if we consider that educational

---

[64] '[non mi si dica che] l'esercitio sia stato dato per condanna della povertà perchè Quintiliano, Seneca e altri antichi dicono non è cosa da uomo il temere il sudore, anzi Galeno riferisce essere stato più' volte in inverno trovato a spezzar legni, pestar orzo e mondare fromento o fare eserciti propri degli'agricoltori. Èlontano dal vero che la nobiltà non si confaccia con la fatica, era in uso presso gli antichi che ogni sorte di persona si esercitasse.' Frediano, *Arca novella*, 155–6.

[65] On this literature see Quondam's introd. to Stefano Guazzo, *La civil conversazione*, 19.

[66] Verrier, *Les Armes de Minerve*, 137–8, 160–3, 174.

treatises were directed to a socially varied readership, not just to people of noble birth, but also to those from educated families at whom the medical advice literature was also aimed.

These ideals were encapsulated in the notions of 'gravity', a word that recurs with growing frequency in the educational literature. It refers to a calm and judicious demeanour characterized by composure of the limbs and facial countenance, moderation in gestural expression, and quiet speech. Initially associated with mature and even old age, this code of physical behaviour was now extended to children and adolescents, who were encouraged to abandon the excitement and unrelenting motion that was typical of their age.[67] This emphasis on physical discipline was justified by the assumption that the bearing of the body was a mirror of the soul; in Sadoleto's words, 'From moderation and the tempering of the soul comes a certain bodily gravitas in every movement and disposition... that corresponds to one's inner gravity.'[68] The domestication of the body could only proceed from a domination of the inner self, a taming of the passions.

This model of composed and dignified physical behaviour that the Church was elaborating in the course of the sixteenth century clearly had a bearing on the redefinition of the nature of exercise that was taking place at the time in both conduct and medical advice literature. The restrained movement expected of the good Christian was to some extent compatible with the graceful nonchalance of the courtier, whilst being diametrically opposed to the heavy breathing, sweating, and flushing produced by the kind of swift and strenuous forms of exercise from which doctors were likewise distancing themselves. But men of the Church were becoming critical even of those more gentle types of exercise that had long been advocated by medical professionals. The game of small ball (*palla piccola*) for example had been much praised, traditionally, as a 'temperate' game, one which exercised all the limbs, without tiring the body, and was seen as ideal, therefore, in a society concerned about overstrenuous activities.[69] However, in his influential treatise Bishop Antoniano expressed strong reservations about its benefits: 'although the game of small ball is highly commended by doctors, to me it seems one makes too much movement, rapidly getting out of breath whereas that which we call billiards seems altogether better to me, and other similar games in which movement and rest are balanced, with due regard for excessive exercise so that strength is not dissipated nor risks to health run in any other way'.[70] Also in the medical field, on the other

[67] Niccoli, *Il seme della violenza*, 105, 117–18, 129–30.

[68] 'dopo questa moderatezza e temperamento dell'animo ne viene una certa *gravità di corpo in ogni moto e atteggiamento*...che corrisponde alla gravità interna' (our emphasis). Sadoleto, *Del ben ammaestrare*, 33.

[69] Benzi, *Tractato utilissimo*, iii^r–iiii^v; Gropretio, *Un breue et notabile trattato*, 359^v; Boldo, *Libro della natura*, 213; Viviani, *Trattato*, 185; and Romoli, *La singolare dottrina*, 264.

[70] 'anche se il gioco della palla é molto commendato dai medici a me sembra che vi si faccia un moto troppo continuato che presto commuove il traspiro, onde quello che si chiama il trucco mi par il migliore, *ed altri simili che sono temperati di moto e di quiete*, dovendo aver riguardo per il troppo esercizio le forze non si dissolvano e non si incorra in altra guisa in alcun pericolo della salute' (our emphasis). Antoniano, *Dell'educazione*, 399–400.

hand, playing small ball was beginning to be seen as an exhausting game and its advantages for health were questioned.[71]

Clerical opinion also contributed to a redefinition of the forms of exercise considered most appropriate for conferring the male body with the seemingly innate graceful deportment now desirable in a gentleman. Increasingly in the sixteenth century, exercise was no longer understood as preparation for war. Instead, the ideal of military preparedness was eclipsed by one of public display and performance, as men aimed to be admired for their physical elegance and dexterity of movement rather than for their strength and success in combat. As a result, recommendations concerning the acquisition of military skills occupy limited space in conduct literature.[72] This increasing distance from military aspirations is also evident in the changing instructions found in treatises for the education of children. Whilst earlier manuals had advocated the physical education of the populace at large for military purposes, the sixteenth century saw a shift to the specific few who would make military life their profession. For example, while Cardinal Sadoleto, writing in 1533, still considered military preparedness as one of the aims of children's daily exercise, in the 1580s Antoniano relegated both military skills, as well as hunting, to 'military youths' (*gioventú militare*) and to those who have chosen 'such a way of life' (*un tal genere di vita*).[73] Equally, as a reflection of this specialization of military activities, horsemanship, wrestling, hunting, and archery are increasingly viewed as special requirements for those entering the army or civic militia.[74]

Some of these activities were still performed by young noblemen but with different aims and in different ways, namely because they enabled young nobles to take part in those equestrian games that remained an exclusive public demonstration of noble class identity throughout the early modern period, in spite of the Church's condemnation of any violent activities that might harm other men.[75] Indeed, although jousts and tournaments continued to take place they increasingly turned into 'sheer spectacles of choreography' in which the performer was appreciated for the elegance of his movements and the splendour of the attire more than for any exercise of strength[76] (see Plate 16).

Martine Boiteux has traced the transformation affecting chivalric games in Rome. In the first decades of the sixteenth century they were already described by moralizing and nostalgic literature as a pale copy of medieval games.[77] In the second half

[71] Lennio for example considers it amongst 'vigorous' exercises. Lennio, *Della complessione*, 37.

[72] Domenichelli, *Cavaliere e gentiluomo*, 313.

[73] Sadoleto, *Del ben ammaestrare*, 29; and Antoniano, *Dell'educazione*, 457–8.

[74] English, 'Physical Education', 257. See also Grendler's analysis of advice on physical activities for students. 'Fencing', 295–319.

[75] For examples of Church criticism in the second part of the 16th century, Antoniano, *Dell'educazione*, 457 and Cobarubias, *Rimedio de' givocatori*, 66, also written by an ecclesiastic. They describe tournaments as prohibited because dangerous, since they cause unnecessary wounds and even deaths, and because much money is spent that should be preserved for more important things. On the attitude of the Church to military games and duels, see Cozzo '"Aliquando necessarium"'. The Council of Trent had also banned the duel, under penalty of excommunication; 'Premessa', in Israel and Ortalli (eds.), *Il duello*, 15.

[76] Bascetta, *Sport e giochi*, 196.   [77] Boiteux, 'Jeux equestres', 141.

of the century, with the introduction of the fencing foil, the games become even less violent and brutal though still not without risk. Later, in the first decades of the seventeenth century, the fighters no longer clash directly but aim to lance the dummy of a Saracen and in some cases the game is between the horses of the nobility (the race of the *berberi*): men are no longer involved.[78]

By the mid-sixteenth century the young noble could exhibit the control he had acquired of his body through the much-tamed war games and a range of other newly popular elite activities such as displays of fencing, dressage, dance, and acrobatic vaulting.[79] This shift in forms of exercise types was noted by contemporaries. The author of a mid-sixteenth-century treatise on ball games pointed out that exercise was no longer energetic and violent, nor intended to make the body robust and fit to fight, but that the new forms of physical education were entirely disconnected from military purposes and aimed to entertain.[80] Indeed, as has been documented by Bascetta in his study of sport treatises, a series of innovations characterize the physical culture of the period: the development of dressage, the emergence of a new type of fencing 'freed from being above all a measure of strength' and of new acrobatic techniques such as vaulting on a wooden horse, are all novelties that develop from the mid-sixteenth century into the early decades of the seventeenth century.[81] The common characteristic of these new forms of exercise is that they emphasize the aesthetic of gesture. Running, jumping, and lifting weights are substituted by more subtle, precise, graceful, and elegant movements. The search for virtuosity, balance, and supple movements is typical of dressage, where the rider has to be at one with his horse and the horse responds not to force or violence, but to subtle signals.[82] In fencing the use of the two-handed sword was replaced by the single-handed management of a lighter sword that promoted agility and smoothness and more and more emancipated fencing from wrestling. Moreover, there was a gradual disappearance of the use of subsidiary weapons (shields or daggers).[83] Likewise, vaulting (see Figs. 5.2 and 5.3) was seen to lend the body a singular grace and refinement—as stated by Giocondo Beluda, who ran the first school of vaulting that opened around 1630 in Bologna, and its benefits for health were regarded as secondary to the forging of a new male body: 'it might also be regarded as rousing the spirit, enhancing judgement and energy, and since it is not violent it is held to be very beneficial for the health of the body'.[84]

The inclusion of dance amongst the techniques that the young noble needed to learn was another important innovation. Dance was valued because it enhanced the ability to control movement and gesture so that youths learned to carry

---

[78] Boiteux, 'Jeux equestres', 147, 152–3, 155, and 160. For similar observations in relation to the French context, see Vigarello, 'S'exercer, jouer', esp. 235–48.

[79] On the various types of academies, their curricula, and extracurricular activities, see Quondam, 'L'accademia', 874–7.

[80] Scaino, *Trattato*, 294–5. See also Grendler, 'Fencing', 308–11.

[81] Bascetta, *Sport e giochi*, 115.

[82] Bonhomme, 'Le Cheval', 338; and Bascetta, *Sport e giochi*, 197.

[83] Bascetta, *Sport e giochi*, 113–18.

[84] 'si puó anche creder che svegli l'animo e accresca il giudizio e la gagliardia e non essendo violento viene riputato molto giovevole alla salute del corpo'. Beluda, 'Trattato dell'arte di volteggiare'. Vaulting schools were opened in Milan, Bologna, Ferrara, Mantua, and Naples; Bascetta, *Sport e giochi*, 342–3. On the 'ennoblement' of vaulting see also S. Schmidt, 'Trois dialogues', 377–89.

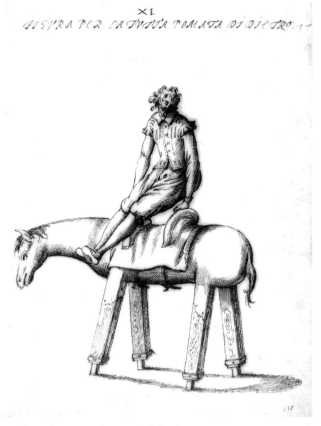

Figs. 5.2–5.3. These drawings, from Beluda's 1659 manuscript treatise on how to use a vaulting horse, capture the principles of grace and composure at the heart of this form of exercise.

themselves with that decorum which is appropriate for gentlemen and perform any physical operation, even the most demanding, with total ease and natural-ness. This makes sense because Renaissance dance, with its strict rules regarding the number of steps but also the position of dancers in a defined space and the reciprocal relation between their movements, embodies the principles of meas-ure, proportion, and geometric order that characterize the aesthetic of the period and could therefore be seen as instrumental to the acquisition of a harmonious use of the body.[85] In 1542 this is clearly acknowledged by Fausto da Longiano who sees among the benefits of learning dance in childhood the fact that 'besides exercising the body it teaches movement in accordance with certain tempos and proportions'.[86]

[85] Castelli, *L'estetica del rinascimento*, 37–8.
[86] 'oltre che esercita il corpo insegna i movimenti con certi tempi e misure.' Longiano, *De lo istituire*, 475.

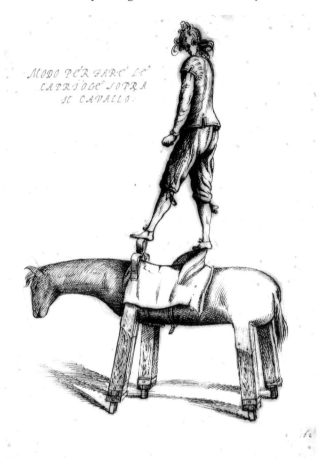

Fig. 5.3.

Dancing lessons, like musical education, were indeed becoming part and parcel of the cultural baggage of the young men of quality but the development courted some controversy. In pedagogical tracts of the fifteenth century dancing had been both recommended 'if done for exercise' and vilified as unworthy, improper, and unseemly, feared as encouraging lasciviousness and for being effeminate.[87] The Church, in particular, had traditionally condemned dance as an occasion for improper physical contact between the sexes and a vain way of spending time that diverted attention from more spiritual occupations. However, as ambivalence about the benefits of dance continued, the focus of anxiety shifted more onto age and its appropriateness in adult men. Both secular and clerical authors argued that though laudable in children it should no longer be pursued in adulthood, because it was seen as effeminizing the souls of mature men to the extent of becoming

---

[87] English, 'Physical Education', 112, 135, and 147.

'indecent, nor can it in any way befit manly gravity and appropriate behaviour'.[88] Those gentlemen who spent days and nights dancing were making fools of themselves. There is a clear parallel with practising music: playing or singing are also criticized in adults for their emasculating effects, so that an adult man should give up singing but could continue to listen to music and songs, though soberly.[89]

Within these age boundaries attitudes to dance appear to have relaxed towards the end of the sixteenth century, perhaps as a result also of the increasingly diverse movements required from men and women in contemporary dance forms. The development of particularly vigorous, lively movements for men reaffirmed gender roles and removed at least the accusation of effeminacy.[90] In spite of some initial resistance, dancing lessons and a musical training were now offered even to the growing number of noble pupils who attended the Jesuit colleges.[91] After the 1560s dance also appears to be considered a form of exercise in the medical advice books, though only marginally.[92] Part of the essential training required of young gentlefolk, dance acquired a new status as it was grouped together with vaulting and fencing amongst what Beluda called 'the chivalrous arts' which were all taught together in the same schools.[93] The links between these physical activities were confirmed in dance treatises. In 1589 Luzi listed among the benefits of dance the fact that 'it endows the limbs and the feet with such grace that it confers great agility on the handling of weapons', and refinement in mounting a horse.[94]

GAMES, OLD AND NEW

Starting with Castiglione's *Courtier* in 1528, civility manuals had not only encouraged the expression of social distinction through gesture and posture, but had repeatedly urged their noble readers to avoid mixing with people of inferior status.[95] This was one of the issues on which both secular and clerical sources agreed and even exercise was to be differentiated according to rank. Bishop Antoniano, for example, argued that exercise types should be different for the peasant, the artisan, the 'middling citizen', and the gentleman. Medical theory, as we have seen, increasingly suggested that physical movement should be differentiated by class as well as by age.[96] As a result the sixteenth century saw the development of several new games which, being less violent, were seen as best suited to gentlemen, whilst changing ways of playing them meant

---

[88] 'sconcio, né puó in alcun modo accordarsi alla gravità virile e ai seri costumi'; Longiano, *De lo istituire*, 119.

[89] Sadoleto, *Del ben'ammaestrare*, 119; and Longiano, *De lo istituire*, 470.

[90] Nordera, 'La donna in ballo', 46–50, 53–5, 138, and 145–51.

[91] Brizzi, *La formazione*, 253; Arcangeli, 'I gesuiti e la danza', 21–37.

[92] See n. 35.

[93] Beluda, 'Trattato del modo di volteggiare', 20.

[94] 'dispone sí graziosamente le membra e i piedi sia di agevolezza grande al giuoco dell'armi'; Lutii, *Opera bellissima*, 6–7, cited in Arcangeli, 'La disciplina del corpo', 434.

[95] See e.g. in Baldassar Castiglione the observation that nobles should 'refrain from mixing with the common people' in the discussion of games and festivities; *Book of the Courtier*, 119; and Quondam, 'Elogio del gentiluomo', 15.

[96] Antoniano, *Dell'educazione*, 52–3.

they were adapted to the needs of gentlefolk. Even separate means of transport appeared that contributed to widen the gulf between the gestational, passive exercise increasingly associated with elite men and that practised by the wider public.

One of the most striking examples of the way in which exercise forms were appropriated by the elite is in the game of *piccola palla* or small ball, versions of which were already popular in the late Middle Ages. It was a game which had traditionally been played in the streets and piazzas as the ball was originally hit with the palm of the hand. Later the use of thick gloves was introduced, which by 1500 were starting to be replaced by rackets. These distanced the player from the dirty ball and reduced the physical impact, making it more suitable for the elites. The use of a cord over which the ball was hit was a further innovation. This led to a variety of different games known as *palla corda*, *palla con raquette*, etc.[97] (See Fig. 5.4.)

Moreover, as De Bondt has documented, during the sixteenth century legislation increasingly prohibited the playing of such games in public, with the result that they

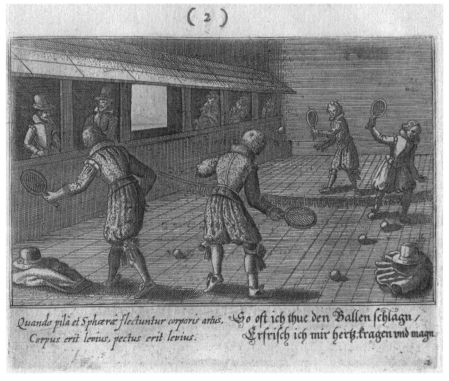

Quando pilà et Sphæræ flectuntur corporis artus, So oft ich thue den Ballen schlagn /
Corpus erit levius, pectus erit levius. Erfrisch ich mir hertz tragen vnd magn.

Fig. 5.4. This engraving, from a seventeenth-century French emblem book, shows a game of *pallacorda*—an early form of tennis in which the ball is hit over a cord hung across the middle of a covered court. The use of raquets and specialized indoor courts characterized the increasing aristocratization of the sport.

---

[97] Nada-Patrone, 'I giochi di palla', 60–1.

were restricted to the new ball courts which were being built within the confines of the palaces of the nobility and of cardinals.[98] Inevitably, these games were increasingly associated with the elite and by 1555 Scaino describes these various small-ball games as providing 'more genteel entertainment' and emphasizes the chivalric virtues of dedication, stamina, and calmness they embodied.[99] He also contrasts them with games played with a larger ball and with *calcio*, an energetic team ball game, all of which he suggests are more appropriate for soldiers. The logic behind this social differentiation perhaps included the fact that the smaller the ball the less effort and strength was required and the more light and graceful the movements employed, which perhaps also explained why during the second half of the sixteenth century we find evidence that women of the nobility played *palla piccola*.[100] Certainly the sport grew increasingly exclusive, played and promoted by rulers which also ensured that it became very much part of elite social spectacle, as the games drew large crowds to the palaces where they were being held.[101]

Although Scaino had suggested that *calcio* was only suitable for soldiers, the game was in fact extremely popular—particularly in Florence—amongst young men of the elite. It was a fast, rough ball game played in teams, with the ball passed by hand somewhat like rugby or netball. The apparent contradiction between such a violent game and ideals of elite deportment was presumably overcome in part by the emphasis laid on the ingenuity and skill required of the players, and in part by the immense social spectacle which surrounded the game: processions of players dressed in splendid liveries, evening banquets, and free festivities for the crowds were all common practice and helped to emphasize the nobility and wealth of the players.[102] Moreover, all accounts suggest that it was played only by the most healthy, strong, and robust of young elite men.[103]

Indeed, a range of sources show that in practice, and not just according to medical theory, there was an increased divergence in the forms of exercise associated with elite men and women of different ages during this period. As we have seen, most medical literature for example forbade ball games to those under 14, or to 'older' men, aged from 35 or 40 onwards and various testimonies seem to bear this out.[104] Doctor Panaroli for example, writing in 1642, criticized parents for 'wrapping their children in cotton wool', by not letting them play ball games which were feared as too vigorous, and only allowing them to play card games indoors.[105] We also learn that mature men indeed stopped playing the game. In the 1620s the nobleman and art collector Vincenzo Giustiniani—then in his sixties—observed

---

[98] De Bondt, *Royal Tennis*, 16–37. He gives a great many examples of the palaces in which they were constructed.

[99] 'Piú signorili trattenimenti.' Scaino, *Trattato*, 311–14.

[100] Scaino, *Trattato*, 55.

[101] De Bondt, *Royal Tennis*, 71–7.

[102] See the numerous 16th- and 17th-century accounts of the game published by Bini, in *Memorie*, 44–6, 86, 89, 90, and 116.

[103] One contributor notes that it was played 'not by craftsmen, not by servants, not by the ignoble, but by soldiers, gentlemen, lords, and princes'. Bini, *Memorie*, 5 (our trans.).

[104] Fonseca, *Del conservare*, 18.

[105] 'E li tengono, come si suol dire...nello scatolino della bombace.' Panaroli, *Abuso*, 10.

that he had greatly enjoyed the *giuoco della palla* 'when I was a lad' and found it benefited his health, although he now considered it to be a dangerously violent and tiring game.[106] A few decades later in a letter to his mother-in-law the Marquis Maidalchini—aged 44—remarks on the fact that he played a ball game during his trip to Rome and comments both on how much it made him sweat and, somewhat nostalgically, on how when playing it he felt that 'he was a boy again', suggesting that he hadn't played it for a long time.[107] However, judging from the accusations made by Doctor Scipione Mercurio in his *On Popular Errors*, not all older men were as easily dissuaded from their pleasures. He admonishes those over 35 (whom he calls the 'young-old') who played for many hours at a time, day and night, despite sweat and exhaustion, and, as he believed, were seriously compromising their health.[108]

Dance was, as we have seen, another activity strictly associated with young people in the conduct literature. It would seem that, at least in the case of women, this was also true in practice. It has been suggested by Nordera that dancing was only practised by young marriageable women, especially in preparation for weddings or amongst themselves, and we find an account which supports this picture. In a letter written by Eugenia aged only 27, but already a remarried widow and mother of three, she recounts with dismay how the evening before she had been persuaded to dance by her young female guests—the three daughters of the Princess of Rossano—and therefore perform an activity she had not practised for at least ten years![109] Overall it seems as if the concerns expressed by clerics and lay commentators about the challenge that physical exercise posed to the adoption of the dignified and measured bodily deportment required of elite parents were taken seriously.

Given that so many forms of exercise were increasingly deemed excessively vigorous it is not surprising to find that several new games were developed, some of which were already popular by the 1550s and which were considered more appropriate for older men, gentlemen, and in some cases apparently women, such as boules, billiards (*trucco*), croquet, ping-pong (*palla maglio da tavolo*), and golf (*pallamaglio*) (see Fig. 5.5).[110] In the seventeenth century for example, *stanze del trucco* (billiard rooms) are found in Roman palaces and in 1658 a surprise visit by her father caught Eugenia Maidalchini 'finishing the day playing *trucco* with the wet nurse'.[111]

Vincenzo Giustiniani, whose favourite game had been *pallamaglio* before ill health prevented him from playing it, provides us with a detailed explanation of

---

[106] Giustiniani, 'Discorso', 326–32.   [107] AST, FSV, B.410, 12.12.1657.

[108] Mercurio, *De gli errori*, 451.

[109] 'la sera si cantò di nuovo e le figlie della Principessa fecero tre balli assai bene e a me ancora mi bisognò fare la Spagnoletta con loro che non so come me ne ricordi più *essendo 10 anni per lo meno che non ho mai ballato*' (our emphasis). ASR, FSV, B.1115, 23.10.1666.

[110] Giustiniani ('Discorso', 328–9) calls them 'Trucco sopra la tavola' and 'in terra'. For the chronology see Oldradi, *Capitolo del palamaglio*, in which the author describes the game and its popularity in a satirical verse asking for it to be banned.

[111] AST, FSV, B.410, 13.4.1658; and B.607, 13.4.1658.

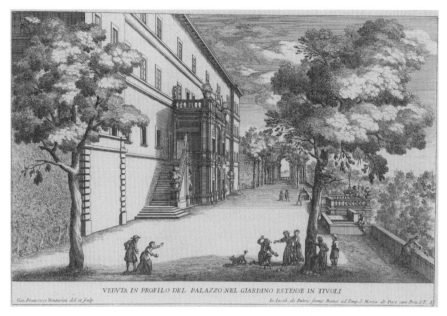

VEDVTA IN PROFILO DEL PALAZZO NEL GIARDINO ESTENSE IN TIVOLI

Fig. 5.5. Boules was approved of as exercise for the elites, including women, since it required little physical effort. This late seventeenth-century engraving—showing people playing the game in the shade at the Villa d'Este at Tivoli—suggests that it was a normal form of recreation for visitors to the garden.

why these games are the most suited to gentlemen of a certain age and status and beneficial to their health. Firstly he notes that they offer the player 'more moderate exercise', with some not even requiring one to move about, although he stresses that they all require a man to exercise his skill and intelligence.[112] In his view pall-mall in particular was 'really suited to gentlemen' because players took moderate exercise but, unlike in boules, billiards, and croquet, they had the freedom to walk about, even to run, and vary their surroundings. Furthermore, players could chat and joke with friends, even do business between strokes. Other advantages which made it particularly appropriate for gentlefolk were that it did not require them to keep their eyes fixed on the ground, nor to bend their backs, nor to dirty their hands—all defects associated with the activities of the lower orders—as even the ball was picked up using a scoop carved into the face of the club and could be replaced when dirty.[113] The success of the game was such that in Rome at least it moved from

[112] Giustiniani, 'Discorso', 328.
[113] Giustiniani, 'Discorso', 329–30. Another game said to have been introduced to Rome in the 17th century from the court of the King of Persia was polo. Giustiniani witnessed the first game played there, and wrote that it required extremely finely trained war horses, and consummate skill, 'grace', and dexterity from the riders, all of which explain why the game was judged to be 'noble'. He recommended however that it was so dangerous for rider and horse alike that it should not be played anymore, advice which was apparently not heeded.

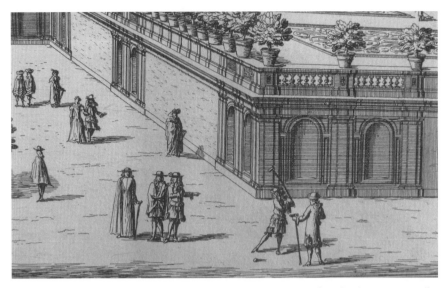

Fig. 5.6. This detail from a late seventeenth-century engraving of a suburban Roman villa, shows a game of pall-mall in progress. The player with the raised club is about to hit his ball along an avenue which had been specially set aside for the game.

the streets into palace courtyards and gardens which were built for this purpose especially in the first decades of the seventeenth century.[114] (See Fig. 5.6.)

Another milestone in the development of a separate culture of exercise and movement was the rise in the use of various types of coaches and litters as the preferred means of transport, not just for gentlewomen (as was the case in the first decades of the century) but for gentlemen too.[115] In Italy this was accompanied sometime in the early to mid-seventeenth century, by a change in the status of horse-riding such that, although it was expected that elite men would learn to be excellent horsemen, riding a horse as a means of transport seems gradually to have been confined to the lower and middling classes. Private correspondence between members of the Spada family shows that men regularly travelled on coaches in the seventeenth century whilst horse-riding was reserved for their male servants. Only in an emergency did the adult men of the house resort to horse-riding as we learn from a letter written in September 1642 when the family had been evacuated to Perugia on the outbreak of the War of Castro. When Cardinal Bernardino heard that a cardinal capable of providing him with first-hand news of the war would be in a nearby town, he and two others jumped on their horses and rode to meet him. It was clearly an exceptional and unexpected adventure and the letter is full of his pride at the prowess he had demonstrated by riding for 5 'miglia di posta',

[114] Waddy, *Seventeenth-Century Roman Palaces*, 54–5.
[115] On the diffusion of coaches in Italy, see Gozzadini, *Dell'origine*, 19–33. On Rome, in particular, see Lotz, 'Gli 883 cocchi'.

(postal miles equivalent to 40 to 50 miles) without spurs or boots and only half a riding whip. On the return journey however, Bernardino, 'exhausted and sweating', was more than happy to accept the offer of a lift from Antonio Benedetti, who was travelling back by litter, accepting what was clearly a more familiar means of transport.[116] This is however the only instance we have encountered in the hundreds of letters we have read of a member of the family horse-riding. Status was by now associated with coaches.

This shift in habits had clearly been under way for several decades and not gone unnoticed among contemporary commentators, nor had it escaped criticism: in the 1540s Fausto da Longiano calls it 'a depraved new Italian custom that gentlemen are allowed to use the coach or carriage!...showing that they have turned into women, having taken up the same forms of exercise'.[117] In reality, even if men, like women, were now travelling in coaches, masculine status was preserved through the different types of coaches they preferred: the *carrozzino*, an open and light coach, faster and more manageable but also more prone to overturn, was a typically male type of coach, used in better weather. Moreover, both gender and age distinctions were reinforced by the fact that women and children tended to travel not by coach but by litter in long journeys, while the adult male members of the household preceded them by coach.[118] We have already seen that doctors were very cautious about the suitability of carriages for young children and women, particularly when pregnant: their delicate bodies could be damaged by the jolting, the unborn child could be shaken out, and the immoderate exercises could cause the body to dangerously overheat. Expedients were therefore adopted to protect the most vulnerable. When an infant was on board and the road was particularly bad the passengers would often get off the coach and walk stretches of the road 'so that the baby wouldn't be shaken about'.[119] The use of a *lettiga* (a litter) was regarded as a much more comfortable and secure, albeit much slower, means of transport for the sick and frail. (See Fig. 5.7.) *The lettiga* had a mattress for the passenger to lie down on as if they were in a bed and they were carried along by either horses or mules.

This shift from horse to coach and litter is particularly relevant to us given that as we saw in the regimens, being driven in a coach or carried in a litter or sedan chair was increasingly being defined as a valid form of exercise even for healthy adult males. This would have provided the theoretical justification for a change in habits that once again separated different social groups even more clearly. Indeed, the impact of travelling on health is described in similar terms to those used when accounting for the negative effects of vigorous exercise. In both cases what was seen as harmful was the ensuing overheating of the body which in turns provoked an excessive build-up of blood and a drying-up of radical heat. Clearly riding exposed

---

[116] ASR, FSV, B.491, 15.9.1642.
[117] 'Depravata consuetudine d'Italia che a gentiluomini sia lecito usar la carretta o il cocchio!...mostrano di esser trasformati con gli esercizi del corpo ne le femmine'. Longiano, *De lo istituire*, 476.
[118] The Spada-Veralli letters systematically illustrate this habit.
[119] ASR, FSV, B.410.21.11.1657.

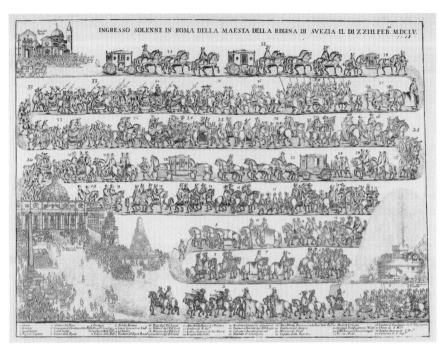

Fig. 5.7. This engraving recording the ceremonial entrance of Queen Christina into Rome in 1655 shows two examples of the restful and comfortable litter commonly used by aristocratic women and children when travelling (top right corner and the middle of the fourth row down).

the body to this risk more than travelling on a coach, although the latter was also seen as an ordeal when protracted for long stretches of time. Contemporary letters quite clearly articulate a similar view. For instance in a letter dated October 1672 the writer attributes a fever to the 'ordeal of the journey' they had previously undertaken.[120] Lay and professionals alike presented travelling by coach or litter as a form of 'exercise', and as such these activities were approved of in moderation but were viewed as harmful if carried to excess.

WALKING AS EXERCISE: THE LAY NARRATIVE

Medical discourse about exercise thus permeated lay narratives. However, if we examine closely the way in which physical activity and its impact upon the body are discussed in seventeenth-century letters we observe that these do not just share but overemphasize the preoccupations surrounding the undertaking of any sort of violent movement in the medical and non-medical advice literature. Letters echo

---

[120] 'patimento del viaggio'; ASR, FSV, B.1115, 8.10.1672.

warnings found in regimens about the dangers of making the blood boil through continuous exercise thereby overheating and exhausting the body, and describe excessive movement as conducive to disease. An ailment that makes her call the doctor in April 1647 and stay in bed for a day is put down by Maria to 'agitation of the blood' caused by 'some little exercise done [while she was away] in Civitavecchia, so one might say that having fun does not agree with her'.[121] The touch of fever that one of her children, aged 6, develops in October 1651, is attributed to the fact that on Friday, when they went to Veceno and Benaro, he walked around quite a bit and as well as walking 'he got up to such high jinks that he wore himself out'.[122] In this and other cases excessive movement is seen as provoking a *scaldamento* (overheating) of the body that leads to the development of a fever. Combined with preoccupations about the impact of exercise on the more mature body, this concern for the damaging consequences of vigorous exercise seems to have led to an overenthusiastic acceptance of walking as the ideal form of physical activity for men and women of adult age. In fact the two terms had been conflated so that in the vocabulary of laymen and women of all classes the word 'exercise' was largely used as synonymous with walking. Certainly for the nobility marriage and maturity corresponded with abandoning more demanding physical activities and exercising just by walking but it would seem that the need to 'exercise' regularly was not a concern alien to the lower ranks.

In 1596 three young men of modest means (two of them enrolled at the Capranica College to become priests, the third just returned to Rome from the war in Hungary) were questioned by the magistrate, on suspicion of theft and swindling. Protesting their innocence, they claimed they had spent the day engaged in activities such as going to a bookshop to buy a book, going to watch horse races, eating meals in their lodgings, and going out for no other reasons than 'to walk around a bit and do exercise'.[123] In the vocabulary of the non-professional, walking was therefore intended as a medicalized activity, clearly related with keeping in good health. The term 'exercise' meaning walking also appears frequently in the Spada-Veralli family letters. Husbands recommend it to wives, mothers-in-law to sons-in-law, and mothers to young married daughters. In March 1659 Orazio Spada wrote to his wife Maria from their country house in Castel Viscardo. She was receiving medical treatment for her lack of appetite and excessive thirst, and he pleaded with her not to tire out either body or mind, to have their son write letters on her behalf, and to take walks 'for God knows your Ladyship has no longer been taking them'.[124] Walking is seen as both a recipe for recovery and a requisite for good health. Two years later, while reminding his wife once again that she should go and walk in the morning 'since exercise does her more good than any kind of medicine', Orazio adds that 'ever since I have been walking all morning I am much

---

[121] ASR, FSV, B.619, 10.4.1647. [122] ASR, FSV, B.619, 3.10.1651.

[123] 'Con intenzione di andare un pocho a spasso et fare essercitio.' ASR, TCG, Costituti, 457, 2.10.1596, 32r.

[124] 'Le lettere non portano buone notizie della salute di VS, inappetenza, sete grande e aver bisogno di pillole. Non dovrebbe affaticare il corpo e la mente e dovrebbe far scrivere dall'abate e fare delle caminate che Dio sa VS non ne ha fatte piú alcuna.' ASR, FSV, B.607, 15.3.1659.

172 *Healthy Living in Late Renaissance Italy*

better'.[125] While Maria is reluctant to do so, other members of the family, like her son Bernardino, aged 23, seem to take the injunction to perform exercise every day very seriously: during a long stay with his newly widowed sister in Viterbo he is said to spend the day reading and taking walks in the evening.[126] Similarly Orazio writing from Castel Viscardo informs his wife that his companion Fra' Giunipero 'is in the best of spirits and takes exercise every day with no fear of gout, only sometimes with displeasure at the wind'.[127]

Whether complying with it or not, people saw walking regularly as a duty. The message found in regimens that exercise should be a daily occurrence seems to have been interiorized, as proven by the many justifications for not exercising found in the correspondence. Replying to an inquiry from her worried mother Eugenia admits that her husband 'has put on some weight but not so much that it can displease, he exercises every morning when the weather is fine and he also gets up early'.[128] And in relation to herself she confesses that she is not too fond of exercise *but* then this is not yet the time (the weather is not suitable?) since it has been raining for nigh on a week, *but* when it is possible she shall do what she can.[129]

These quotes also betray the strong connection between exercise, the warmer seasons, and good weather. Indeed bad weather is regularly signalled in letters as a major factor that reduced people's mobility and hence their opportunities to exercise. Severe wind or copious rain and the fear of getting wet forced them to stay at home for days; the practice of paying regular visits to kin and friends was interrupted and the family had to resort to domestic entertainment.[130] It is striking how the weather affects the life of this aristocratic family—even mass is said at home in times of fierce rain.[131] But even at a lower social level bad weather is perceived as a reason for staying put and indoors. This is a theme for example in several entries of the mid-sixteenth-century diary kept by the painter Pontormo: 'Thursday morning I got up early but when I saw how bad the weather and wind were I did not work and remained at home'; 'Wednesday morning was cold and I stayed at home.'[132] The advice found in educational treatises, that 'in bad weather it is better to stay indoors than to take exercise outside...you know the reasons why and you will find them out from the physicians', is closely echoed in these records.[133]

---

[125] 'perché l'esercitio le giova piú di qualsivoglia medicamento...di che vado a piedi tutta la mattina sto assai meglio e piú anche adesso che ho cavato il sesto dente che fu hier mattina.' ASR, FSV, B.607, 2.8.1661.
[126] 'Il sig. Bernardino non parla più di andar via e io lo compatisco che qua non ha nulla di svario e passa tutta la giornata in leggere e la sera va a camminare.' ASR, FSV, B.1115, 7.9.1662.
[127] 'sta allegramente e fa esercizio ogni giorno e non teme di podagra solamente gli dispiace qualche volta il vento.' ASR, FSV, B.607, 25.3.1659. In another letter he refers again to the friar as a model for his wife, admonishing her that she should do exercise frequently; B.607, 1.4.1659.
[128] 'si è ingrassato è vero ma non tanto che possa dispiacere, esercitio quando è bontempo lo fa ogni mattina e anco si leva di buonora.' ASR, FSV, B.410, 11.4.1657.
[129] 'l'esercizio non le piace troppo e poi adesso non è ancora tempo che son una mano di giorni che sempre piove ma quando se potrà farò quel che posso ...'; ASR, FSV, B.410, 13.9.1656.
[130] e.g. ASR, FSV, B.1115, 2.11.1666, 9.11.1666, 14.11.1660; B.410, 11.9.1656; and B.607, 6.8.1661.
[131] ASR, FSV, B.410, 19.11.1656.
[132] Pontormo, *Diario*, 22 and 27, entries 21.3.1554 and 17.4.1554.
[133] Lombardelli, *Il giovane studente*, 39.

Outdoor exercise is therefore seasonal, largely relegated to the warmer seasons, but in cities it is also difficult to perform in good weather due to the heat and to the dusty roads that also restrict movement.[134] Moreover, the habit of going about in a carriage is ingrained: by the seventeenth century this is the usual means of transport for well-off men and women alike. Orazio's walks in Rome are occurrences rare enough to be recorded in letters. Gender prejudices make exercise in cities particularly unlikely for well-off women who, for reasons of decorum, cannot go out on foot but only in carriages and only accompanied either by an elderly woman of their rank or by a mature married or widowed maid entrusted to watch over their mistress's reputation and clearly identifiable by the veil they wore.[135] When Eugenia's matron quits her service this poses real limitations to Eugenia's movements and the urgent need to find another suitable companion occupies considerable space in her correspondence with her mother.[136] Things get even more complicated in the numerous periods in which women are pregnant. Letters make clear that 'exercise' meaning walking is highly recommended in the ninth month but completely banned at the beginning of a pregnancy: Marchesa Vittoria (Maria's daughter-in-law), who suspects that she is pregnant, does not leave the house.[137] In the early stages of a pregnancy exercise is understood as damaging the foetus: 'there is no news regarding the pregnancy, and until I can be sure that I am not I cannot exercise, and now it seems that whenever I move about a little I have some spots of bleeding again, and this week I have had it twice even if I take none'.[138] As for the intermediate months the advice seems contradictory. Eugenia is constantly rebuked by her mother for going out either too much or too little. Her husband is also very anxious about her movements: he does not want her to travel in a carriage and fears she could fall even when walking, hence visits to the villa are also banned.[139] Things do not seem to have changed a great deal since the late sixteenth century: in a letter written in October 1593 Giulia Veralli, pregnant, reassures her husband that, 'As for my going out, be assured that I do not fail to obey you, for I never leave the house … and were it not for the matter of coming here to the new house I should not have stirred out at all.'[140] As a result pregnant women of the higher orders are confined to the house for very long stretches of time. There were times during the frequent periods in which she was pregnant when Eugenia did not leave the house for up to fifteen days, and periods in which she only went out on Sunday, to go to church.

---

[134] ASR, FSV, B.1115, 9.10.1669.

[135] In Rome this figure took the name of *matrona* but elsewhere in Italy *citella* or *donna di velo e di rispetto* because she wore a veil. Spinola, cited in Gallo, 'Le livree', 79.

[136] ASR, FSV, B.410, 27.9.1656, 10.10.1656, and 31.3.1657.

[137] ASR, FSV, B.618, 20.9.1678.

[138] 'della gravidanza non c'è niente di novo e sino che non mi asicuro di non essere non posso fare esercitio, e adesso pare che quando fo un poco di moto mi torni un poco di segno quando apariscie e questa settimana l'ho avuto due volte e pure io mene astengo.' ASR, FSV, B.1115, 3.8.1661.

[139] ASR, FSV. B.410, 3.1.1656.

[140] 'Circa al mio uscire, sappia che non manco di obbedirla perché non esco di casa … et se non fosse stato l'occasione del venire qui alla casa nova non mi sarei mossa.' ASR, FSV, B.449, 23.10.1593.

When going out was impossible galleries and picture galleries offered the patricians, including the Spadas, the opportunity to exercise indoors. As recently outlined by art historians, galleries in the Italian palace evolved in the sixteenth century from the open loggia and portico, and were designed with the explicit purpose of providing a space for walking when the weather was cold.[141] Their value for health was stressed by architects like Serlio and Scamozzi who highlighted the positive effects on both the body and the mind of contemplating cheerful paintings often representing landscapes, and the sight of plants while walking back and forth along these structures (see Plate 17).[142] In the case of galleries of antiquities the experience of strolling in these spaces offered a full immersion in the vestiges of ancient civilizations that equally delighted the soul.[143]

But galleries were also a flexible space and at certain times of the day could become the theatre of more mundane physical activities like children's play and exercise. For example, the gallery of the Maidalchini palace in Viterbo offered the young Count Innocenzo a space where he could experiment with walking and running on his own under the proud and amused eyes of his mother and her *donne*.[144]

Especially in the case of women, however, exercise mainly took place in the villa that most well-off families owned, by 1600, in the countryside or on the hills surrounding the city, during the long season of the *villeggiatura* (this in Rome lasted from May to the end of October). There is plenty of evidence that *villeggiatura* represented for women an opportunity to take physical exercise and for a less segregated style of life. In October 1659 Maria Spada writes from Tivoli that she is happy to send back the carriage, she will only need it for returning to Rome 'since here she enjoys walking'.[145] A few years later, her daughter Eugenia, writing from Giove (a locality still regarded as one of the hidden gems of central Italy), where her newly married second husband held his land, recounts how 'On Wednesday, all morning and then the afternoon we went out and about around these avenues which are truly beautiful, some way in the carriage and some way on foot.'[146] In another letter she comments that 'the place is very beautiful and there are lovely walks'.[147]

But shady walkways, courtyards, and porticoes were not intended purely for the benefit of their owners. David Coffin has shown how all or part of the gardens surrounding the great villas built in and around Rome were often intended for use by the public, as a place to walk and take the air. Latin inscriptions placed over the public entrance and on the walls confirmed this ideal of offering open access for all, provided they respected the grounds.[148] Those living in Rome and not privileged enough to own a villa could therefore take their exercise by walking in the magnificent gardens which surrounded villas such as that of Cardinal Caraffa on the

---

[141] Frommel, 'Galleria'.   [142] Gage, 'Exercise', esp. 1172 and 1188; and Prinz, *Galleria*.
[143] On galleries of antiquities, see Riebesell, 'Sulla genesi delle gallerie'.
[144] ASR, FSV, B.1115, 31.7.1658.
[145] 'che qua a lei piace camminare'; ASR, FSV, B.619, 17.10.1659.
[146] 'Il mercoledì tanto la mattina come il giorno si andò a spasso per questi stradoni che veramente son belli e si andò un pezzo in carrozza e un pezzo a piedi.' ASR, FSV, B.1115, 23.10.1666.
[147] ASR, FSV, B.1115, 16.10.1666.   [148] Coffin, *Magnificent Buildings*, 164–89.

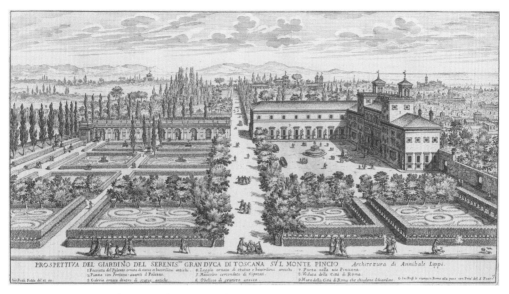

Fig. 5.8. From the sixteenth century villas were provided with formal gardens that included long *viali* (avenues lined with plane trees) where residents and guests could walk sheltered from the sun.

Esquiline Hill, Palazzo Cesi in the Borgo, Villa Giulia, Villa Borghese, or, further afield, Villa Lante at Bagnaia and Villa d'Este at Tivoli (see Fig. 5.8). This trend continued well into the seventeenth century.[149] Moreover, the hilltops preferred as locations for *villeggiatura* also included *viali* where walkers could stroll contemplating nature and enjoying nice views of the countryside.[150]

The countryside could therefore be a destination for groups of women, also for day outings from the city: in September 1678 for example, Maria, now 62 years old, went to walk with the nuns and her daughter Eugenia to the Balduina, a locality on the southern side of Monte Mario, the highest part of Rome. Both young and elderly, lay and religious women (in spite of the prohibitions against leaving the convent!) were therefore seeing the benefits of walking in the country and greatly enjoyed it.[151] As we see in Chapter 6 a specific expression even designated this type of exercise: *moto di campagna* (country movement), good for health on account not just of the physical movement but also of the positive emotions the contact with the pure air and the beautiful landscape of the countryside would foster. Ready-made female shoes specific 'for walking' (*da camminare*) also seem to have existed. In 1657 Eugenia asks her mother in Rome to provide her

[149] Russell, 'Girolamo Mercuriale's *De arte gymnastica*'.

[150] See e.g. the letter in which a mixed group of younger and older ladies and their maids take the fresh air along a *viale* more than a quarter-mile long. ASR, FSV, B.491, 9.5.1638; and Coffin, *The Villa d'Este*, 11, 14.

[151] ASR, FSV, B.618, 28.9.1678.

with a pair of such shoes.[152] Historians of fashion have stressed the constraints imposed upon women's mobility not just by restrictions dictated by reasons of decorum and modesty but by a craze for impractical footwear that obliged them to walk on platform shoes (chopines or *pianelle*) clearly unsuited for long walks, and, later, on high heels. The evidence from letters, however, complicates the picture, suggesting that more comfortable female shoes were also used by gentlewomen.[153] The inventory of one early seventeenth-century prostitute who left the profession to enter a convent shows that she owned a range of types of shoe: she had two pairs of 'felt slippers', two pairs of 'Spanish shoes', four pairs of the raised *pianelle*, and finally two pairs of 'women's shoes' which perhaps were unremarkable practical shoes.[154] Clearly, these more prosaic examples of footwear have not been preserved in museum collections but elements of it have been recovered in archaeological excavations.[155]

Walking was therefore enjoyed as an extremely common pastime, and understood as providing exercise, whether for the body or as 'recreation' for the soul. And by the mid-seventeenth century, walking for the sake of doing exercise was a frequent occurrence even for women, in spite of the various restrictions that decorum and modesty imposed upon their movement. Letters reveal how women had appropriated this activity and followed the rare exhortations found in the medical literature that they should walk. It is worth noting that this contrasts with the instructions found in conduct literature which indicated that household chores were the most appropriate exercise for women. The tradition of household management books systematically promoted the idea, even the enlightened religious reformer Aonio Paleario (1503–70) argued in his mid-sixteenth-century treatise that in cities 'young women...should in the morning, after prayers, take exercise by tidying up the room, making the bed, shaking out clothes, brushing their father's, mother's, and brothers' clothes'.[156] Nearly eighty years later the treatise published in 1629 by Bishop Frigerio but still reprinted in the 1650s, reiterated that women's appetite, health, and beauty would benefit greatly from their doing moderate physical exercise at home such as 'drawing water, sometimes washing linen, making bread, shaking out clothes, tidying up, inspecting the house'.[157] People of the time however did not conflate women's exercise and domestic work. The distinction emerges with evidence in the letter that Orazio, in Rome, writes to his wife in their villa in Tivoli in July 1661: 'If the days were a whole week they

---

[152] ASR, FSV, B.410, 12.12.1657.

[153] Semmelhack, *On a Pedestal*; and Laughran and Vianello, '*Grandissima gratia*'.

[154] Beatrice Mendoza Hispana, ASVR, MCI, vol. 198 (Vecchia Segnatura), 1605–6, 5.4.1605.

[155] Melli (ed.), *La città ritrovata*, 146–8 and 150–4.

[156] 'le fanciulle...perchè sieno sane e gagliarde e atte alla generazione...in città potranno la mattina dopo le orazioni esercitarsi assettando la camera, facendo il letto, scuotendo i panni, spazzando la vesta del padre, della madre, dei fratelli e appresso desinare che avranno letto e scritto, e fatta alcuna ragione, consumare il resto del giorno e buona parte della notte coll'ago e col fuso.' Paleario, *Dell'economia*, 64.

[157] 'Le donne, se faranno moderati esercizi corporali in casa come cavar acqua, lavar talvolta le biancherie, fare il pane, scuoter le vesti, tener in ordine, visitar la casa e simili mangeranno con più appetito, saranno più sane e pareranno più giovani e belle.' Frigerio, *Arte*, 41.

would seem short to Your Ladyship since she likes to do in a day what takes a whole week but if she does not take a little exercise in the morning and the evening Your Ladyship will not feel the benefit of this air that in the experience of other years exercise has marvellously given her. But if she goes for a walk in the morning before settling down to work and considers that she has risen an hour later, so in the evening she may imagine that night has fallen a little earlier and everything will go well with her.'[158]

The health benefits of walking gave women an opportunity to expand the extremely limited range of exercise options considered appropriate for them by physicians and the writers of conduct literature and they enthusiastically embraced it. This presents a picture very different from that which emerges from recent histories of walking and footwear based on English and French sources. These have suggested that prior to the eighteenth century walking was neither considered as having any health connotations, nor as an appropriate activity for members of the upper classes, associated as it was with being too poor to ride in a carriage.[159] Furthermore, it is argued that poorly maintained roads, lack of pavements, and fears of encountering people from the lower orders discouraged and restricted the mobility of pedestrians around early modern cities.[160] By 1600 however, in Italian cities such as Rome men and women frequently took walks, whether in the gardens of their villas, the galleries of their palaces, or around town. Even in the city itself new spaces were designed for walking. In the seventeenth century considerations of health and comfort led Pope Alexander VII to order the planting of huge numbers of trees even along the streets and piazze of Rome to protect pilgrims, visitors, 'street sellers', and those going out for their evening strolls from the hot sun.[161]

CONCLUSION

As correctly perceived by critical commentators such as Longiano, commonly held definitions of exercise were profoundly modified in the sixteenth century and early decades of the seventeenth century to accommodate new patterns of gentility. The new idea of the male body elaborated in conduct literature for gentlefolk justified the abandonment of strenuous forms of exercise or at least their transformation into spectacle and choreographed celebrations of class identity. The emergence of socially exclusive new sports, such as *trucco* and golf, which as well as being less physically demanding, were performed in socially segregated spaces and in ways that symbolically expressed class distinctions, further widened the gulf between

[158] 'Se i giorni fossero una settimana intiera a VS riuscirebbero corti perché ella vuol fare in un giorno quello che porta tempo una settimana intiera ma se non fa un po' di *esercizio* la mattina e la sera VS non sentirá il beneficio di questa'aria che pure per l'esperienza degli altri anni esercisio le conferisce mirabilmente. Pero' vada a camminare la mattina prima di mettersi al lavoro e faccia conto d'essersi levata un'hora piú tardi, cosí la sera si figuri che si sia fato notte un poco prima e le riuscirá ogni cosa'; ASR, FSV, B.607, 24.7.1661.

[159] Riello, *A Foot in the Past*, 60–2.

[160] McNeil and G. Riello, 'The Art', 177–9.   [161] Krautheimer, 'Roma'.

plebeian and aristocratic pastimes. Definitions of exercise now praised activities, such as dance, that conferred elegance and grace on the body of the aristocrat. Though some of these transformations were also occurring elsewhere they seem to have taken place particularly early in Italy.[162] The early development of a genteel, urban culture, conversant with courtly values, and long detached from military ideals, provided the context for the emergence of what many saw as a debased notion of exercise, no longer a preparation for war but increasingly social entertainment. The religiously inspired educational treatises that also flourished in the second half of the sixteenth century gave another slant to this process, emphasizing ideals of *gravitas* that made vigorous movement particularly incompatible with the physical dignity expected in men of quality, especially of mature age. From the mid-sixteenth century medical advice about exercise was also subtly redefining its paradigms, placing a greater emphasis on gentle movement and on the dangers that energetic exercise represented for the refined body of the gentleman. Only those aged between 21 and 35 were unreservedly encouraged to engage in more demanding physical activities, and even then there were many exceptions. Compared to their medieval predecessors, doctors also stretched the boundaries of what constituted effective exercise, praising the advantages of exercising eyes, mouth, and chest through singing and speaking loud, and the limbs through dancing. They increasingly promoted gestational movement as a valid form of exercise for all, thus legitimizing the habit of riding by carriage or litter rather than on horseback that was becoming increasingly common among the prosperous classes. And by depicting walking as the most appropriate form of moderate exercise, irrespective of age, gender, and class, they gave impetus to the fashion for walking which, within a matter of decades, was enthusiastically embraced by both men and women.

The comparison of regimens, conduct literature, and letters thus highlights a relationship of mutual influence between change in medical attitudes to exercise, new models of male physicality, and new customs developing in society. Although medical ideas were affected by general shifts in values and by change in the actual customs of the leisured classes, it is also worth noting that this was a two-way exchange: lay testimonies present an understanding of the notion of 'exercise' and its effects on the physiology of the body and its health that is profoundly affected by the language and contents of the medical advice literature. The dangers of immoderate exercise however were conceptualized in lay narratives in terms that actually exacerbated the tones found in the medical discourse: laypeople seem to have taken to the extreme the recommendations of doctors to avoid energetic exercise, especially in adulthood, and exaggerated the potentially damaging effects of overheating the body and the blood. As a result their attitude towards physical activity was extremely cautious: once married, all that was left for them was to go for walks for their exercise. Even within these limits however, one should note that the medical injunction to exercise regularly, even if just in the form of walking, was taken very seriously, by men and women alike.

---

[162] Tlusty, *The Martial Ethic*, ch. 7.

6

The Well-Tempered Man

In 1550 a new regimen appeared for the Italian market written in conversational style, as a dialogue between a certain Theophrastus, and his friend Poligolo.[1] Aptly named after the eminent Greek physician, Theophrastus is the principal speaker as he takes it upon himself to explain to Poligolo the importance of adopting a healthy lifestyle if he wants to avoid premature death. Theophrastus then works his way systematically through the Non-Naturals until he finally reaches what he calls 'the sixth thing, the accidents of the soul, called passions by the ancient Greeks'. At this point Poligolo interjects, not without some irritation since he is clearly getting rather bored, and demands to know what the passions have got to do with the rules of healthy living. Theophrastus patiently replies that they are very important 'because they conserve or destroy health', adding just a little despondently 'which is what we have just been talking about'. Poligolo's perplexity as to why the passions should have any bearing on the topic of health is intriguing. As a rhetorical device it appears to be an attempt by the author to 'hook' the reader, enabling him to identify with the character, by reassuring him that he is not alone in being mystified by the link between passions and health. This suggests that it was perhaps considered by the author to be a hard topic for readers to grasp and possibly less obviously connected to health than the other Non-Naturals, or merely that the topic was less well known. Certainly, he shows a consideration for his readers which was not shown by all our authors as they tackled an issue which by the mid-sixteenth century was fraught with complexities and contradictions.

The relationship between the so-called 'passions of the soul' and the health of the body had been explored since antiquity by physicians, moral philosophers, and subsequently, by theologians. Each discipline contributed substantially to early modern understandings of the strong correlation between body and soul, providing physicians with a range of techniques and 'languages' for describing and managing what we would call 'emotions', but which were then known mainly as 'accidents', 'perturbations', 'affects', or 'passions' of the soul, according to one's frame of reference.[2] One of the key challenges for physicians in sixteenth- and seventeenth-century Italy lay in reconciling these different traditions which apportioned varying degrees of importance to the role played by bodily (somatic) qualities in disturbances of the soul.

---

[1] Pictorius, *Dialogi*, 75–6.
[2] On the idea of these different 'languages' for discussing mental states see J. Schmidt, *Melancholy*, 4.

The Galenic medical tradition understood the passions as being caused by changes to the balance of humours within the body, or alterations to inner heat caused by the movements of spirits as they reacted to external events or objects. A renewed interest in Galenism coupled with Vesalian anatomy over the sixteenth century led to more materialist explanations of the spirits and their operations, as physicians sought to locate the spirits in relation to the organs—head, heart, and liver—and to identify their passage through the body, whether via the blood or nerves. Coupled with this was uncertainty about how to describe these spirits. Whether they were material or immaterial; whether 'vapours' of the blood or a material part of the soul; and whether the spirits were merely the instruments of the intellective and immortal soul or, as was increasingly being argued by physicians, were actually part of the organic soul. The Galenic view was already a worryingly 'materialist' explanation for the emotions, but one of the implications of this new understanding was that the emotions were driven by physiology, not by the intellect and reason; and that there was therefore a separate 'material' soul linked to the specific individual, rather than just an immortal, 'intellective' soul.[3]

These views also came into direct conflict with the teaching of the Catholic Church on the nature of the soul. Based on the teachings of Aristotle, elaborated by St Augustine and St Thomas Aquinas, the Church asserted that there was only one immortal, immaterial soul which could be divided into three parts; ruling all was the intellective rational soul; below this was the animal or sensitive soul responsible for sense perceptions and 'appetites'; most lowly of all the vegetative or nutritive soul, governing growth and generation. According to this scheme there was broad agreement that the passions could be divided into 'inappropriate passions of the lower appetite directed towards worldly objects and appropriate affections, or movements of the will, directed towards goodness, truth and, ultimately God'.[4] So although there was but one soul, this was an account which stressed the duality of mind and body and saw the passions and appetites in extremely negative terms, as rebellious and disobedient, over which the rational and moral part of the soul had to assert its authority.[5]

The moral philosophy of the Stoics offered the third of the most influential accounts of the passions. The philosophical teachings of the Hellenistic school known as the Stoics had been transmitted by early Christian theologians, through the newly published writings of Seneca, Cicero, and Plutarch and then popularized by the Flemish philosopher Lipsius, with the publication in Latin in 1584 of his 'Book of Constancy'. Stoics were deeply concerned by a desire to control the passions for the benefit of the health of the soul. They saw common emotional responses not as physiological movements of the spirits (like Galen) nor as involuntary and rebellious movements of the soul (Augustine and Aquinas) but as 'mistaken value judgements', 'evils' of opinion, or 'tempests' of the soul, to be calmed through

---

[3] For an account of the organic soul see Park, 'The Organic Soul'.

[4] We draw here on Thomas Dixon's account of classical Christian psychology in *From Passions*, 26–46; this sentence is based on St Aquinas, quoted at p. 27.

[5] Dixon, *From Passions*, 29.

willpower, in the quest for peace of mind.[6] It was the duty of the rational man, who hoped to attain 'tranquillity' or constancy of the soul, to temper these 'judgements'. Thus in order to avoid sorrow he should cultivate indifference, accept his fate calmly, expect the worst, avoid ambition, and avoid pursuit of material and worldly success. In Christian neo-Stoicism these often extreme views were tempered by Christian faith and religious devotional practice. One should turn to Christ for solace, as the source of true comfort; accept misfortune as an expression of God's will; and ask for God's help in accepting one's lot in life.

Corresponding to these three understandings of the passions, we also have three potentially different approaches to management of the soul. One medical, based broadly on managing the body's physiology and spirits; one religious, intent on disciplining and dominating the rebellious appetites; and one philosophical, based on redirecting ones thoughts and bringing the 'passions' under the 'strict control of the intellect'.[7] There was however much blurring between the latter two approaches as Counter-Reformation theology and practice, driven particularly by the Jesuits, focused extensively on cultivating self-discipline through control of the imagination and the passions (which were seen as closely linked) as part of the religious devotion of both laity and clergy alike.[8]

Given the range of the authorities which contributed to debates on the passions and the delicacy of the questions central to these debates, it is not surprising to find evidence of some confusion in the regimens. Indeed, as the sixteenth century progressed, medical accounts of the passions of the soul became more complicated, riven by internal contradictions and inconsistencies, as physicians sought to reconcile the reinvigorated Galenic tradition with the demands of Catholic orthodoxy, overlain with Stoic and Catholic techniques for emotional control. In this chapter we will outline the Galenic explanation for the impact of the passions on the body and health, before discussing the range of techniques offered by the regimens for managing the passions and explore the extent to which the Church and neo-Stoicism influenced the advice given by physicians. We also question the importance of melancholy in discussions by Italian physicians. In the second half of the chapter we shift the focus to cheerfulness; examining advice given on how readers could promote *allegrezza* and asking whether and how these recommendations were implemented and incorporated into daily life.

LINKING 'ACCIDENTS OF THE SOUL' TO ILLNESS

The terms 'accidents', 'perturbations', and 'affects' of the soul, which tended to be used by medical writers even until the seventeenth century, corresponded to the Galenic principle by which the vital spirits reacted to external objects or events in

---

[6] Kraye, 'The Revival', esp. 99–102 (101); Kraye, 'Moral Philosophy', esp. 364–74 (372); Kraye, 'Philologists and Philosophers', esp. 151–2; and Dixon, *From Passions*, 50.

[7] Dixon, *From Passions*, 51; Kraye 'Philologists and Philosophers', 152.

[8] On Jesuit discipline and Loyola's spiritual exercises see Janelle, *The Catholic Reformation*, 124–35.

a predictable and essentially 'passive' manner.[9] The number of 'accidents of the soul' discussed and the order in which they were presented in regimens varied.[10] Benzi's early regimen gives the following fairly comprehensive list: love/hate; cheerfulness/desperation; desire/fear; hope/anger; compassion/fury; courage/boredom; hate/envy; and sadness/jealousy.[11] However, some might only mention cheerfulness, anger, fright, fear, melancholy, and envy.[12]

Explanations of the accidents of the soul in regimens focused on the movements of the spirits and in particular their relationship with the heart.[13] The spirits transmitted heat and vitality around the body, and were therefore responsible for the temperature of the heart which, as the body's 'furnace', should ideally always be maintained at a constant temperature. The spirits however were believed to be very volatile and at the slightest provocation from 'accidents' they changed their behaviour, albeit in predictable ways, and it was these changes in movement of the spirits which resulted in the bodily symptoms associated with fear, anger, joy, and so on. Whilst most authors considered that in moderation the passions were generally healthy, because they stimulated the spirits, all viewed long-term or sudden reactions of the spirits as potentially being very dangerous, resulting in fluctuations in the temperature of the heart which, if moderate, triggered illness but if severe could result in sudden death known as *morte subitanea*.[14] Conveying this to readers was one of their main concerns, as they illustrated their point with grim tales of sudden death caused by joy, sorrow, and anger drawn from classical antiquity.

According to Galenic physiology, however, the movements of the spirits were secondary to one's underlying constitutional, humoral predisposition.[15] As explained by Lennio for example, the ideal complexion, with evenly balanced humours, gave a 'well-tempered' person whose spirits would not react too quickly nor too extremely to emotional triggers. Excessive choler made the body hot and dry, making for a more fiery, inflammable character, rather like straw, one author explained, which catches fire quickly, but also quickly burns out. Those with excessive black bile were slower to anger and clung to their anger, because the bile was dry and cold, and they were known as melancholics. The phlegmatic, their heads filled with cold damp phlegm, were barely able to sense any 'motions of the soul', which explained why they remained so unmoved; it was also thought to be a sign of their lack of intellect and perhaps not coincidentally, women were generally associated with this complexion. Finally those with excess blood, the sanguine, were filled with damp heat, which predisposed them to fun, parties, and pleasures.[16] In addition

---

[9] This insight from the introductory essay on the passions by García Ballester and McVaugh in their edition of Arnaldi, *Regimen sanitatis*, 803.

[10] According to Dixon, there has 'rarely been any consensus on the number of passions…nor which of them are principal', and this also holds true for our regimens; *From Passions*, 18.

[11] Benzi, *Tractato utilissimo*, 35–6.

[12] e.g. in Pictorius.

[13] See Bound Alberti, 'Emotions', 1–21, esp. 3–7.

[14] For a comprehensive discussion of changing understandings of sudden death see Donato, *Morti improvvise*.

[15] Bos, 'The Rise and Decline', esp. 36–7.

[16] This summary is based on Lennio, *De gli occulti miracoli*, 55–7.

to these underlying predispositions the body might also experience temporary humoral imbalances. The heat of the summer produced more *collera* in the body, the autumn was feared since it led to excessive production of black bile, and in winter the cold weather could result in closing of the pores, which trapped humours within the body, leading to their putrefaction and excessive amounts of phlegm. In all these cases the resulting overproduction of certain humours weakened the body and spirits, making them more likely to overreact to external stimuli and more vulnerable to the effects of accidents of the soul.

In addition to the individual's constitution, the acute reactions of the spirits were understood as falling into two broad categories, those which involved a withdrawing inward towards the heart, such as fear and sorrow, and those which caused a moving outwards, away from the heart, as in joy and anger. All the other 'accidents' such as pride and shame were explained in similar ways, but as composed of varying combinations of centrifugal and centripetal forces. In joy and anger the movement of the spirits away from the heart resulted in increased body heat and vitality, accounting for example for the flushed colour of the cheeks. However, it was widely thought that excessive hilarity or joy could overstep the limits of health, causing the spirits to rush so excitedly out of the body that they left it denuded and empty of spirits. This loss of heat and vitality would lead to a sudden chilling down of the body and heart, possibly resulting in sudden death.[17] Likewise, whilst the gentle heat brought on by mild anger was thought quite healthy, prolonged anger was linked to a drying-out of the body, leading to white hair and wrinkles. More dangerously, extremes of rage and fury caused the spirits to heat up so much that they became inflamed, to the extent that the heart could actually catch fire with fatal consequences.[18] (See Fig. 6.1.)

In emotions such as fear, sorrow, and melancholy the spirits reacted in the opposite way. When presented with something fearful the spirits recoiled immediately back into the heart, thereby constricting it. This resulted in a loss of spirit movement, depriving the body of vital heat and causing the pallor, chill, and stillness associated with fear and sorrow. Indeed, in extreme cases fear caused the blood to freeze so rapidly that it resulted at best in temporary paralysis of the limbs and at worst the fleeing spirits suffocated the heart, extinguishing its flame totally which caused sudden death. These explanations presumably account for the expressions still in use today, such as 'I froze with fear' and 'I nearly died of fright'. Moreover fear was regarded as being particularly dangerous in children because their constitutions are weaker, so their bodies were more vulnerable to fright. This could result in earache, joint pains, and fevers, and therefore had implications for child-rearing advice. Two authors warned that children should never be frightened and adults should coax them and defer to them rather than try to threaten them.[19]

The ideal state for a healthy body was therefore one in which the spirits travelled around the body in a calm, peaceful, but purposeful way—distributing natural heat evenly throughout the body. The only accident of the soul which corresponded

---

[17] Petronio's *Del viver* was unusual in its refutation of the dangers of *allegrezza*.
[18] Anguillara, *Vaticinio*, 24.
[19] See Petronio, *Del viver*, 265; Fonseca, *Del conservare*, 113.

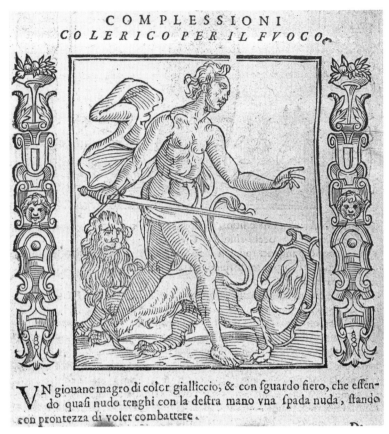

Fig. 6.1. A representation of 'Colerico' (Anger) from Ripa's emblem book for artists (1st edn. 1593). He cites Galen to explain that the youth is thin because the heat of his body—symbolized by the flame on his shield—has dried him out. This distemper leaves him vulnerable to sudden reactions of the spirits carrying heat, leading to impetuous, unpremeditated actions, denoted by the drawn sword and his nakedness.

to this model was called *allegrezza*, which we could translate as cheerfulness or happiness or mirth. It was understood as a calm, tranquil happiness, the result of something which 'delighted' the spirits, making them 'expand towards the outer parts of the body' so as to embrace it, in which movement the spirits gently heated the body.[20] *Allegrezza* also increased the total number of spirits in the body, thereby increasing overall body heat and vitality.

Cheerfulness has been widely neglected in historical scholarship on emotions, which has tended to focus on the socially disruptive states of anger and pride, or on melancholy, which in the course of the sixteenth and seventeenth centuries came to be seen as the most problematic of the 'accidents of the soul' to prevent and cure.[21] However,

[20] Based on Traffichetti, *L'arte*, 117–18.
[21] The most relevant discussion of *allegrezza* in this medical context is Ludke Finney, 'Music'.

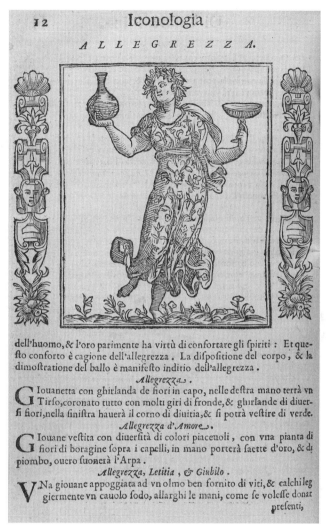

Fig. 6.2. A representation of 'Allegrezza' (Mirth) from Ripa's emblem book for artists (1st edn. 1593). He explains that the glass of red wine alludes to red wine's power to 'cheer men's hearts' and the gold of the goblet comforts the spirits, both producing mirth. He adds that musical instruments and dance may be included in the iconography.

medically speaking *allegrezza* was the ideal 'default' emotion for the body, both as general health preservative and as a remedy and its significance should not be underestimated since it was ultimately the goal of all the advice on the management of the passions. As one author writes in its praise: '*Allegrezza*...is consolation and repose...filling the body with good nourishment keeping the senses vigorous, conserving the intellect whole, maintaining and increasing health and prolonging life.'[22] (See Fig. 6.2.)

---

[22] '*Allegrezza è... consolatione, eriposo...empie il corpo di bonissimo nutrimento, tiene vigorosi tutti li sensi, conserva intiero tutto l'intelletto, mantiene, e accresce La sanità, e prolonga La vita.*' Petronio, *Del viver*, 348.

MELANCHOLY

The state known as melancholy in some ways resembles what is now termed 'depression', but it had its own complex symptoms and pathology. Melancholy was feared particularly because it took various forms, was a chronic condition associated with a range of somatic disorders, and was considered extremely difficult if not impossible to remedy, unlike extremes of joy, anger, shame, and fear which were generally more acute and transitory problems.[23] As well as resulting from humoral imbalances, fear and sorrow could act as triggers, since they both led to lessening of spirit movement, causing mental and bodily torpor. This resulted in cooling and drying of the body which if prolonged provoked melancholy. Excessive crying impeded the digestion and resulted in spirit loss, impairing the functions of the brain and in cases of extreme and sudden grief the movement of the spirits could actually suffocate the heart, another cause of sudden death.[24] (See Fig. 6.3.)

Although there were discussions of melancholy in ancient texts and melancholy had been mentioned in late medieval regimens, it was not dealt with extensively until the 1489 Latin publication of Ficino's *De vita libri tres*. This was a healthy-living guide which instructed elderly scholars on how to avoid succumbing to melancholy and was to become the standard reference work on the subject. Ficino explained that melancholy was principally produced by excessive black bile (known as 'the other bile'), which is 'always pestilent and abominable' and was caused particularly by a sedentary lifestyle, lack of sleep, and overexertion of the mind.[25] It was associated with the drying and cooling of the body and loss of vital heat, compounding tendencies already present in the bodies of the elderly. Excessive black bile also obscured the intellect and animal spirits and weakened the brain, with clear implications for scholars and intellectuals. Ficino devotes twenty-four of the twenty-six chapters of his regimen to suggesting ways of avoiding or mitigating its terrible effects whilst he only briefly describes a 'very rare' form of 'natural bile' which, drawing on Aristotle, is described as beneficial to the intellect, discussed in two short chapters.[26] Much has subsequently been made of these allusions to the links between melancholy and 'men of genius', contributing to the fascination of the topic for historians not only of medicine, but of literature, music, and art. It is also used to explain melancholy as a 'popular' and 'fashionable' ailment in the late

---

[23] Although there were chronic conditions linked to other states: anger for example could become vendetta. There were three main kinds of melancholy, many subspecies, and many linked disorders which gave physicians grounds for much speculation, most famously in Robert Burton's *Anatomy of Melancholy* (1621). There is a vast bibliography on the topic from differing perspectives. We have consulted Gowland, *The Worlds*; J. Schmidt, *Melancholy*; Carrera, 'Understanding Mental Disturbance'; and Carrera, 'Madness'.

[24] See e.g. [Maineri], *Opera utilissima*, 47–9; Durante, *Il tesoro*, 44–5; and Paschetti, *Del conservar*, 228.

[25] 'Percio che ella è cosi pestifera, e abominevole', Ficino, *De le tre vite*, 8ʳ.

[26] For the beneficial effects and the links with great minds, Ficino, *De le tre vite*, 4ᵛ–8ʳ. Aristotle observed that great statesmen, philosophers, and authors were melancholic or suffered from black bile in his so-called *Problemata*, 30.1; *Aristotle on the Parts*, 376–85. Kaske and Clark however consider that Ficino writes 'at length' about the positive intellectual value of melancholy; see their edition of Ficino, *Three Books on Life*, 6–12.

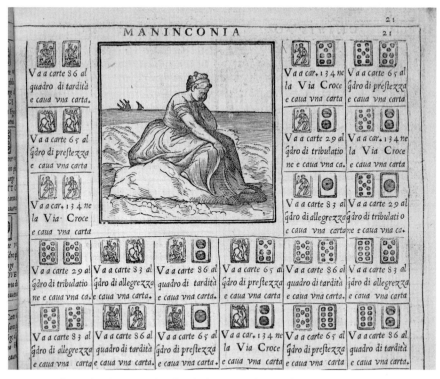

Fig. 6.3. This stylized image of Melancholy was used as an illustration in a 1550 collection of games of chance. The boat in the background alludes to Christian notions of melancholy as a state in which the soul is adrift without a helmsman.

sixteenth and seventeenth centuries. This, along with the publication of treatises on the topic in England, Spain, and France, has led to a characterization of the period by some as an 'age of melancholy'.[27]

However, our study of discussions of melancholy in Italian regimens does not support the perception that there were any positive aspects to melancholy (i.e. genius), nor that it was a topic of particular interest to Italian physicians or readers, at least not any more than were anger or joy.[28] Had they perceived melancholy as a particularly threatening disease one would assume that they would have written more on the subject in Italian in their preventive regimen, given that all agreed there was little one could do to cure it. As it was, apart from the Italian translation of Ficino in 1548, vernacular regimens by Italians simply included melancholy in

---

[27] e.g. Velásquez, *Libro del melancholia* (1585); Bright, *A Treatise of Melancholy* (1586); Du Laurens, *Discours de conservation* (1597); and Burton, *Anatomy of Melancholy* (1621). Arikha focuses on melancholy as a particular characteristic of Renaissance culture in *Passions and Tempers*, 113–24. Behringer (*A Cultural History of Climate*, esp. 115–20) draws on climate data and a range of literary and artistic sources to support his account of this period as one dominated by despair, melancholy, and suicides.

[28] See also Piers Britton's critique of a tendency to glorify melancholy in art historical scholarship in 'Mio malinchonico', 674–5.

the context of their general discussions of the passions. There are only two notable exceptions: Petronio in his regimen *Del viver*, and Paolo Zacchia in his *De mali hipochondriaci*—which was not strictly speaking a regimen—published in 1638.[29] The only other works in Italian specifically on melancholy were three translations of Du Laurens's treatise, the first of which appeared in 1626.[30]

Petronio's work was particularly innovative, as he developed his own insights and clinical techniques for managing a condition he calls *fiachezza*. *Fiachezza* means something like exhaustion and weakness, and is an ailment which not only shares many symptoms with melancholy, but which he later refers to again under the rubric of the passions, clearly linked to that disorder.[31] However, he saw *fiachezza* as being a particularly 'Roman' form of melancholy, given his strong Hippocratic emphasis on locality. In keeping with this he offered a new and distinctive interpretation both for its causes and cures. Contrary to Ficino's account of melancholy as caused by excessive cold and dryness which produce 'the other black bile', Petronio regards it largely as a condition of excessive dampness. This he attributed to the damp dense air and winds in Rome, and the damp foods which filled the body with excess humours, leading to bloating, fullness, weakness, and fatigue.[32] However, he also cites the effect of psychological factors, specifically linked to the competitive social environment of Rome, such as the ambition for wealth, and pride and the 'annoying trials' of a litigious society.[33] But rather than embroiling himself in a traditional discussion of the spirits he focuses on the way these 'griefs'—which he does however imagine as somehow being corporeal—'penetrate' into the deepest part of the soul. Having their 'root fixed high', they lead to *rammarico* (bitter sorrow), and prevent men from sleeping and eating and produce strange, restless, and fearful behaviour.[34] Just over half a century later Paolo Zacchia published his volume describing a range of conditions which, following Galen, he subsumes under the general term of disorders of the hypochondria, with particular attention to the condition known as 'Hypochondriac melancholy'. Also discussed by Du Laurens in his treatise on melancholy, this condition manifested itself both through physical symptoms related to excessive flatulence, with burning sensations in the belly, and symptoms normally associated with melancholy, such as excessive worrying, fearfulness, sadness, and tearfulness. It appears to have become an increasingly significant problem in seventeenth-century Italy, one which physicians evidently struggled to identify, categorize, and explain.[35]

[29] Zacchia, *De mali*.

[30] Du Laurens, *Discorsi della conseruatione*. Also under Ferrari, *Democrito et Eraclito*. The third was Du Laurens, *Il tesoro*.

[31] Petronio, *Del viver*, 199–229, 342–8.

[32] Petronio, *Del viver*, 205–6.

[33] 'C'habbia origine solamente dall'animo', and a few lines earlier he says it 'depends on' the imagination. Petronio, *Del viver*, 225. In this imagery he had possibly been influenced by Fernel, or Fracastoro, both of whom had written on contagion using the metaphor of a seed or foreign body which implants itself within the body.

[34] 'Essendo penetrato questo rammarico nelle piu intime parti del cuore', and 'Hanno fissa alta la radice'; Petronio, *Del viver*, 206 and 343.

[35] Zacchia, *De mali*.

ILLNESS AND THE PASSIONS IN DAILY LIFE

Despite the complexities of medical accounts of the passions, contemporary cor-respondence provides considerable evidence that the link between emotional turmoil and illness was widely accepted at the time amongst the laity. In letters sent by the agents of Cardinal Hippolito d'Este in the 1560s to his nephews, for example, we find evidence of the ways in which anger was thought to have caused his gout.[36] The cardinal's gout had spread rapidly up his legs, making him very ill, and he had also become very thin. Although he wanted nothing more than to go into his garden, which he loved dearly, he had been prevented from getting out for six days before he finally insisted on being allowed to be taken out in a chair. The agent explained that 'all this derives from the great rage he gets into because he is not allowed to go out and about looking at all his delights [meaning his beautiful garden, with its grottos, fountains, flowers and animals].' And this point is later reiterated, writing that his illness stems 'from choler and his anger about his things'.[37]

Turning to the Spada-Veralli correspondence a hundred years later, we find a letter in which Eugenia recounts how her husband had become extremely irritated with several artisans who had come to see him to insist on being paid for the previous two to three years' work. That evening he fell ill, and she attributed his illness to the fact that he had finally 'lost his temper' with them.[38] The following autumn his haemorrhoids started hurting him, and he suffered from *alterazioni* and Eugenia writes 'I think it is because he is so upset by the death of Sig. Olimpia [his aunt]'.[39] Worrying (*affanni*) was also viewed as a cause of illness, as when Eugenia commented that after the death of her uncle, the Cardinal Bernardino Spada, her husband was worrying so much about what would become of the car-dinal's possessions she was concerned that he would fall ill.[40]

Melancholy was certainly also perceived as an important threat, understood as arising from humoral ill-balance, disturbed emotions, and boredom. When Eugenia Spada-Veralli informed her mother that the Bishop of Sulmona, Mons. Carducci was ill in the autumn of 1654 she explained that 'People say that the illness is more melancholy humours than anything else.'[41] The link between bore-dom and becoming melancholic was also made explicit: in June 1653 Eugenia writes that the bad weather has limited their activities and prevented them from getting out, so that 'not knowing what to do with ourselves' it has caused melan-choly.[42] In one letter there are references to the upsetting events which cause Eugenia's

---

[36] These letters are reprinted in Pacifici, *Ippolito II D'Este*.
[37] 'Et tutto questo viene da tanta collera che esso se piglia de non possere ire il dí a spasso a vedere le sue delitie... Per collera et rabia che esso ha delle sue cose.' Anonymous agent to Alfonso II d'Este, Tivoli, 29.7.1571; Pacifici, *Ippolito II D'Este*, 349.
[38] 'Prese collera' and 'Cosí la sera per questa cosa si sentiva male'. ASR, FSV, B.410, 21.6.1656.
[39] 'E penso sia perchè si prese gran disgusto alla morte della Sig. Olimpia.' ASR, FSV, B.410, 30.9.1657.
[40] ASR, FSV, B.1115, 15 or 25.1.1662.
[41] 'Il male dicono sia più humor malinconico che altro.' ASR, FSV, B.619, 15.10.1654.
[42] ASR, FSV, B.619, 7.6.1653.

husband to be 'very melancholic'.[43] Hypochondriac melancholy is also understood. In 1678 Maria Veralli writes describing her state of health to her husband, expressing her fear that she has been experiencing effects of hypochondria 'triggering more than usual worries about melancholy'—although some of those around her suggest that it could even be of benefit to her, whilst others make her anxious about it. These 'sensible' people have advised her not to move about and to rest 'so as to banish these worries about melancholy'.[44] The frequent references to melancholy in the Spada-Veralli correspondence, along with even more frequent references to the need to be 'cheerful', suggest on the one hand that melancholy was a concern amongst the late seventeenth-century elite, and on the other that there was a clear sense of what should be done to prevent it: invariably correspondents emphasize the importance of seeking out variety, diversions, cheerful company, and making the most of the natural environment. As we shall see, these were amongst the classic prescriptions offered by medical writers for the avoidance not only of melancholy, but of all other negative emotional states.

GOVERNING THE PASSIONS: MANAGING BODY AND SOUL

Traditionally, doctors had three approaches to offer readers needing advice on protecting their health from accidents of the soul. Firstly, physical therapies could be adopted so as to prevent imbalance in the humours, which had formed the basis of pre-fifteenth-century advice, and which remained constant over the following two centuries, albeit with some modifications. Older regimens had commonly recommended treatments such as heroic purging and vomiting to remove excess choler or black bile; whilst rehumidifying and warming baths might be suggested for rebalancing the dry and cold bodies of melancholics.[45] A similar approach was advocated by Lennio who explained that when corrupt humours were trapped within the body, it caused the imagination 'to conceive of alien and lewd fantasies, at times leading to madness, mania, frenzy' and so on.[46] On Galen's authority he advocated vomiting, bloodletting, and unstopping blocked haemorrhoids, whilst Petronio suggested bloodletting as a remedy for grief.[47] These were however the exception, and in general milder evacuatory techniques appear to have been preferred, as in Auda's mid-seventeenth-century suggestion to wash and purge the eyes and fumigate the brain 'so as to purify the intellect'.[48] Instructions on diet also continued to play a significant role well into the late seventeenth century. Cornaro for example assured his readers that the passions in particular 'do not really have much force, nor can they do much damage to a well-regulated body', by which he

---

[43] ASR, FSV, B.410, 24.9.1656. [44] ASR, FSV, B.618, 5.11.1678.
[45] See Ficino, *De le tre vite*, 20ʳ, 25ʳ⁻ᵛ, 55ʳ. [46] Lennio, *Della complessione*, 8.
[47] Lennio, *De gli occulti miracoli*, 58–9. Petronio, *Del viver*, 347.
[48] Auda, *Breue compendio*, 253.

meant a body subject to a strict and parsimonious diet.[49] As we have seen, Petronio stressed the role played by watery cold foodstuffs in causing *fiachezza*, whilst as late as 1652 Auda devoted a separate chapter to the ten foods which were most likely to generate melancholy, demonstrating the importance with which diet was still regarded.[50]

A second method, particularly favoured in late medieval regimens, was to avoid potentially disturbing sights or situations such as for example looking upon flagellants or the destitute.[51] However, if one failed to avoid exposure to upsetting sights or experiences, and 'sad things enter the soul' then the only resource left was willpower to 'make a great effort … with strong virile will, to preserve yourself, so these sad things don't impress themselves on the mind'.[52] This advice drew on beliefs of the power of the imagination over the body, based on the understanding that sensory impressions held by the imagination retained the qualities of the original object; so imagining something fearful had the same damaging effect on the body as actually seeing it, causing prolonged agitation of the spirits and appetites.[53] The role played by distractions and diversions in turning one's attention away from such disturbing recollections was much emphasized and continued to underpin advice in the sixteenth and seventeenth centuries.

From the mid-sixteenth century onwards a third approach to the passions became prominent. This was based on a Christianized notion of the spirits as a substratum of the higher rational soul, and therefore subject to the will, whose sphere of action was located in the brain. Thus it relied on notions of dominance and governance of the spirits and passions, not just avoidance. However, this approach collided with the more corporeal Galenic notion of the spirits as involuntary movements of the organic soul, centred in the heart, discussed earlier. As a result there is no overall coherence of approach, as each physician seems to negotiate his own particular route through this confusing inheritance of philosophical, medical, and theological texts, ancient and modern.

We can see this shift at its most obvious in the changing terminologies adopted by the writers of our regimens. For example some authors adopted Christianized terms like 'lusts' with strongly negative connotations to replace the more neutral medical term 'appetites' and some focused on the Christian vices such as greed, ambition, selfishness, and cruelty, which were described as 'passions'. Bertaldi even added drunkenness and abuse of tobacco to the list.[54] Concomitant with this, some portrayed the spirits as wilfully unruly, acting in defiance of the rational parts of the soul. Paschetti for example explained that men were 'infested' with passions,

---

[49] 'Non han per il vero molta forza ne possano far molto danno a i corpi regolati.' Cornaro, *Trattato*, in Milani (ed.), *Scritti*, 85.

[50] Petronio, *Del viver*, 297.

[51] Benzi, *Tractato utilissimo*, 38ᵛ.

[52] '*bisogna sforzzarsi quanto si può per la conservatione della sanitade e con forte e virile animo reservarsi dallo impressione tristabile*'. Benzi, *Tractato utilissimo*, 37ʳ.

[53] On the role of sight and its relationship to the imagination and rational faculties see Quiviger, *Seeing*, esp. 17–19. For an example, see Fonseca, *Del Conservare*, 112.

[54] Fonseca, *Del conservare*. The others who use these terms are Lennio, *Della complessione*; Bertaldi, *Regole della sanità*; and Paschetti, *Del conservar*.

echoing Lennio's account of the spirits as supernatural agents, demons, capable of inciting one to unreasonable passions. For him they were 'incorporeal spirits', assailing the body and 'inciting' it to libidinous thoughts, even 'pushing the melancholic to envy' and hate.[55] Not all physicians went to these extremes however. Petronio, despite being a papal physician, did not noticeably defer at all to notions of vices or appetites and with the exception of his discussion on melancholy, retained a strong focus on the traditional physical explanations of the actions of the spirits.

Another sign of the acceptance of a more spiritual notion of the passions was in the debate on the efficacy of physically based cures and the role of the physician in curing the passions. We have already noted the persistence of a humorally based paradigm for moderating or even curing disorders of the spirits, whether through evacuations, diet, or medicines. However, such a physical approach represented an implicit challenge to a more spiritually based interpretation of the relationship between the spirits and the soul. Petronio acknowledged these tensions quite bluntly when he wrote that some would, 'quite reasonably, be doubtful, asking how such a medicine can remove melancholy whose origins are purely in the soul'.[56] He then went on, however, to affirm that white hellebore did indeed cure 'simple' melancholy, but his explanation of the reasons why it could, relied on a clever analysis of the psychological effects of strong medications on the rational faculties. Bertaldi was less subtle, asserting that one must prevent the soul from being agitated by the passions, not with drugs, drinks, 'compositions', or other medicines, 'but with words and reason'.[57]

The notion that physicians were qualified to give advice on governance of the soul as well as of the body was not new. Moderation and temperance had implicitly underlain the whole concept of a regimen since antiquity, although recommendations had been limited mainly to distraction and avoidance. However, the prevailing view in late medieval regimens was that it was up to moral philosophers to correct the 'habits' of the soul, and the duty of the doctor to correct the 'accidents' of the soul.[58] Benzi for example had clearly voiced disquiet at the idea that he should 'make his patients more virtuous'.[59] However, we can see that by the late sixteenth century physicians were placing even greater emphasis on the role of the will over the 'passions', evident even in their choice of vocabulary.[60] Traffichetti for example advised that if reason 'governs' the passions one can 'resist' all the accidents of the soul. As a result one will avoid sorrow, hate, and envy altogether.[61] Indeed, it appears

---

[55] Fonseca, *Del conservare*, 220: 'infestato'; Lennio, *Della complessione*, 18–19 and 44: 'spiriti incorporei' and 'incitano a commetter le sceleragini. Bertaldi (*Regole della sanità*, 9) similarly argues that the concupiscent part of the soul makes it ill with the mud of carnal filth, temporal delights, and the dishonesty of the senses and that the passionate soul creates putrid fevers.

[56] 'Uno ragionevole dubio, come possa tale medicamento levare la melancolia c'habbia origine solamente dall'animo.' Petronio, *Del viver*, 225.

[57] 'ma con...parole e ragioni.' Bertaldi, *Regole della sanità*, 10.

[58] [Maineri], *Opera utilissima*, 47.

[59] Benzi, *Tractato*, 36.

[60] Galen's *On the Passions* was also often cited by physicians. e.g. Traffichetti, *L'arte di conservar*, 124.

[61] Traffichetti, *L'arte di conservar*, 125ᵛ.

that towards the end of the sixteenth century doctors were forging a new role for themselves as moral and even spiritual counsellors to their patients, drawing on a combination of neo-Stoic philosophy and religious discipline in their advice on moderating the passions. They were helped in this process by the Counter-Reformation emphasis on using introspection and confession as the tools for attaining spiritual health. Hence Fonseca stresses that to attain the 'tranquillity of the soul' which is necessary to protect our health one must 'Know thyself', desire nothing too deeply, and avoid worldly ambition.[62] We can see many parallels between his advice and that given by the humanist writer Lombardelli, in his tract *Della tranquillità dell'animo* (On the Tranquillity of the Soul) probably written for intellectuals and scholars. The difference is one of emphasis. Whilst Fonseca advises cultivating serenity in order to attain health, Lombardelli presents it as a goal for its own sake, with good health as one of its positive side effects, asserting that 'the man who studies tranquillity will live a long and healthy life'.[63]

Sermons given by Carlo Borromeo to nuns in the monastery of St Paul in the late sixteenth century also illustrate the similarities between the goals, techniques, and vocabulary of the Church and those of physicians. The only difference was that the nuns were aiming to attain spiritual good health rather than bodily health, but everyone was aiming for *allegrezza*. Prayer and spiritual exercises enabled the sisters to avoid all strong emotions and cultivate complete detachment from worldly cares. Moreover, once achieved, their spiritual good health would be visible to all, through the 'angelic *allegrezza*' illuminating their faces.[64]

Perhaps the readiness of some physicians to assume the role as adviser on moral matters can also be attributed to the stress placed on the importance of turning to a trusted person who could point out one's failings, in both religious and philosophical teaching. This was certainly echoed in the advice meted out by physicians to those seeking greater control over their passions. Good friends were recommended by some authors; upright, sober citizens by others. Some even suggested that best of all were 'Priests, theologians, and confessors'.[65] However, doctors were also included as helpful role models and advisers, and Petronio took this role very seriously. He explained that when dealing with a patient afflicted with a form of *fiachezza* caused by the passions, it was very important to know how 'deeply' it had penetrated the soul; this he said was so difficult to determine that 'there is nothing in [a doctor's] training' which can help them recognize it.[66] He then offers his readers a technique which he had developed, based on a mixture of self-revelation from the patient, and 'psychological' analysis and confrontation by the doctor, aimed at getting the patient to acknowledge the roots of his problem—anticipating the principles of psychoanalysis. There was, he stressed, no other remedy 'than finding

---

[62] 'Conoscer se stesso'. Fonseca, *Del conservare*, 114.

[63] 'Lo studioso di tranquillità si mantien sano della vita lungo tempo.' Lombardelli, *Della tranquillità*, 46.

[64] 'Letizia e gaudio spirituale' and 'Angelica allegrezza'; Borromeo, *Sermoni*, 29.

[65] Bertaldi, *Regole della sanità*, 10 and 817; Traffichetti, *L'arte di conservar*, 124; and Petronio, *Del viver*, 220.

[66] 'Che con l'arte non s'è potuto fin'hora arrivare a questa cognitione'. Petronio, *Del viver*, 220.

the hidden causes, which so secretly trouble the patient', and having found this, it is often possible to rectify the problem, depending on the severity of the case.[67] Fifty years later when Frediano wrote his regimen, he evidently, in contrast to Benzi, relished his role as moral adviser. He even observed apologetically that he could 'hear' someone reminding him 'that I am getting swallowed up in virtuous precepts and dealing more with morality than with physic, am more a philosopher than a medic'. Despite this moment of insight, he carried on with another eighty pages of pious advice on how to control the passions.[68]

By the seventeenth century discussions of the passions in the regimen genre as a whole were riven by glaring contradictions. Physiological explanations of the accidents of the soul were followed by the advice to govern the spirits with reason: recommendations on diet and purges are found alongside the exhortation to renounce all cures for the passions except for 'supernatural remedies, Christian examples and morals'.[69] Nor is there any one dominant tendency. Authors such as Lennio, Frediano, and Bertaldi appear to have been more strongly influenced by a religious outlook. Traffichetti and Fonseca seem to combine a Galenic with a neo-Stoic approach. Petronio, despite being papal physician, makes no mention of the consolation of Christ and, despite the gap of some fifty years, the extremely popular mid-seventeenth-century regimen by Auda remains firmly entrenched in the Galenic tradition. What was constant, however, and shared by all authors throughout the period, was the focus on promoting *allegrezza* of the spirits. *Allegrezza* was both a preservative and cure, as by nourishing and delighting the spirits their balance, harmony, and health were restored. This resulted in increased body heat and vitality overall, thereby preventing or protecting the body from the negative consequences of unexpected accidents of the soul. In the next sections we will therefore explore the various ways in which one could promote *allegrezza* and stave off the many disorders resulting from being physically 'dis-tempered', focusing particularly on the flowering of villa culture and looking at the various ways in which villa life comforted the spirits and encouraged good cheer.

DELIGHTING AND COMFORTING THE SPIRITS

Although authors of late medieval regimens were certainly aware of the importance of *allegrezza*, and made brief mention of this as an ideal, it was Ficino who first emphasized the importance of 'delighting', 'comforting', 'fortifying', and 'refreshing' the spirits, and explored the various ways in which this could be accomplished, with

---

[67] 'trorar la causa nascosta, la quale cosi secretamente travagliava l'infermo'. Petronio, *Del viver*, 221.
[68] 'Che esco el proposito, mentre m'ingolfo ne precetti della virtù, e tratto più da morale, che da fisico, più da filosofo che da Medico.' Frediano, *Arca novella*, 221.
[69] Lennio a good case in point. In his *De gli occulti miracoli* he explains at length why it is he is 'pursuaded that the humors are the causes of the passions' (pp. 54–8). Yet, elsewhere and in his *Della complessione*, as noted earlier, he also stresses the need for self-control and mentions the role of evil spirits.

particular stress on delighting the senses.[70] By the mid-seventeenth century the importance of *allegrezza* was so evident that Auda considered it to be one of the three most important health precepts for anyone caring for their health without the aid of a doctor. He explained:

> One must be cheerful, since happiness excites natural heat, tempers the spirits, makes them purer ... prolongs life, sharpens the intellect, and puts man in a state of readiness for his business dealings.[71]

The broad outlines of how this could be done had not changed since the late Middle Ages: all recommended invigorating and cheering the spirits, as well as offering diversions from sad thoughts. This was achieved through the fusion of pleasant physical activities and mild intellectual stimulation. Savonarola's list was comprehensive, advocating such activities as singing, music, dancing (sometimes with 'women' and sometimes with 'ladies'!), triumphs, games, novels, and 'disputing matters divine, philosophical and human'.[72] Lennio stressed cheerful banquets and gatherings of 'joyful family members', with the accent on 'wonderful meals and benign and generous wine'.[73] Anguillara and Petronio emphasized the value of pleasant conversations, the latter focusing also on the sporting pleasures and diversions of men of his class: amusing dogs, expensive horses, sailing, and fishing.[74] Durante not only recommends these pleasures, but explains that exercising the mind by singing psalms and listening to 'theological stories' will delight and invigorate the soul and spirits, which will help the body to better resist infirmity. Possibly he was just echoing Savonarola, but perhaps he was also influenced by the increasingly sober models of the pleasures appropriate to a Christian gentleman in the late sixteenth century.[75]

As noted by Ficino, those devoted to a life of the intellect in particular had to be careful not to overstrain the animal spirits since this led to them withdrawing, drying out, and consuming natural heat, which contributed to the onset of melancholy.[76] Fonseca was very specific about how to avoid this danger, and suggested that scholars place a limit of two hours' study in the morning and two in afternoon, with the rest of the day dedicated to exercise, eating, and honest pleasures and discussions.[77] Only Lombardelli however, in his 1594 advice manual for students, specifically mentions Ficino's *Delle tre vite*: he asserts that it is 'something all students should have', and he too stresses the importance of seeking out cheerful

---

[70] Aldobrandino for example just mentions 'joy, delight'. *Le Régime du corps*, 31–2. Alderotti (*Libello*, 7) suggests wearing beautiful clothes which will 'cheer the soul'.

[71] 'Si deve stare allegramente, imperoche l'allegrezza eccita il calor naturale, e contempera li spiriti, li rende più puri ... prolonga la vita, acuisse l'intelletto, e rende l'huomo piu atto alli negoti.' Auda, *Breue compendio*, 252.

[72] 'Hor con donne, hor con signorie ... hor con disputationi di cose divine, e filosofiche, e humane.' Savonarola, *Libreto*, 54–5; Boldo, *Libro della natura*, 276.

[73] 'Conviti, festivi, giocondi famigliari, ... mense geniali; benigno generoso vino.' Lennio, *Della complessione*, 3–4.

[74] Anguillara, *Vaticinio*, 23–4; Petronio, *Del viver*, 222–3.

[75] Durante, *Il tesoro*, 45–6, 18. [76] Ficino, *De le tre vite*, 3ʳ–4ʳ.

[77] Fonseca, *Del conservare*, 117.

diversions.[78] For example, after dinner students should take a walk or stroll slowly by the fire (depending on the season), 'talking cheerfully, for half an hour, with the family, or read or listen to a novel, or other such cheerful but honest things'.[79] It is a measure of the diffusion of these ideas that even a late sixteenth-century treatise for artists mentions that since they lead a largely 'intellectual' life they should take care to incorporate physical exercise and cheerful discussions with friends into their daily routine as a way of avoiding melancholy.[80]

Whilst the vital spirits in general were responsible for overall heat and vitality of the body, it was thought that the animal spirits, particularly those which mediated between the senses and the intellect, played a particularly important role in maintaining the health of all the intellectual and perceptual faculties. Since all the spirits were thought to be nourished and strengthened by inhaling aromatic and sweet scents there was an emphasis on seeking these out, particularly in gardens. This was based on the premise that scents and the spirits were made of similar substances—i.e. of vapours—and that inhaled scents provided nourishment for the spirit.[81] Ficino cited the Arab author Avicenna, saying that just as sweetness was particularly needed for fattening the flesh, so aromatic scents fattened the spirit.[82] These ideas still pertained a hundred years later when another scholar, also drawing extensively on Arab sources, described scents as 'food of the soul', delighting and strengthening the natural heat and spirits, fortifying all the senses, and comforting the sight and hearing.[83] Indeed, the recommendation that one should ensure the regular inhalation of nourishing sweet airs to help prevent disorders of the passions, complemented the advice regarding two of the other Non-Naturals: exercise and air. Thus Petronio advised elderly men to exercise 'especially in the open air which will purify their spirits, cheer them, and make them more robust'.[84]

Advice on ways of promoting the health of the spirits responsible for sight went back to the Aristotelian theory of optics and was given particular prominence by Ficino.[85] He explained that the spirits (or 'rays') of the eyes are the most important of all the animal spirits, and by *re-creating* (nourishing) them one is helping one's spirits overall. This is achieved by gazing on shiny flat surfaces, such as pools and mirrors, which 'delight' the eye-rays, 'hold' them, and prevent them from

---

[78] 'Ficino *de la Vita* da tenersi per gli studenti'; Lombardelli, *Il giovane studente*, 41.

[79] 'Doppo cena, se sia di state, passeggiarete mez'ora, o più, o caminerete per lento esercizio, di verno, al fuoco, ragionerete allegramente, per'una mez'ora, con la famiglia, o leggerete, o farete leggere una novella, o altre cose allegre ma honeste.' Lombardelli, *Il giovane studente*, 30.

[80] See Pino, 'Dialogo', 135–6.

[81] Avicenna wrote that 'aromatics...feed the breath'; *The Canon*, 548. Thanks to Iolanda Ventura for sharing her paper 'Cultural Interpretation of Perfumes in Early Modern Scientific Literature' where she mentions his emphasis on aromatics and the heart (paper given at the Sixteenth Century History Conference, Geneva, 2009).

[82] See Ficino, *De le tre vite*, 56ᵛ–57ʳ.

[83] 'cibo dell' animo' and 'confortino la vista e l'udito', Anguillara, *Vaticinio*, 23, 10–12. Anguillara acknowledges his debt to Arab texts in the title of the book.

[84] 'Si purificano più, si fanno più allegri e più gagliardi.' Petronio, *Del viver*, 294.

[85] Carol Rawcliffe explains medieval theories of optics, as well as discussing the health benefits of gardens in the context of medieval England in '"Delectable Sightes"', 1–21, esp. 11–12.

dispersing.[86] Alternatively, the eye's spirits are attracted by that which is green, therefore expanding and moving out towards that colour. In turn the 'greenness' 'moves out towards them, resists them gently, stops them from dissipating, returning them back (*refreshed* and *comforted*) to the eye'.[87] The return of spirits is a key concept, since loss of spirits is always negative, and in excess light they disperse, certain sights 'break' them, and darkness and shadows cause them to flee. These ideas on sight were very familiar in late sixteenth- and seventeenth-century Italy. Durante for example advises that one wear green glasses 'to corroborate one's sight', and, on the basis that pleasurable sights will delight the eyes, he suggests wearing expensive clothes in lovely colours, advice which was later elaborated upon by Du Laurens.[88] A hundred and fifty years after Ficino, Auda was still recommending that in order to restore one's sight one should look at clear, transparent water, whether found in fountains, wells, cisterns, or rivers, drawing on the notion that the dampness of water and greenery pleases and somehow affects the crystalline humours of the eye. He also includes the suggestion that one should particularly gaze on greenery and water in the morning, to strengthen the eyes after the dark of night.[89]

The spirits of the ears likewise were believed to benefit greatly from beautiful sounds, in particular from music, birdsong, and running water, although we find no coherent explanations in our sources of how this affected the spirits. This must be attributed to the fact that auditory or 'musical' therapy had not been part of the 'regular armoury' of the Galenic or Hippocratic physician in ancient times and was not a tradition inherited by Renaissance physicians.[90] However, biblical references to the healing power of music and works by the late medieval philosopher Boethius on the music of the spheres meant that there was a Christian precedent, whilst texts showed that the ancient Greeks had different musical 'modes' which were said to create particular effects on listeners, although the musical styles of the Greeks had been lost. Therefore explanations and beliefs on the power of music were drawn from the Arabic medical tradition, although as is clear from the lack of explanations offered, the theory behind this was not well understood by our medical authors.[91] Furthermore, although Ficino had made extensive claims for the power of music to cure the soul in the third part of his book *De vita libri tres*, this section had been condemned by the Church and there is no evidence that his comments were known or accepted by the authors of our regimens.[92] This may explain why our medical authors did not make any detailed comments on the power of music to influence the passions, limiting themselves to vague if enthusiastic comments that those suffering from melancholy would benefit from listening

---

[86] 'E tengono i liquidi raggi de gli occhi'; Ficino, *De le tre vite*, 48[r-v].

[87] 'Resiste e va ad incontrare i raggi de gli occhi, senza offendergli, e gli ferma, perche non vagando di lungo, si vengano a dissipare.' Ficino, *De le tre vite*, 47[r]–51[r], esp. 48[r].

[88] *'occhiali verdi per corroborar più la vista'*. Durante, *Il tesoro*, 46. Du Laurens suggests gazing on jewels; *A discourse*, 192.

[89] Auda, *Breue compendio*, 256.

[90] Horden, 'Commentary on Part I', and 'Commentary on Part II'.

[91] For a detailed discussion of this problem see Burnett, ' "Spiritual Medicine" '.

[92] On the fortunes of the third book see Kaske and Clark's edition of Ficino, *Three Books on Life*, 56. However, music scholars view Ficino as having laid the foundations for discussions of the relationship between music, the body, and mind from the 17th century onwards. See Gouk, 'Raising Spirits'.

to cheerful and 'sweet' music, by keeping birds, since such things 'cheer the soul, recreate the spirits and chase away sadness'.[93]

Musicians, music theorists, and composers were more certain about the links between music and the passions and were specifically engaged during the late sixteenth century in a quest to re-create a form of music which would express the passions and move the affects of their listeners ever more powerfully. At its height, this style was exemplified in the dramatic madrigals of Gesualdo and the first operas by Monteverdi around the turn of the century.[94] However, one commentator, a bishop and administrator of one of Rome's largest hospitals, was unconvinced by the new style. He argued against it on the grounds that it completely lacked the power to 'move' and moderate the affects of the soul whereas, according to him, in antiquity the impact of music on the soul had been immediate:

> What wealth there was, and efficacy, so that through singing someone who was lazy and slow became speedy and impetuous; someone who was choleric became happy and content...he who was afflicted was consoled and cheered up whilst he who was so excessively happy became sad.[95]

Another source in which the power of music over the affects of the soul is discussed in depth is Piccolomini's 1552 advice book on raising children. He argues that if one gets accustomed to listening to certain (appropriate) kinds of music, one can control and moderate the affects, even giving specific recommendations as to how to do this. He explains that the airs played in Lombardy 'inflame' the soul with courage and fury, whilst Neapolitan airs sweeten and even make it 'effeminate and soft'. The vehemence of French airs make the mind sour, Spanish airs subdue and tame the soul, and so on. As to the kinds of instruments used, he suggests that the lyre, viols, or lute, 're-create the spirit' whilst playing wind instruments is dangerous to one's health, since blowing through the instrument 'forces' the spirits, weakening the chest. Worse, the resulting 'agitation of the spirits makes them very unwilling to moderate behaviour'.[96]

Beliefs in the positive effects of music on the health of one's spirits, and the certainty that it could moderate one's passions for the better, were surely amongst the many forces which drove the surging popularity of domestic music-making over the sixteenth century. Evidence from across the social spectrum testifies to the growth in popularity of music books, and instruments, whilst stylistic and formal

[93] *'quali rallegrano l'animo e ricreano gli spiriti e cacciano la tristitia'*. Bertaldi, *Regole della sanità*, 863. See also Anguillara, *Vaticinio*, 23–4; Durante, *Il tesoro*, 46; Du Laurens, *A discourse*, 192.

[94] See Penelope Gouk on the 'fundamental redefinition of the goals of music' taking place at the time, in 'Raising Spirits', 92. On the use of music to ward off melancholy see also her 'Music', and Austern, 'Musical Treatments'.

[95] 'che ricchezza era quella, che con l'efficacia di cantare, uno che stava pigro, e lasso, facevasi accelerato e impetuoso; chi stava colerico, diventava lieto, e contendo;...si consolava e allegrava chi stava afflitto, si affliggeva chi stava soverchiamente allegro.' Franco, *Lettera*, 14–17. It was addressed to Cavaliero Gualteruzzi who writes a reply. The bishop was administrator of Santo Spirito in Sassia in Rome.

[96] 'E in parte effeminato, e molle lo rendano' and 'Sforzato il fiato et lo spirito,...et che peggio è per il conturbamento, et concitatione de gli spiriti, si rendano manco disposti alla moderation de' costumi'. Piccolomini, *Della institutione*, 59[v]–62[r].

developments resulted in the hugely popular madrigals and motets which were sung by several voices.[97] Music-making was commonplace and mobile; it took place in the home, in gardens, even in the streets. Whether listeners and performers were actively using music for its medical benefits remains a subject for research, but an indication of just how pervasive these beliefs were is made evident in the inscriptions placed on keyboard instruments. These were often beautifully decorated with a motto placed in a prominent position—usually near the keyboard.[98] Amongst the many different kinds of motto used, a great many alluded to music's power to 'cheer' the spirits or 'refresh' the heart such as: 'Sweet song refreshes sad hearts'; 'Music composes and softens the heat of angers'; and 'Music is the companion of joy, the medicine of sorrows'.[99]

By the mid-sixteenth century therefore, recommendations about how to promote the health and *allegrezza* of the spirits shared a common emphasis on providing the key senses of sight, scent, and hearing with a range of sensory stimuli, and the intellect with stimulating but pleasurable diversions. In the following section we will see how these therapeutic pleasures were extremely closely linked with time spent in gardens and particularly with time spent at the suburban or country villa.

ALLEGRIA AT THE VILLA

What can I say of the tremendous satisfaction we draw continually whilst re-creating our spirits in this sweet air, which, as well as always conferring admirable *allegria* on us, calms our minds, purges our intellect, makes the spirit tranquil, and corroborates the body. Who could estimate the great contentment we derive from feeding our eyes whilst we look and consider the view of high mountains, the pleasantness of hills, . . . the green of the fields.[100]

As we have seen in Chapter 2, the delights of villa life, long since extolled by Pliny, had started to become part and parcel of the way of life of the Florentine elite in the early fifteenth century.[101] By the mid-sixteenth century they were no longer simply country estates supplying key agricultural goods to the family but a fashionable locus of sociability, pleasure, and good health and a great many dialogues and encomiums were written in its praise.[102] A range of sources demonstrate that

[97] See Dennis's account of the huge expansion of domestic music-making in 'Music', 228–43. Also Spagnuolo, 'Gli atti notarili'.

[98] See McGeary, 'Harpsichord Decoration', 1–2.

[99] McGeary, 'Harpsichord Decoration', 23–7.

[100] 'Che dirò io poi della grandissima satisfatione che continuamente prendiamo nel ricreare gli spiriti nostri con questo suavissio aere? Il quale oltre le mirabil allegria, che ci presta sempre, ci rasserena la mente, ci purga l'intelletto, si tranquilla lo animo, e ci corrobora il corpo. Appresso chi potrebbe mai estimar il gran contento che pigliamo . . . nel pascere gli occhi, mentre che miriamo, e consideriamo le prospettive de' monti altissimi, l'amenità de' colli, . . . la verdezza dei prati. Etc.' Gallo, *Le dieci giornate*, 146ᵛ–147ʳ.

[101] See Lillie, *The Florentine Villa*, 24–5.

[102] See e.g. Giamboni, *Capitolo*; Lollio, *Lettera*; Scamozzi, *Intorno alle ville*; and Taegio, *La villa*.

by the mid-sixteenth century members of the elite clearly linked the controlled natural environment of the villa or garden with a clear set of medical benefits.[103] It was healthy not only because of the benefits of good air and the provision of appropriate places for exercise, as discussed in Chapters 3 and 5, but because it was a place where specific colours, scents, vistas, and sounds were intended to have a positive impact on the well-being of the animal spirits. Moreover the association made between time spent at the villa—*villeggiatura*—and laughter, informality, and good cheer was specifically conceived of to divert people away from pernicious states such as anger, anxiety, boredom, and melancholy with all their attendant health complications. Hence a contemporary noted that Pope Pius IV appreciated staying at the Villa Massimo not just because of its healthy location, but because it was 'so cheerful'.[104] This link between villas and health was also emphasized for users as for example through an inscription over a villa entrance which stated that it was a place of 'continuous salubrity', or through the positioning of statues of Aesculapius and Hygeia, the Greek god and goddess of health, which were intended not just to ornament but 'signify the particular properties of plants or water where they stood'.[105]

The study of the layout of almost any contemporary villa, coupled with research by garden historians, shows how closely the overall design of villas met the health requirements specified in regimens regarding exercise, the passions, and the air. We have already noted the provision made for strolling in the shade. But in addition planting schemes in these very formal gardens relied heavily on rows of scented plants which added to the sweetness of the air all year round. Thus espaliers of citrus trees, and hedges of myrtle, laurel, juniper, and cypress were extremely common. Rosemary, lavender, hyssop, and again citrus could be used for the low hedges in parterres. Bitter orange trees (*melangoli*) seem to have been particularly favoured— with orange gardens at the Vatican Villa Belvedere, Castel Sant'Angelo, and the garden of Cardinal Orsini.[106] (See Fig. 6.4.) At Palazzo Spada in the 1630s Bernardino Spada had six bitter orange trees planted when he redesigned the garden, whilst he had the walls of the courtyard entirely covered with espaliers of mixed citrus trees.[107]

Judging from a description of the grounds of Villa Aldobrandini, the overall layout was also conceived of with an awareness of the beneficial effect of certain kinds of views on the eyes.[108] The author rates particularly highly those views which allowed the eye to sweep across a view, or look down an uninterrupted vista, as if following Ficino's advice on not allowing the sight to be 'broken' by harsh angles.

---

[103] On villas and health see also Coffin, 'Pope Innocent VIII'.

[104] 'Si per essere allegrissima'; the architect Domenico Fontana's observations, cited in Massimo, *Notizie istoriche*, 41.

[105] The inscription was over an entrance to Cardinal Carafa's villa on the Quirinal Hill, from about 1483; cited by Coffin in *Gardens and Gardening*, 245. On the statues see Lazzaro, *The Italian Renaissance Garden*, 137.

[106] On planting schemes, see Coffin, *Gardens and Gardening*, 195–203.

[107] Neppi, *Palazzo Spada*, 269.

[108] The author is purportedly Cardinal Aldobrandino himself, but Onofrio argues that it was probably actually written by his secretary, Agucchi. D'Onofrio, *La Villa Aldobrandini*, 75–83.

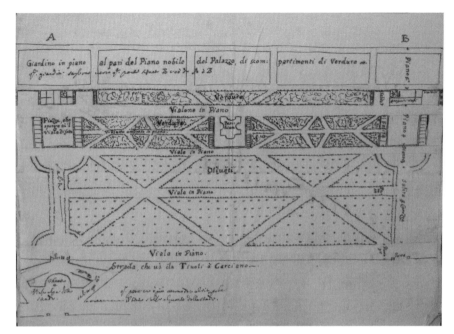

Fig. 6.4. This plan of the garden at the Spada villa in Tivoli, possibly by Orazio Spada, indicates that there was 'greenery' in the borders and 'a little flat shady walkway' as well as a fishpond; the gardens had a view out over olive groves—all key elements in a 'healthy' garden. (See companion sketch at Fig. 3.4.)

Instead the view from the house across the landscape is designed so that the eye does not 'tire itself', nor become 'discomforted', but seems as if it 'can go on as far as it likes'.[109] The view of the countryside beyond is such that it 'confers *vaghezza* on the eye, and the sight has much space in which to roam'. Finally in the view towards the north there is a gap in the mountains 'so as not to annoy the eye'.[110]

These optical theories were also applied to interior decoration as the distinction between outdoors and indoors could be blurred by artistic illusions and there was a tradition dating back to Pliny of regarding representations of landscapes as an adequate replacement for a real view. Indeed, one painter put particular stress on the fact that frescos painted in loggias overlooking gardens should depict 'stories of joy and happiness that contain not even a hint of melancholy'.[111] Likewise in his 1656 regimen Pietragrassa mentions that walls should be decorated with paintings and tapestries, whose beauty will 'satisfy...the sensory powers'. They should be covered in scenes with many figures, 'enjoying themselves out hunting, in forests and

[109] 'Non si stancha et non receve incomodo...che tanto vada inanzi quanto a punto egli desidera.' D'Onofrio, *La Villa Aldobrandini*, 88.
[110] 'Che vaghezza gli recha, le vista ha gran spatio di spatiarvi'; 'Anco per non infastdiir l'occhio'; D'Onofrio, *La Villa Aldobrandini*, 89.
[111] Witte cites many examples to this effect, including the physician Giulio Mancini, in *The Artful Hermitage*, 48–51. The artist was Gian Paolo Lomazzo; *The Artful Hermitage*, 50.

fishing or in orderly battles and sieges', which he notes gives people something to talk about, thereby also stimulating their intellect.[112] (See Plate 18.)

Another common practice was that of lining galleries, courtyards, and loggias with brightly painted and moulded vases of flowers and citrus trees. This combined the beneficial effects on the spirits of views and scents with those of exercise. In his description of contemporary villas Agostino Del Riccio notes that these areas provide a place where one can walk about in all weathers, particularly in winter 'which is the salvation of our bodies', and that the sight of the fruits of these plants, red amongst green fronds, 'greatly comforts our sight'.[113] Such practice is confirmed for us by Maria Veralli writing in late November 1678 when she describes having gone to visit a villa and walked through a long windowed gallery, wide enough to walk four abreast, which was lined with rows of citrus trees in huge coloured vases.[114]

Villa life provided for the auditory spirits through the natural presence of birdsong, the provision of the sound of running water from fountains, and the emphasis on music-making. A contemporary account of Villa Aldobrandini refers to its fountains as a 'delight which men hold so dearly', and noting that instead of being located in the woods, wherever one was, whether in bed, or walking, and particularly when eating, 'one can see this water emerging, with all the effects which this produces', therefore also referring to the sound of the water.[115] Music-making on the other hand was an integral activity in the daily 'routine' at the villa. In his albeit idealizing account of villa life, Gallo notes that during the hours when it was too hot to go outside, visitors to the villa entertained themselves by reading, playing card games, singing, and playing instruments, and again in the evening when they leave the garden they play the 'lute, viol, other string instruments, and dance'.[116] (Plate 19.)

Starting in the late fifteenth century, villa life was increasingly associated with providing the ideal setting for lively intellectual gatherings and conversations with friends, initially modelled on the symposia and *conviti*—or banquets—which ancient Greeks and Romans were known to have held in their gardens.[117] The positive impact of such events on health was remarked on by one participant in 1550 after a particularly pleasant evening. In his letter the next morning he notes how 'it *invigorates* the limbs, *restores* the humours, *re-creates* the spirits, *delights* the senses, and awakens reason' (our emphases).[118] This association between time spent at the

---

[112] 'Appaghino con le vaghezze degli oggetti le potenze sensitive…massime se rappresentano diverse figure che nelle caccie, foreste e pescagioni si trastullano e in ordinate battaglie e assedi.' Pietra-grassa, *Politica medica*, 411–12.

[113] '*ch'e di gran salvezza a' nostri corpi*'. And '*molto ci confortano in vedere…*' Riccio, *Del giardino del re*, 45ᵛ–46ʳ.

[114] ASR, FSV, B.618, 26.11.1678.

[115] 'Si vede nascer questa aqua con tutti gli effetti che fa…questa delitia che alli homini sole esser tanto cara.' D'Onofrio, *La Villa Aldobrandini*, 102.

[116] Gallo, *Le dieci giornate*, 148ᵛ–149ʳ.

[117] On the Roman academies and their activities in gardens, see e.g. Rowland, *The Culture*. See also Price Zimmermann, 'Renaissance Symposia'; and Gnoli, 'Gli orti'.

[118] Letter from M. Claudio Tolomei, Rome, 1550, published in MacDougall, 'L'ingegnoso arti-fizio', 13–14.

villa, *allegria*, good company, intellectual pursuits, and health forms the premises of a dialogue written in 1558 called 'The Banquet of the First of August'.[119] Written as a preface for a translation of Galen's work on the passions, it is set in a villa to which a group of friends has repaired to pass the 'boring and scorching' month of August and to celebrate the festival of Ferragosto. The term 'Ferragosto' is explained as meaning 'Seize August', to be interpreted as 'living together cheerfully with one's friends' in pleasant conversation, eating cooling delicate foods and wines as a way of counteracting the heat and boredom of the month so that August 'can do us no damage'.[120] And the eminent interlocutors—amongst whom were several leading contemporary clerics—were introduced as wearing an expression of 'joyful hilarity and heartfelt good cheer'.[121] Rather than merely setting the scene for a light-hearted dialogue, implicit in these comments is the idea that an appropriately cheerful disposition was an important personal and social attribute for men of the educated elite.[122]

This use of the villa garden as a place of 'intellectual' conviviality was also reflected in the physical structures which appeared in the sixteenth-century garden such as a small building known as a *diaeta*, which offered a peaceful and verdant retreat from duties and relaxing conviviality. There are references to *diaete* as early as 1518 in Raphael's plans for the Villa Madama, placed so as to be protected from unhealthy winds and to receive sunlight all day, making the room 'very cheer-ful...a truly delightful place to spend time in winter with gentlemen'.[123] And a description of Isabella d'Este's isolated garden *studiolo*, loggia, and garden at Man-tova emphasizes its influence on the passions, able to 'invite every sorrowful soul to put aside his melancholy humour and dress in gladness'.[124] And when there was not the space for placing *diaete* in a garden they can be found as towers, like the 'Tower of the Winds' described in Chapter 3.[125] According to Elizabeth MacDou-gall even the design and contents of the garden itself were 'expected to provide nourishment for the mind'.[126] A seventeenth-century description of the statuary and facade of Villa Borghese in Rome supports her analysis, explaining that 'Here one's sight and intellect must really get to work, exercising its speculative faculties

---

[119] Firmano, *Convito del Primo di d'Agosto*.

[120] 'Ch'altro non era che convivare allegramente con gli amici.' Firmano, *Convito del Primo di d'Agosto*, 2–3. Ferragosto is still celebrated, but on 15 August, to coincide with the Feast of the Assumption.

[121] 'Gioconda hilarita, allegria di cuore'; Firmano, *Convito del Primo di d'Agosto*, 2.

[122] Claudia Lazzaro observes that whilst the garden had long had connotations of paradise, arcadia, and as a *locus amoenus*, the Renaissance emphasis on play and freedom was new. *The Italian Renaissance Garden*, 137.

[123] Napoleone (ed.), *Villa Madama*, 62. Napoleone includes translations of Raphael's letter as well as of Pliny's influential account of his Laurentian villa.

[124] Alberto Cavriani writing 6 May 1525, to Isabella d'Este, cited in Witte, *The Artful Hermitage*, 48: 'Invitano ogni animo mesto a deponere lo humore malanchonico et vestirese de letitia'.

[125] Witte notes that the influential architect Scamozzi's interpretation of the *diaeta* is as a tower on top of a villa; Witte, *The Artful Hermitage*, 46. For other examples see *The Artful Hermitage*, 44–50.

[126] MacDougall (ed.), *Fons sapientiae*, 3–5. She also notes the role of 'robust, ribald, comic relief' provided by the games and diversions which took place.

in the statues and busts of significant people.'[127] MacDougall views garden fountains as 'the most important feature of Renaissance gardens', designed to please the
spirits of both the eyes and to stimulate the intellect by providing onlookers not
only with something lovely to gaze upon, but with the challenge of deciphering the
complex mythological and allegorical references embodied in the statuary and
nearby topiary. Even the complex mechanisms of the fountains themselves provided the onlookers with food for thought.[128] Other sources focus on the fun to be
gained from fountains and other water features. In 1574 Agostino Gallo praised
water for the beauty and for the '*allegria* which it always confers on us', and he
observes that 'there is no greater pleasure to be had' than seeing old and young,
men and women, 'cheerfully' entering the pools, attempting to catch fish and frogs,
falling in and generally getting splashed and wet. He even concludes that at such a
sight 'I know of no man so melancholic that he wouldn't burst out laughing…and
truthfully I know of no other remedy like it for banishing sad humours.'[129] In the
rest of his account there is an almost relentless insistence on the fun and joy entailed
in every activity which occurs at the villa: there are jokes, tricks, and witticisms:
they speak of 'cheerful things', some so funny that everyone was 'rolling around on
the floor'.[130] Even here, the medicinal value of all this laughter is celebrated in a
passage which makes a play on the double meanings of the word 'humour': 'This
is really being in a good humour, even though, admirable as it is, it is no more
important than the other humours; but it is highly medicinal for so many humor-
ous people like myself.'[131]

If Gallo's account seems over-idealizing, it is useful to compare it with the vivid
account of a visit to the gardens of the Villa d'Este in Tivoli by the Dominican
priest and garden writer Agostino Del Riccio who died in 1598.[132] He describes
seeing young women and their families lured into a grotto to listen to mechanical
songbirds only to find water first dripping, then trickling, and finally cascading
down from the roof whilst their exit route has been cut off by a 15-foot-wide strip
of water jets. He describes the women's various reactions as panic, anger, and
hilarity as they try and decide what to do before rushing out, soaked to the skin,
through the jets. Del Riccio concludes blithely: 'I who have seen this thing, was
quite cheered up and it made me laugh to see such a pleasant thing.'[133] This account
and his suggestions as to how to create a garden feature that would send one's

---

[127] 'Qui ha ben la vista, dove impiegarsi e l'intelletto, dove esercitar la speculazione, nelle statue e nei
busti de persone insigni.' Manilli, *Villa Borghese*, 25.
[128] MacDougall, 'L'ingegnoso artifizio'.
[129] 'Oltre le dette acque ci sono di molta satisfattione per la bellezza e per l'allegria, che tuttavia ci
donano…Entrando allegramente nel vaso tutti…non so qual'huomo si malinconico che non scopi-
asse da ridere. Che per verita io non so qual ricetta si trovasse pari a questa per scacciare i tristi humori.'
Gallo, *Le dieci giornate*, 141[r].
[130] Gallo, *Le dieci giornate*, 149[v].
[131] 'Questo è ben'humore, non pur sopra a gli altri humori mirabilissimo, ma molto medicinale per
tanti humoristi pari miei.' Gallo, *Le dieci giornate*.
[132] Del Riccio, 'Del giardino', 73–4.
[133] 'Io che ho visto tal cosa, mi sono rallegrato e risomi di cotal piacevolezza.' Del Riccio, 'Del
giardino', 87. MacDougall publishes a letter by Claudio Tolomei from 1550 which gives a similar
account of the amusements provided by fountains in *Fons sapientiae*, 13.

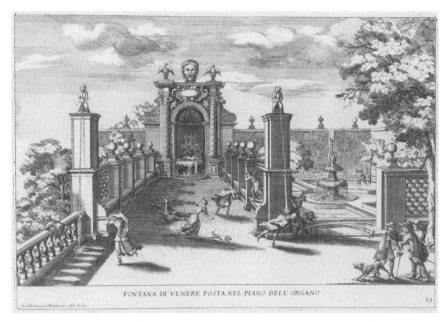

FONTANA DI VENERE POSTA NEL PIANO DELL' ORGANO

Fig. 6.5. This engraving of a fountain at the Villa d'Este in Tivoli, is one of several in which Falda shows visitors surprised by jets of water and onlookers laughing at them. Dated to the 1670s, about one hundred years after our first textual references to fountains as sources of *allegria*, this image suggests the longevity of these ideals.

guests tumbling into a moat (albeit with no danger of them drowning), suggest that practical jokes involving water to create general amusement were central to the conception of some of the fountains. We can even see these jokes 'in action' illustrated for us in several of Falda's engravings of the villas around Rome. These show unsuspecting visitors running away from sudden jets of water, the expressions on their faces of surprise and dismay, raising the question whether those on the receiving end of these jokes found them as funny as the onlookers (Fig. 6.5).

Half a century later, we find no change in attitudes as the Spada-Veralli correspondence furnishes us with numerous examples of the importance attributed to finding ways of keeping oneself occupied, distracted, and cheerful and the links—sometimes implicit, often explicit—which this had with good health. In the autumn of 1666 Eugenia seems concerned about her mother's health. Writing to her when she is in Rome, Eugenia twice urges her to find some 'diversions': 'Go out and about for a stroll a little and amuse yourself,' she writes, 'and don't let yourself get upset about things—leave them to God's will.'[134] A few years later there is an exchange of letters between Eugenia and her mother who has gone to Castel Viscardo with Eugenia's younger sister Virginia. Virginia must have been

---

[134] 'Si abbia cura e vada un poco a spasso e si svari e non si pigli fastidio ma lasci fare a Dio.' ASR, FSV, B.1115, 16.10.1666.

quite ill and had probably been sent away to the country for her health, since Eugenia suggests that 'What with the variety and the exercise she will return to Rome fat', meant as a sign of good health and well-being.[135] In the same series of letters we also note the considerable emphasis placed on the different forms of entertainment arranged for those who have gone to the castle, and the expectation that a large group of people will ensure a cheerful stay. 'I am glad to hear you are all keeping well and happy,' writes Eugenia; 'there are many of you and it is impossible for you not to be cheerful.'[136] And after nearly a month away it appears as if Virginia 'is cheerful and this holiday in the country has done a great deal of good for her health'.[137]

In October 1666 it was Eugenia's turn to be out of town, staying at Giove in Umbria, country seat of her new husband the Duke of Giove. From her letters to her mother in Rome we are given a flavour of the variety of ways in which she kept herself busy. On the one hand she must have mostly been outside in the garden or on walks and visits since she notes: 'I am enjoying every last moment here, and am never inside.' And when the Princess of Rossano arrives with her daughters and female attendants they spend a day 'out and about on these lovely roads', partly travelling in the carriage and partly walking, followed by an evening's singing and dancing, all of which ensured that they were 'very cheerful'.

The exhortation to seek out *allegria* resonates throughout the Spada-Veralli letters, and is often spoken of in the same breath as health, although it does not come with explicit causal links to health. For example, when signing off her letters Eugenia often writes something like: 'Keep cheerful, and keep in good health.'[138] Or, as in a letter which Eugenia wrote in 1669 to her mother who was travelling between their properties, she starts by thanking her for her letter and the news that they had 'arrived well and were all in good spirits'.[139] Later in the letter she notes that she is 'cheered' by the news that more people will join her mother at the castle, 'because you will be more cheerful, because there can be no melancholy wherever the Marchese Carlo Francesco finds himself'.[140] Even when she switches to the subject of finding a possible wet nurse for the baby she is carrying she asks her mother to check whether a particular wet nurse's youngest children 'are lovely and cheerful' ('se son belli allegri'), presumably as an indication of their health and the quality of the woman's milk.[141] And echoing the advice in regimens that wearing beautiful clothes cheers one's spirits, after her young son Andrea had been seriously ill, we read that in order to cheer him up and help his recovery she got him dressed.[142]

---

[135] 'E io credo che tra il svario e l'esercitio tornerà a Roma grassa.' ASR, FSV, B.1115, 12.10.1669.

[136] 'Godo di sentire che tutti stanno bene e allegramente...che loro son tanti ed è impossibile che non si stia allegramente.' ASR, FSV, B.1115, 12.10.1669.

[137] 'E la signora Virginia che è venuta fora stia allegramente e questa villeggiatura li ha da fare gran servitio alla salute.' ASR, FSV, B.1115, 19.10.1669.

[138] For example, when she exhorts her mother and those around her to be cheerful and eat well; ASR, FSV, B.1115, 25.9.1669.

[139] 'Arrivati bene e stavano allegrammente.' ASR, FSV, B.1115, 25.9.1669.

[140] 'Perchè staranno più allegri perchè dove vi è il march. Carlo Francesco non vi è malinconia.' ASR, FSV, B.1115, 25.9.1669.

[141] ASR, FSV, B.1115, 25.9.1669.

[142] 'Andrea oggi l'ho vestito un poco per rallegrarlo.' ASR, FSV, B.1115, 23.7.1662.

CONCLUSION

When Maino de Maineri wrote his regimen back in the mid-fourteenth century he noted that it was the duty of the moral philosopher to correct the habits of the soul and the duty of the doctor to correct the accidents of the body to keep men healthy.[143] For Maino and other physicians until the mid-sixteenth century it seems that dealing with the passions meant recognizing the uncertain boundary between body and soul, whilst noting the reciprocal impact one had on the other. Their approach was to limit themselves to a few sensible remarks about the need to avoid vice, to guard against excess, or make a great effort to protect oneself from potentially thoughts saddening and images.[144] And it was this question of the extent to which a doctor could stray into morality and advise his patients on their conduct which was to become the single most significant change in the preventive advice given by some of our authors, and which accounts for the greatest disparities between them. So whilst some of them barely acknowledged the whole problematic area of the accidents of the soul, and others virtually ignored the 'moral turn', about half of them seemed to relish their chance to stray into the territory of the moral philosopher, and exhort their readers to restrain their appetites and be governed by reason.[145]

Those authors who did embrace the 'moral turn' were on the whole less likely to recommend physical remedies for the passions, even when their explanations still relied on the same Galenic paradigm of overheating, dramatic cooling, loss of spirit movement, and the build-up of pernicious humours. However, the success of Auda's regimen, with its emphasis on a dietary approach to the passions, is a testament to endurance of the humorally based paradigm and a reminder that despite the new emphasis on the soul, old understandings did not simply melt away but continued to influence medical thinking.[146]

We have argued here in favour of a greater emphasis on the whole notion of *allegrezza*, and Petronio's lengthy discussion of it, and his refutation of the belief that one could die from too much joy, was perhaps not unconnected to a more widespread sixteenth-century re-evaluation of the importance of *allegrezza*, which emerges here not only in regimens, but from other literary forms and correspondence.

This is not to say however that melancholy was ignored by our physicians. Rather, that it was more of a minority interest. Following Ficino it seems initially to have been considered a problem only for those who spent too much time in 'speculation and contemplation', although the group of those who might be affected by this was gradually extended. Petronio implied that all men caught up in the ambitious and litigious environment of Rome were susceptible to *fiachezza*, and Viviani (1626) added orators and merchants to the ubiquitous figure of the

---

[143] [Maineri], *Opera utilissima*, 47.
[144] 'guardare dau' [Maineri], *Opera utilissima*, 49; Benzi, *Tractato utilissimo*, 37ᵛ.
[145] Traffichetti, *L'arte di conservar*.   [146] Auda, *Breue compendio*, 263.

scholar.[147] Furthermore, the fact that early seventeenth-century physicians were seeking to understand the disorder termed 'hypochondriac melancholy', perhaps also suggests the 'appearance' of a form of melancholy which could be explained for a much broader section of society, given that the traditional account only really recognized it as an illness of intellectuals and the elderly.

Above all, what is interesting is the impact this advice seems to have had on the perceptions and activities of the lay elite. On the one hand we find no indications that the precepts of moral philosophy and religion regarding the need to control and dominate the passions had any significant role to play in the daily lives of our correspondents. On the other, it is clear that they feared the impact of emotional turmoil, worry, and particularly boredom upon the body. Hand in hand with this there is also a wealth of material-culture evidence to show that ideas about the importance of pleasant sights, sounds, and amusements had penetrated many aspects of interior decoration, room design, and especially of garden and villa layout not to mention the activities which filled the daily lives of those who lived and visited there.

---

[147] Viviani, *Trattato*, 175–7.

7
'Salute!' (Cheers!) Drinking to Your Health

During antiquity, food and drink and their interactions with the trio of exercise, sleep, and evacuations had been put at the heart of discussions of healthy living, such that by the sixteenth century, they were surrounded by a battery of regulations and prohibitions Even though the other Non-Naturals acquired more importance over time relatively speaking, this attention to diet remained significant in regimens throughout the sixteenth and seventeenth centuries, tending to account for the longest sections of some of the texts. Thus Petronio's regimen, which in its original Latin version was entitled *On Roman Food*, and Paschetti's 1602 *Del conservare la sanitá* devoted about half of their texts to the subject; and four-fifths of Durante's *Il tesoro di sanitá* (1586) was on food. However, this can be attributed not to novelty in approach but to the fact that authors systematically analysed the medical properties of each foodstuff one by one.[1] Most of the contents of these sections had remained virtually unchanged over centuries.[2]

From the late fifteenth century a growing interest in diet was also reflected in the appearance of food writing as an autonomous genre.[3] Whether as recipe books, instructions for courtiers on banqueting, or books on single food categories, such as fish, salads, and wines, these books often included elements of medical dietary advice, thereby contributing to the further dissemination of this knowledge. This development was stimulated by the emphasis on courtly dining and banqueting which spread through the princely courts of late fifteenth-century Italy.[4] The multifaceted history of food and diet, in particular the complex relationship between food and the body and the rules attached to eating during the Renaissance, has already attracted considerable scholarly attention over the last thirty years.[5] In view of this, our intention here is to briefly summarize the medical framework underlying these dietary precepts before turning to focus instead on three less familiar aspects: the relationship between prescription and practice, the Lenten diet, and the debate on hot and cold drinking.

---

[1] Marilyn Nicoud describes the emergence of this genre of 'encyclopaedic' regimens in *Les Régimes*, 269–79.

[2] See Petronio's apology for 'lifting the same passages' from earlier authors; Petronio, *Del vivere*, 91.

[3] See Grieco, 'La gastronomia'.

[4] Girard, 'Du manuscrit à l'imprimé'.

[5] For a recent survey and bibliography of the history of alimentation see Redon and Laurioux, 'Histoire de l'alimentation'. For late medieval regimens see Nicoud, *Les Régimes*, esp. 159–64, 257–79, 300–4. For a comprehensive discussion of digestion, foodstuffs, and regimens see Albala, *Eating Right*.

In the face of the barrage of complex advice on what one should and shouldn't eat, it is surprising that relatively few historians have speculated on the relationship between prescription and practice as regards dietary regulations.[6] The most sustained exploration of this issue so far appears in Nicoud's case studies of the Sforza court in the late fifteenth century, which show the difficulties experienced by physicians attempting to influence the dietary choices of their royal patrons.[7] In view of this we were intrigued to find the extent to which the Spada-Veralli letters show that food intake was constantly being monitored, advised upon, and reported within the family. Thus we use them here to explore the advice given amongst family members to see whether or how it relates to official prescription, and to assess how seriously dietary advice was taken. However, from the mid-sixteenth century onwards, devout Catholics also had to contend with the additional complexity of Lenten food regulations, as the importance of fasting for spiritual and bodily health was reaffirmed by the Counter-Reformation Church. As yet a marginal topic in histories of food, Lent has been considered mainly in the context of the contrast between the extremes of feasting and fasting, or the rivalry between religious confessions. More recently Gentilcore has explored the precepts and practices linked to the rising power and influence of the Jesuits.[8] Yet our discovery of two regimens written specifically to rebut criticisms of the unhealthiness of the Lenten diet has prompted us to ask whether our correspondents were also critical of the rigours of such diets and to examine the extent to which they observed it.

The remainder of the chapter shifts from eating to the much less well-researched topic of drinking, but in particular, the debate on what was known as 'hot' and 'cold' drinking. This burst onto the medical world in the latter decades of the sixteenth century, becoming an entire subgenre of medical advice. Fascinated by the almost vitriolic intensity of the debate, we look at why it occurred, examine the terms of the debate, and using a variety of sources we explore the extent to which cold drinking was practised. Contemporary concerns with the health implications of objects used in drinking also prompt us to ask whether or how health considerations might have shaped the material culture of drinking.

HEEDING THE PHYSICIAN'S ADVICE?

Another of the reasons for the disproportionate length of the sections on foods lay in the complexity of the advice, since foodstuffs were thought to affect the body in a variety of ways. Foods were categorized according to a range of qualities. The 'complexion' of the food (i.e., whether it was hot, cold, moist, dry, or a combination of these) determined whether it was of nutritional benefit for the individual. The quantity of food ingested and the relationships between different foodstuffs

---

[6] See e.g. Flandrin, 'Introduction' and 'From Dietetics', esp. 363–4; and Gentilcore, *Pomodoro*, 27–30.

[7] See Nicoud, 'Les Médecins', 210; 'Les Pratiques diététiques', 401; and 'Les Savoirs diététiques'.

[8] Gentilcore, 'The *Levitico*'.

also all had to be calibrated so as to keep each individual's constitution in perfect equilibrium, taking into consideration criteria such as one's age, the amount of exercise taken, and the season.

Another set of considerations were the effects which certain foods had on the digestive process itself, something which was thought to be extremely delicate and in need of constant vigilance. Drawing on an ancient simile, food and wine were likened to the oil one puts in a lamp to maintain a steady flame: the flame was one's inner heat which had to be kept at a constant temperature, neither burning too quickly nor feebly.[9] Meanwhile, the process of turning the food into fuel appropriate for the lamp was crucial. The stomach was envisaged for readers as a kind of stove, where food was 'cooked' or 'concocted' before being distributed through the body by the blood ('digestion') in a several-stage process. Failing to 'concoct' and then digest one's meal fully left so-called 'raw' or poorly digested foods to fester in the stomach, producing dangerous fumes and vapours and leading to blockages in the body's evacuatory pathways, all of which could contribute to any number of ailments. To facilitate concoction doctors therefore had to consider the texture of food, which affected how 'digestible' it was, as well as the effect of foods on the digestive processes overall.[10] For example some foods such as certain raw vegetables helped stimulate appetite by 'opening' the stomach; others, such as dried fruits or cheese, served to 'close' the top of the stomach, enhancing the first phase of digestion. Thus the order in which foods were eaten was crucial. A mid-seventeenth-century household advice manual also confirms that this kind of information fell firmly within the remit of the *scalco* (the steward in charge of the table in the noble household): the author notes that 'the *scalco* has the life of his master in his hands' and to ensure his good health must only prepare those few foods which were suited to his master's complexion, so long as he liked them.[11]

Regimens included advice about how to ensure whether the body was 'ready' to eat, having expelled the residues from previous meals, and this included discussion of the relationship between eating, exercising, and sleeping. For example, one should only eat when hungry and not before; only take vigorous exercise before meals—but not if very hungry—and take very gentle exercise after eating, so as to ensure the descent of food to the bottom of the stomach without diverting heat away from it. The rules governing eating and sleeping sought to ensure the best conditions for digestion; therefore for example they recommended sleeping two hours after eating, and changing position whilst asleep to facilitate the descent of food.[12]

The simplest message imparted by the regimens—that foods have a direct impact on health, and that some foods were good, some bad, and that one needed to eat foods in a 'regulated' way—was certainly understood by our correspondents in the Spada-Veralli family. There was even an expression for what we term 'junk' foods:

[9] For an example of this see Petronio, *Del vivere*, 315.
[10] For a full discussion of digestion and particularly textures see Albala, *Eating Right*, 91–8.
[11] 'Lo scalco ha in mano la vita del padrone.' Frigerio, *Arte d'acquistar*, 85.
[12] See Ch. 4 for more detail.

porcherie. Thus when writing about the Marchesa Pacifica, her mother-in-law who had been gravely ill, Eugenia observes to her mother that a recent setback in her recovery is thought to have been nothing more than indigestion because 'she eats well and wants some junk foods'. This does however suggest that rather than avoiding *porcherie* completely, the marchesa considered them something she could eat when well.[13] Furthermore, on more than one occasion, presumably in response to a question or reminder from her mother, the pregnant Eugenia reports that she is 'eating well' and not having any 'rubbish'.[14] Interestingly, though, in one of these letters she is not quite clear which kind of *porcherie* her mother means since she adds 'and I think you must be referring to fruit, which this year I don't like very much and am eating very little of'.[15]

Fruit, like vegetables, were medically problematic, considered to be cold, watery, viscous, and difficult to digest. Our correspondents were clearly aware of this, although they are most worried about grapes which some medical writers seem to regard as the most benign of fruits.[16] 'There is no danger I'll fall ill from eating grapes this year, as I've seen neither vines nor grapes,' announces Giulia Benzoni to her husband in 1599. Eighty years later Maria Veralli put her servant Paradiso's ill health down to his poor constitution 'accompanied by eating too many grapes'.[17] These comments suggest that whilst attempting to heed medical advice, there was a tension between strong lay beliefs about foods and medical doctrine.

Advice on not drinking excessive amounts of wine, which was considered to be 'heating', also seems to have been heeded. When the wet nurse hired for Eugenia's first child is ill, Eugenia reports to her mother that the wet nurse 'is not eating foods which heat her and she waters her wine very well'—thereby reducing its heat.[18] Several years later and suffering from a prolonged inflammation in the arm (understood as resulting from overheating), Eugenia herself is nonetheless allowed to continue drinking wine since she 'drinks so little of it and those I do drink are so light'.[19] Giulia Benzoni earlier in the century was also careful not to drink too much wine, though what she did drink was 'as black as ink'.[20] It is not clear whether or not Giulia was pregnant at the time, but certainly the regimen written by the uncle of the family physician, Doctor Rodrigo Fonseca, explained that pregnant women could drink small quantities of black wine, considered to be extremely nutritious.[21]

---

[13] 'Perchè mangia bene e vol qualche porcheria.' ASR, FSV, B.1115, 19.10.1669. See Nicoud's observations on the ignoring of food regulations when healthy; 'Les Pratiques diététiques', 401.

[14] 'Mangio bene e non porcherie', ASR, FSV, B.410, 18.10.1656; and 'Porcarie non ne mangio', B.410, 14.3.1657.

[15] 'Perchè li frutti che questi credo che voglia dire quest'anno non mi piacciono troppo e ne mangio pocchissimi.' ASR, FSV, B.410, 18.10.1656.

[16] Boldo describes grapes as the 'best' amongst autumn fruits; *Libro della natura*, 87. Petronio however warns that mature fresh grapes 'disturb the belly' and if eaten in quantity 'bloat the stomach'. *Del viver*, 129.

[17] 'Sarà stato anco accompagnato da mangiare troppo uva.' ASR, FSV, B.618, 1.10.1678.

[18] 'Non mangia cose che riscaldino e il vino lo anacqua bene.' ASR, FSV, B.410, 22.7.1657.

[19] 'Ne bevo tanto poco e sono leggieri.' ASR, FSV, B.1115, 26.7.1662.

[20] 'Negro come ch'inchiostro ma di questo puoco me ne curo.' ASR, FSV, B.449, 10.4.1603.

[21] Fonseca, *Del conservare*, 28.

The accounts of the death of Cardinal Bernardino Spada however offer consider-able contrast. Unlike the women of his family, he blithely ignored advice on leading a carefully regulated life. Thanks to his hereditary healthy constitution he was rarely ill, but the suggestion is that in his last few years he fatally overstepped the limits: rather than resting when on *villeggiatura* at Tivoli he took twenty-two cases of books for his work; instead of sleeping well he worked late into the night; and in the years before his death 'he never restrained his disorderly eating habits, always choosing the most unhealthy things, with the sweetest of wines'.[22] Eventually his 'living without rules' caught up with him and during the grape harvest in 1661 he gorged heartily on snails, 'ignoring the *cappone* and other substantial foods'. This triggered vomiting and illness and led them to suspect his disordered eating as the cause of his death.[23]

VEGETABLES, LENT, AND HEALTH

When imparting dietary advice another factor which had to be taken into consid-eration and has not yet been mentioned, was that certain foods had been thought to be more or less digestible according to the social class of the body consuming it. Grieco has explained the basis for the late medieval belief that every plant or ani-mal could be placed on a vertical hierarchy according to which, the higher a plant or animal grew or lived, the more it suited the bodies of the nobility and vice versa: so birds and fruit were more easily digested by the wealthy, whereas pork and root vegetables suited the bellies of the poor.[24] However, despite their original connota-tions as a food for the poor, scholars agree that vegetables became an increasingly familiar sight on the tables of the elites over the sixteenth century, even becoming 'a sign of distinction and a delicacy'.[25] This was a change which defied traditional medical perceptions that vegetables offered little nourishment and could even be damaging. Boldo for example writes in 1575 that unless conserved in salt and vinegar for a year, green vegetables are all 'very obviously of little nourishment, generate bad juices and for the most part, damage the stomach'.[26] Petronio was more forgiving, explaining that although 'herbs' offered 'poor nourishment' alone, they were actually very effective at 'tempering the blood' in all ways, as long as they were eaten with bread and 'good' foods.[27] Recent evidence suggests that his views

---

[22] 'Anche nei vitto non si temperò mai del suo consueto di vivere senza regola, e di attaccarsi sempre al peggio con vini di tutta dolcezza.' ASR, FSV, B.463, cap. XXXII.

[23] 'Lasciando il cappone e altri cibi di sostanza, ne mangiò con gusto.' ASR, FSV, B.463, cap. XXXII.

[24] See esp. Grieco, 'The Social Politics'; 'Food and Social Classes'; and 'From Roosters to Cocks', 89–140. Albala however argues that class only became really important in dietary tracts during the 16th century; Albala, *Eating Right*, 184–216, esp. 190.

[25] On the shift towards vegetables, see Flandrin, 'From Dietetics', 418–32; Grieco, 'La gastrono-mia', 147–8; Gentilcore, *Pomodoro*. The citation is from Jeanneret, 'Ma salade et ma muse', 212.

[26] 'Tutti gli herbagi che si mangiano, come é cosa manifestissima, oltra che danno al corpo poco nutrimento, generano ancora cattivo sugo, e la miglior parte sono nocivi allo stomacho.' Boldo, *Libro della natura*, 39.

[27] 'Che tutte le erbe sono di cattivo nutrimento...ma...se vede che non si convertono tutte in cattivo ma in buon sangue, pur che pero si mangino e con il pane e con gli altri buoni cibi.' Petronio, *Del viver*, 93.

were more in line with social trends, since by the end of the seventeenth century vegetables of all kinds formed 'a significant part of the diet' in almost every meal taken at the Jesuit colleges in Rome.[28]

Increased fruit and vegetable consumption can be linked with the growing cultural influence of religious reform, as abstinence, sobriety, and self-discipline in matters of diet were increasingly seen as the hallmarks of the devout Christian gentleman: indeed Boldo even criticized those who undertook excessive 'fasts, vigils, and programmes of abstinence' out of a desire to appear more devout than others.[29] Albala notes a shift in 'tone' in dietary advice after the mid-sixteenth century which he describes as the decline of the 'pleasure' principle.[30] Previously, hunger had been regarded as an important sign of physical readiness for the next meal. Furthermore, what tasted good was considered to be beneficial and physicians were expected to heed a patient's desires in respect of food.[31] According to Albala, this acceptance of pleasure was replaced by a new mistrust of appetite, now connoted with greed and gluttony.[32] Although to some extent expressed as polemical comments directed against the courtly milieu, the change in tone was just another facet of the Counter-Reformation's emphasis on restraint and discipline of the body in general, and the unruly appetites driving sexuality and gluttony in particular.[33] None of our authors embraced the Church's call for sobriety and restraint in diet as ardently as the mid-seventeenth-century doctor Frediano whose section on food and drink was entirely reshaped by the religious agenda. Completely omitting any discussion of individual foodstuffs and their medical effects on the body, he devotes over a hundred pages to pious advice on cultivating an appropriately sober attitude towards food and eating, making explicit the linkage between sobriety in one's diet and sobriety in civil and political life. He includes instructions on how one should eat 'calmly, slowly, and decently'; he has a horror of 'being sated' or 'gorged'; and when warning against the pleasures and dangers of being ruled by 'taste' rather than simply choosing foods which nourish the body he warns his reader to 'moderate this tyrant', and ignore anything which 'delights' the palate.[34]

Fasting had historically been regarded as an ideal opportunity for believers to 'purge' their body and soul, and the mid-sixteenth-century physician Rangoni vouched for it as being more effective for health than the medically induced purges which had long been popular.[35] The intended effects of these various foods on the

---

[28] Gentilcore, 'The *Levitico*', 103.

[29] 'Certe astinentie e vigilie, e altri digiuni.' Boldo, *Libro della natura*, 280.

[30] Albala, *Eating Right*, 177–8. See also Montanari, *Convivio*, p. xxiii.

[31] For a discussion of the conflict between pleasure and rules in diet in the late 15th century see Nicoud, *Les Régimes,* 367–75. Also see the introd. and ch. 10 of Bartolomeo Platina's regimen, *On Right Pleasure*, 101–3, 115.

[32] Albala, *Eating Right*, 31–2, 177–8.

[33] Pictorius for example in his regimen chides courtiers for ignoring the rules on keeping fish and meat separate; *Dialogi*, 27–8.

[34] 'Con quiete, con decente lentezza.' Frediano, *Arca novella*, 89. On how to eat, 90 ff.; on temperance and on dangers of aromatic seasoning and the palate, 102–3, and on sobriety and civil life, 134.

[35] Fourteenth-century Florentine preachers stressed the purificatory benefits of fasting; Ciappelli, *Carnevale e Quaresima*, 48. 'Conserva sani più sicuramente i corpi che le purgazioni.' Rangoni, *Consiglio*, 33.

body and spirit were evidently common currency, as expressed succinctly in the rhyming couplets of a 1604 poem by the late sixteenth-century satirical poet Giulio Cesare Croce:

> Then fish was tried
> to keep us mortified
> and make men docile
> humble and quiet.[36]

However, the medical benefits of fasting were questioned in the seventeenth century, as the Catholic Church tightened up its expectations of the faithful. The importance of fasting during Lent had been reaffirmed first by the Council of Trent and then in the 1570s by Carlo Borromeo. Believers were called upon to use abstinence as a way of expressing penitence, dominating their physical appetites, and heightening their intellectual and spiritual acuity.[37] For six weeks a year (in addition to regular fast days on Wednesday, Friday, and Saturday, monthly fasts, and fasts on saints' days) the faithful were expected to eat only one main meal a day, although a light *collation* was allowed in the evening. The image in Fig. 7.1 illustrated for the faithful not only the correct foods for Lent, but the appropriate physical and psychological demeanour of the penitent.

Yet there were evidently some who voiced serious concerns about the healthiness of the Lenten diet, with sufficient force to require a response from the Church. One such text was *On Lenten Foods*, by the eminent physician Paolo Zacchia, first published in 1636. After emphasizing that the 'mother' Church cared implicitly for the health and well-being of the faithful, exemplified particularly through exemptions from dietary regulations for certain categories of people, Zacchia then examines and refutes the medical criticisms evidently advanced against fasting.[38] One observation for example was that although two meals a day were considered healthiest for the digestion, only one full meal a day was permitted in Lent. The prohibition on meat, eggs, and dairy products meant that people ate mainly fish and vegetables, although they were believed to generate unhealthy cold and damp humours. Moreover, it was suggested that the sudden and dangerous change of dietary routine in Lent went against the Hippocratic view that maintenance of the body's normal habits was absolutely key to healthy living. Zacchia responded to these observations in detail. He explained that the reason for reduced meal times, taken at a set hour, was so as to assert one's control over hunger and unruly appetites. He pointed out that Lent took place during springtime, which was the season in which the body was presumed to be filled with superfluous 'bad' humours and excess blood. By reducing the most nutritious foods, particularly meat, one reduced the production of blood and diminished body heat and by extension the number and vitality of the spirits. This made it easier to curb the impetus of 'libidinous'

---

[36] (Our trans.) Croce, *Comiato*, unnumbered: 'Poi il pesce fu trovato | Per tener mortificato | L'huomo, e farlo mansueto, | In tai tempi, e humile, e quieto.'

[37] See Vanasse, 'Le Jeûne'; de Boer, *The Conquest*, 76–7, 174–5; Grieco, 'La gastronomia', 148.

[38] Zacchia, *Del vitto quaresimale*. e.g. those under the age of 7, the 'old', the ill, those who fatigue themselves whether intellectually or manually, and, significantly, men 'required' to perform their conjugal duties; *Del vitto quaresimale*, 9–15.

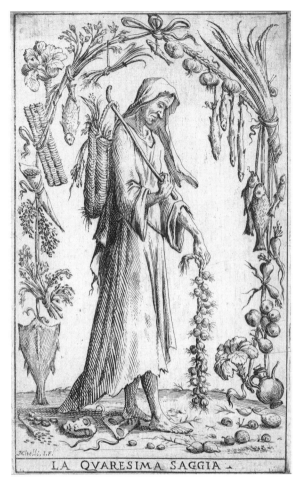

Fig. 7.1. This seventeenth-century didactic print conveys information about both the foods and the grave demeanour appropriate to the observance of Lent.

spirits, and 'appetites'.[39] By reducing surplus humours one also eliminated those vapours which clouded and diminished the powers of the intellect, thus promoting the ability to focus on spiritual matters. Furthermore, by eating less and avoiding rich foods, more 'spirits' were kept available for the demands of the intellect rather than the body and it was this link between correct diet and the 'health' of the soul which was the central purpose of Lent.[40] Yet, despite ripostes by the likes of Zacchia, as late as 1652, Giò Francesco Giuliani's text suggests that there was still a widespread sense that fasting was dangerous for health.[41] Written as a dialogue between

[39] These principles are explained in Zacchia, *Del vitto quaresimale*, 2–8.
[40] Jeanneret, 'Ma salade et ma muse', 218–19.   [41] Giuliani, *Dialogo*.

a doctor and his patients who were seeking dispensations from Lent on the grounds of ill health, he argued that virtually every ailment his patients were suffering from could actually be cured by the Lenten diet, rather than exacerbated by it.

Given the awareness of the relationship between food and health which we have already documented, it is perhaps not surprising that the Spada-Veralli family also expressed grave concerns about the unhealthiness of the Lenten diet, which is particularly significant given that two close family members were cardinals. Albala has framed his discussion of texts like Zacchia's in the context of Protestant–Catholic polemics, attacks on ritual practices by reformers, and the role of fasting in upholding Catholic confessional identity.[42] Yet these letters suggest we give more weight to the resistance offered by the devout themselves, torn between the deeply engrained precepts of Galenic dietary advice and the rigidity of Lenten requirements. Furthermore, the chronology suggests that the reassurance offered by physicians like Zacchia and Giuliani as to the healthiness of the Lenten fast had not prevailed over more traditional medical concerns. Writing in February 1678, for example, Maria Veralli echoes Zacchia's advice not to overeat during Lent, whilst attributing her husband's stomach problems to Lenten foods: 'Be careful not to eat too much since this undermines the complexion, since they [Lenten foods] are of such little substance.'[43] A couple of weeks later she notes that the household is observing Lent, eating 'leafy vegetables and foods of no consequence'.[44] Later on when her husband is suffering from haemorrhoids she again explains it as deriving from 'these Lenten foods and the time of year'.[45] At the end of Lent in 1678 we read of her relief that everyone has come through this dangerous period unscathed: 'I am very pleased to hear that Lent has treated you so well that you are not suffering its after-effects.' She adds however that her children are well but 'have pale complexions'—presumably thanks to the lack of nourishing foods—and she goes on to warn her husband to 'be careful over Easter, or the sudden change in foods will trouble you'.[46]

Yet far from any attempts to avoid Lent, the Spada-Veralli women seem to have been deeply reluctant to abandon it, even when we might suppose they had good reason. The letters between Giulia Benzoni and her husband Giovan Battista Veralli were written during Lent in 1601 against a background of marital disputes over money, Giulia's grief at having recently suffered a miscarriage and her anxiety to produce an heir, as well as worries about her general ill health. Over the course of several letters Giulia laments how hard it is for her to fast when Giovan Battista is sending her so little money that she cannot afford fish nor (unspecified) other produce which would make it easier for her to keep Lent. Giulia also marvels—ironically—that she has managed to keep Lent so far, considering that 'there isn't even a cabbage leaf here,

---

[42] Albala, 'The Ideology', esp. 49–51. Likewise Vanasse, 'Le Jeûne'.
[43] 'E si guardi di non fare di trapassi che sono di pregiudizio alla complessione, per essere questi di poco sostanza.' ASR, FSV, B.618, 26.2.1678.
[44] 'Herbe e bagatelle'; ASR, FSV, B.618, 12.3.1678.
[45] 'Li cibi di quaresima e la stagione'; ASR, FSV, B.618, 26.3.1678.
[46] 'Ho molto gusto di sentire che la quaresima l'habbia trattato così bene che non se ne senta', ASR, FSV, B.618, 6.4.1678; and 'si guardi dalla Pasqua, che nel mutare de' cibi no la travagli', ASR, FSV, B.618, 28.9.1678.

let alone anything else', in reference to the fact that her husband had allowed the kitchen garden to be left unplanted. Moreover, she reminds him she doesn't eat legumes—that other Lenten staple. Despite all this she stresses that she is managing 'not to eat until 20 hours'—about 1 or 2 p.m.—and that she is 'still keeping Lent, and I want to last as long as I can'.[47] Giulia seems to be threatening that unless he sends her the wherewithal to get better food, probably fish, she will probably break Lent, and one presumes, from her tone, that this would reflect badly on their honour as a couple, or perhaps particularly on his honour as husband and 'ruler' of his wife.

In 1647 we find similar tensions in letters between Maria Veralli and her uncle, Cardinal Bernardino Spada. Maria had evidently been ill and Bernardino must have ordered her to stop fasting. In her letter she replies that although she was reluctant to do so, she had been on the verge of obeying his instructions but fortunately on waking up that morning she had suddenly felt better, and therefore no longer needed to break Lent. Some twenty years later it was her daughter's turn to write to her, in rather a similar vein, describing how despite fearing that she has suffered a miscarriage, she didn't want to break her Lenten fast so she had stayed in bed and eaten soup and eggs, which presumably she was allowed either because she had been pregnant, or because she had miscarried.[48]

From these letters it would appear that members of this elite, clerical family had to negotiate a course between the pleasures and the demands of fashionable, social eating, the restrictions imposed by medical advice, and the notions of renunciation and bodily discipline emphasized in Counter-Reformation theology and conduct guides. They also provide evidence of the interiorization of the Lenten duty, or perhaps that this had become an important social duty for members of their class— possibly, as Boldo indicated, observed with some ostentation. Meanwhile, the critiques of Lenten restrictions per se show how pervasive Galenic prescriptions still were, although possibly Giuliani's attack on those who sought to evade Lent may highlight social fractures in the extent to which the Lenten obligation was accepted.

COLD DRINKING

Compared to the astonishing variety of foodstuffs discussed in some regimens, water and wine were the only drinks mentioned, since any other forms of drink, such as infusions of herbs and cordials, were regarded as medicines rather than beverages[49] (See Fig. 7.2).

---

[47] 'Adesso è Quatragesima et io non ho un quatrino per comprarmi un'oncia di pesce, hora vedete come mi posso trattenere a dar Quatragesima et sa V.S. come ha lassato l'horto et io non magno legumi.' ASR, FSV, B.449, 20.3.1601. 'Rengratio poi infinitamente V.S. della diligenza ch'ha fatta di farme gustare Quatragesima et fin adesso io l'ho fatta senza pesce e quando V.S. mi mandarà le robbe la farò più che posso, et quando non posso più qualche santo me agiutarà, che V.S. puol considerare come si possa fare Quatragesima da queste bande, non essendoci manco una fronde de cavoli, nonché altro'. ASR, FSV, B.449, 27.3.1601.

[48] ASR, FSV, B.1115, 20.4.1661.

[49] They might be called decoctions, cordials, distillations, juleps, etc. They were usually made with added honey or sugar and sometimes drunk hot, as well as prescribed externally.

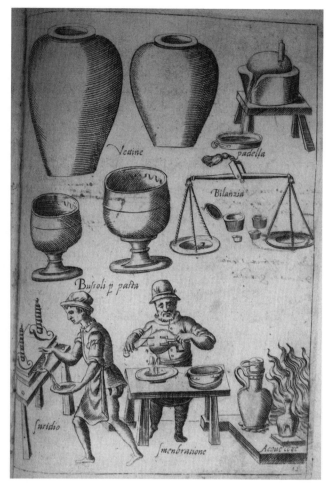

Fig. 7.2. This engraving in Bartolomeo Scappi's celebrated 1570 cookbook illustrates equipment and procedures used in the kitchen. The kind of 'cooked waters' contained in the vessels on the bottom right would have been medicinal infusions of flowers and herbs.

How much and when one should drink, whether before or after eating, and which types of wine to drink according to one's constitution formed the core of this advice, but the intricate detail of the matter meant that it could run to scores of pages.[50] Great emphasis was also placed on the quality and quantity of wine drunk, since it was considered a very special element of the diet; nutritious, humidifying, heating, and so on according to its colour, sweetness, acidity, and density. Generally speaking, provided the appropriate wine for one's constitution was consumed in moderation and suitably diluted, it was thought to confer a multitude of benefits on the body as well as playing an important role in assisting digestion. Nevertheless, all

---

[50] Durante has the most succinct list of twelve rules on drinking wine; *Il tesoro*, 312–16.

wines interacted differently with different food types so they must be selected accordingly. Furthermore, it was agreed that wine should very rarely be drunk 'neat', but diluted with water, according to the variety and strength of the wine.[51] The topic was so complex that the sixteenth century saw the proliferation of volumes exclusively on the nature of wines from different localities and their respective medicinal properties.[52] One regimen even provided tables indicating the correct proportions of water to dilute various wines, according to the desired results. (See Fig. 7.3.)

This said, several pages could easily be devoted to the dangers of excessive wine consumption and most authors noted that the ancient Romans had forbidden wine to men and women under the age of 35, and caution was advised although the only total prohibition on wine in medical texts was applied to babies, children, and youths.[53] One author described the 'terrifying effects' of allowing children wine, and Durante forbade it to those under 25.[54] It was deemed that in their case wine 'added fire to fire', overheating their already 'hot' constitutions and producing vapours in the head, 'igniting anger and libido', and preventing them from learning 'a trade or science'.[55] Moralists and pedagogues, anxious about women's dangerous libido, also urged women to drink with caution, or even forbade wine to women too.[56]

The mid-sixteenth century also witnessed a lively public debate between physicians, historians, and public health officials as to how best to provide sufficient good-quality drinking water for the rapidly expanding population of their cities, stimulated by the prominence given to water in Hippocrates' *Airs, Waters, and Places*.[57] Regimens also began to include far more comprehensive instructions on how to identify the best possible drinking water, discussing the virtues and drawbacks of sources such as rain, snow, springs, wells, lakes, and rivers, concluding that fountain and spring water were the most healthy. Authors were also concerned with how 'heavy' or 'light' the water was, how dirty it was, and the effect of the winds and sun upon it, and some included extended discussions about the merits of the various springs, fountains, and watercourses in their respective cities.[58] Importantly however, it was noted that if one had doubts about the water quality it could always be 'cooked' (i.e. boiled) or distilled, as had been practised by the 'ancients', as 'cooking' the water purified it, and made it 'lighter' and more

---

[51] Thus, throughout the early modern period, the Republic of Venice supplied workers such as shipbuilders at their workplace with several litres a day of what was known as the 'workers' beverage', wine diluted with water at the ratio of 1:2. Davis, 'Venetian Shipbuilders', esp. 59, 61, and 68.

[52] For an introduction to wines and bibliographical references, see Grieco 'La gastronomia'; and Malacarne, *Sulla mensa*.

[53] e.g. Mercurio, *De gli errori*, 350–2.

[54] 'Spaventevoli effetti'; Panaroli, *Abuso*, 13. Also see e.g. Durante, *Il tesoro*, 315–16; Fonseca, *Del conservare*, 30; and Paschetti, *Del conservare*, 331.

[55] 'Perche si aggiungerebbe fuoco a fuoco.' Durante, *Il tesoro*, 315–16. and Paschetti, *Del conservare*, 332.

[56] e.g. Frigerio, *Arte d'acquistar*, 24.

[57] On these debates see Siraisi, *History, Medicine*, esp. 168–93. On the provision of new water supplies for Rome, see Wentworth Rinne, *The Waters*.

[58] See Petronio, *Del viver*, 38–45; and Paschetti, *Del conservare*, 318–22.

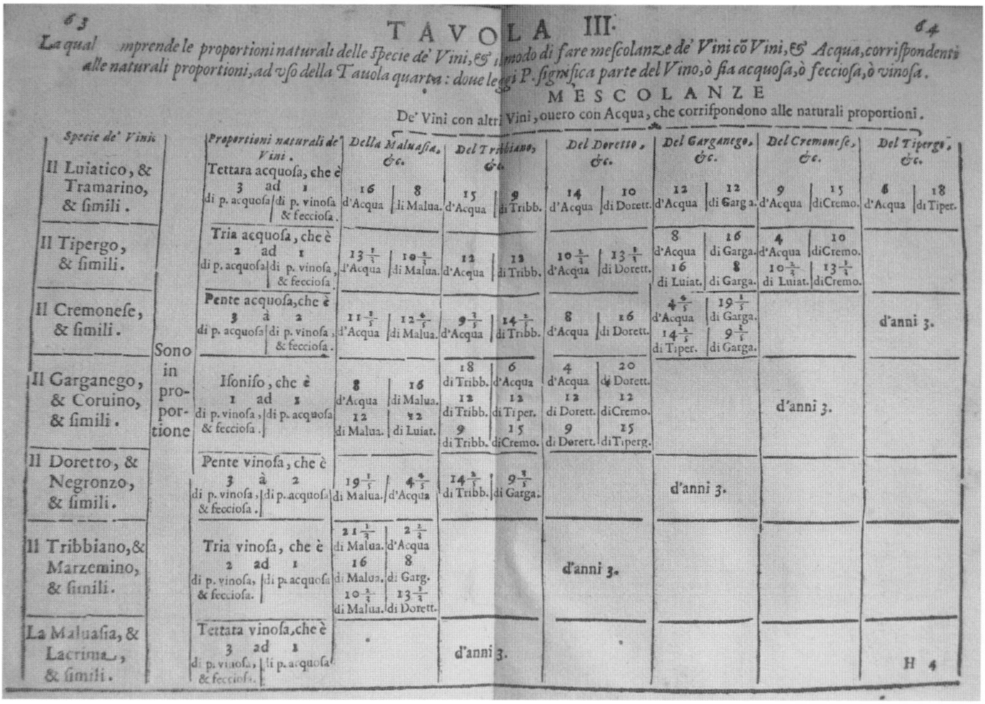

63 TAVOLA III. 64

La qual comprende le proportioni naturali delle specie de' Vini, & il modo di fare mescolanze de' Vini cō Vini, & Acqua, corrispondenti alle naturali proportioni, ad uso della Tauola quarta: doue leggi P. significa parte del Vino, ò sia acquosa, ò fecciosa, ò vinosa.

MESCOLANZE

De' Vini con altri Vini, ouero con Acqua, che corrispondono alle naturali proportioni.

Specie de' Vini.		Proportioni naturali de' Vini.	Della Maluasia, &c.	Del Tribbiano, &c.	Del Doretto, &c.	Del Garganego, &c.	Del Cremonese, &c.	Del Tipergo, &c.
Il Luiatico, & Tramarino, & simili.	Sono in proportione	Tettara acquosa, che è 3 ad 1 di p. acquosa | di p. vinosa & fecciosa.	16 d'Acqua | 8 di Malua.	15 d'Acqua | 9 di Tribb.	14 d'Acqua | 10 di Dorett.	12 d'Acqua | 12 di Garga.	9 d'Acqua | 15 di Cremo.	6 d'Acqua | 18 di Tiper.
Il Tipergo, & simili.		Tria acquosa, che è 2 ad 1 di p. acquosa | di p. vinosa, & fecciosa.	13 1/3 d'Acqua | 10 2/3 di Malua.	12 d'Acqua | 12 di Tribb.	10 2/3 d'Acqua | 13 1/3 di Dorett.	8 d'Acqua | 16 di Garga. 16 di Luiat. | 8 di Garga.	4 d'Acqua | 10 di Cremo. 10 2/3 di Luiat. | 13 1/3 di Cremo.	
Il Cremonese, & simili.		Pente acquosa, che è 3 à 2 di p. acquosa | di p. vinosa, & fecciosa.	11 1/5 d'Acqua | 12 4/5 di Malua.	9 3/5 d'Acqua | 14 2/5 di Tribb.	8 d'Acqua | 16 di Dorett.	4 4/5 d'Acqua | 19 1/5 di Garga. 14 2/5 di Tiper. | 9 3/5 di Garga.		d'anni 3.
Il Garganego, & Coruino, & simili.		Isoniso, che è 1 ad 1 di p. vinosa, & fecciosa. | di p. acquosa	8 d'Acqua | 16 di Malua. 12 di Malua. | 12 di Luiat.	18 di Tribb. | 6 d'Acqua 12 di Tribb. | 12 di Tiper. 9 di Tribb. | 15 di Cremo.	4 d'Acqua | 20 di Dorett. 12 di Dorett. | 12 di Cremo. 9 di Dorett. | 15 di Tiperg.		d'anni 3.	
Il Doretto, & Negronzo, & simili.		Pente vinosa, che è 3 à 2 di p. vinosa, & fecciosa. | di p. acquosa	19 1/5 di Malua. | 4 4/5 d'Acqua	14 2/5 di Tribb. | 9 3/5 di Garga.		d'anni 3.		
Il Tribbiano, & Marzemino, & simili.		Tria vinosa, che è 2 ad 1 di p. vinosa, & fecciosa. | di p. acquosa	21 1/3 di Malua. | 2 2/3 d'Acqua 16 di Malua. | 8 di Garg. 10 2/3 di Malua. | 13 1/3 di Dorett.		d'anni 3.			
La Maluasia, & Lacrima, & simili.		Tettara vinosa, che è 3 ad 1 di p. vinosa, & fecciosa. | di p. acquosa		d'anni 3.				H 4

Fig. 7.3. These tables from Peccana's 1627 treatise on cold drinking show the correct proportions of wine to be mixed with water according to the type of wine used. On another page he shows the results. For example, half water and half wine produces 'the drink of truth'.

'digestible'.[59] Water storage was also a topic of interest, and the merits of different types and materials used for vases, cisterns, and piping were thoroughly debated.[60]

It was not just the quality of the wine and water which mattered to physicians, but the temperature at which they were drunk. The norm was to drink one's wine and water at room temperature or that of a cellar, but in the mid-sixteenth century a fierce controversy arose over whether the increasingly popular practice of chilling one's drinks 'artificially' with snow, ice, or even (much disapproved of) saltpetre was healthy or indeed safe.[61] Chilling drinks and fruit was not an entirely new phenomenon since snow and ice had been used by elites in the Italian peninsula to cool their food and drinks more or less without interruption since the Roman Empire.[62] Over the sixteenth century it became increasingly fashionable

[59] 'Che egli sia bene a cuocere ogni sorte d'acqua.' Bacci, *Del Teuere*, 128. See also Fonseca, *Del conservare*, 30; Paschetti, *Del conservar*, 315–16. Even Lombardelli refers to the quality of drinking water, *Il giovane studente*, 39.

[60] Boldo discusses the dangers of oil conserved in copper vessels in *Della natura*, 284. Tanara specified there should be no lead used in piping in *L'economia*, 6–7.

[61] The debate extended to the temperature at which fruit was consumed too. Interestingly, the use of snow and ice to preserve foods is not mentioned.

[62] This is pointed out by Scotoni, 'Raccolta', 60–1.

and the subject of an energetic printed debate. By 1627 Peccana declared that there was 'No house, whether in a city or elsewhere, . . . that in summer does not cool at least with water, if not with snow and ice.'[63] Criticism was aimed initially at the nobility and the courtly milieu, amongst whom, according to one contemporary critic, the fashion had become so extreme that 'they wouldn't know how to eat even a cherry, . . . even in mid-winter which wasn't frozen or chilled with snow or salt-petre'. Some gentlemen, he continues, 'even take their medicines with ice'.[64] By well before 1600 this increased consumption of snow and ice was enabled by sophisticated systems of collection, supply, and storage, regulated and taxed by the papal authorities so as to ensure that the city never ran short of this precious commodity.[65] Perhaps unsurprisingly, the production of polemical tracts on the subject coincides precisely with this shift from cold drinking as a minority luxury to being a widespread phenomenon even amongst lower social groups.

As Waddy has pointed out, snowfalls were not uncommon even in and around Rome in the sixteenth and seventeenth centuries.[66] Snow falling in the nearby mountains was gathered and kept in 'snow pits' (*conserve* or *pozzi*) then delivered on specially designed conveyances which were pulled by night along regularly maintained 'snow roads'.[67] The nobility had their snow delivered to private snow and ice pits which were being incorporated into their palaces by the 1550s (see Fig. 7.4).

For those without such facilities, by the early seventeenth century there were as many as thirty-nine authorized 'snow shops' in Rome.[68] As Scipione Mercurio complained in 1603:

> Once snow was only used by princes and the greatest prelates. Now it has finally passed down even to plebeians, and now there is so much available in the city that it is sold on the piazzas at such ridiculously low prices, that for a *baiocco*, you can buy enough for one person's lengthy dinner.[69]

In reality the debate as to whether or not cold drinks were healthy was not a new one. In his *Airs, Waters, and Places* Hippocrates enumerated the damaging effects of cold water, attributing to it a range of illness from catarrh and phlegm to barrenness in women and madness in the old.[70] Galen's approach to the subject was more ambiguous, not only permitting cold drinking in particular cases but actually

---

[63] 'Non è casa in città over in altro luogo dentro e fuori d'Italia dove di state non si raffreddi almen con acque, se non con neve e ghiaccio.' Peccana, *Del bever*, 12.

[64] 'Non saprebbono alcuni mangiare una ciregia, ne' frutto alcuno, etiando di mezza vernata, che non fosse aghiacciato o rinfrescato con la neve, o co'l salnitro.' Bacci, *Del Teuere*, 138–9.

[65] By 1608 it generated 13,500 *scudi* in taxes annually; Scotoni, 'Raccolta', 61 and 69. Also *Regesti di bandi*. This register documents the numerous laws issued to regulate the trade.

[66] Waddy, *Seventeenth-Century Roman Palaces*, 15.

[67] Scotoni, 'Raccolta', 60–70.

[68] On private snow pits, as in the Villa Giulia, or Pitti Palace, see David, *Harvest*, 1–30, esp. 9–10. On snow shops Scotoni, 'Raccolta', 61 and 69.

[69] 'L'uso della neve era solo frequentato da prencipi e prelati maggiori. Ogni ciavatino vuol la neve. poiche in detta città ve ne concorre tanta copia, che si vende per le piazze a vil mercato, quando per un baiocco se n'ha tanta che basta per una persona ad ogni lungo disnare.' Mercurio, *De gli errori*, 538.

[70] Hippocrates, *Airs, Waters, Places*, esp. pt. IV, 150; pt. VII, 152.

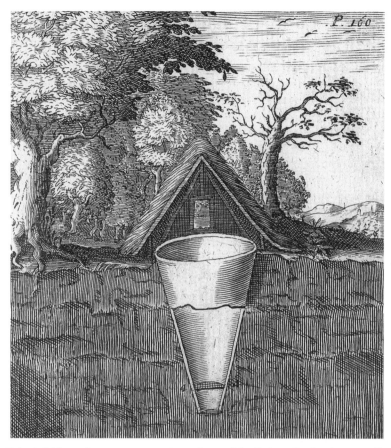

Fig. 7.4. A fairly rudimentary snow pit as observed by Robert Boyle when travelling in Italy in the mid-seventeenth century. More permanent structures were often built into the premises of suburban villas.

preferring it.[71] Over the intervening centuries authors had swung between these two points of view, cherry-picking arguments apparently at random or steering to an ambivalent middle ground. By the early Renaissance however the medical literature was, in de Planhol's words, 'in a horrible muddle' over whether cold water was safe to drink or not.[72] In 1558 the first text to appear in Italian on the topic by the physician Bacci made clear his disapproval of cold drinking for Mediterranean peoples.[73] The 1574 publication of a tract by a physician from Seville who enthusiastically praised the virtues of snow sparked an escalation in the debate which, spilling over the boundaries of the regimen, found its voice in individual tracts,

[71] We are indebted here to de Planhol's careful analysis of the evolution of antique medical thought on this topic; *L'Eau de neige*, 215–24.

[72] 'Un horrible melange'; de Planhol, *L'Eau de neige*, 223.

[73] Bacci, *Del Teuere*.

creating a kind of subgenre of health-advice literature.[74] In the following hundred years, with particular concentration in the decades before 1630, at least eleven tracts were published for or against cold drinking in Italian alone. This debate was also conducted in Latin, and a seventeenth-century text attests to its transformation into a scientific dispute about processes and phenomena involved when liquids were frozen. The whole issue of the beneficial effects of cold on the body more generally was central to the wider eighteenth-century debate on 'cold regimen' which particularly preoccupied the English.[75]

Disagreement about the effects of cold drinks focused on four areas or functions of the body. The first was body heat. Those against cold drinking argued that a sudden wash of cold liquid could cool the body down to the point of potentially extinguishing the flame within, whilst those in favour argued that cold drinks reduced excessive body temperature and fevers, particularly in the summer, as well as maintaining one's natural inner humidity.[76] They also claimed that the lassitude and weakness felt by the body during hot weather occurred because natural heat had been 'exhausted' which could only be corrected by a cold drink which 'reawakened' and stimulated body heat to return.[77] The brain was the second concern. Those against cold drinking claimed that it ultimately led to the spawning of cold humours around the brain, fuelling fears that the damage caused accumulated over a lifetime, leading to forgetfulness and imbecility in the old.[78] This belief certainly troubled one reader who noted in the margin of Bertaldi's regimen: 'drinking with snow may not harm in the short term but does over time'.[79] This was however ridiculed by supporters of cold drinking, who argued that on the contrary, during hot weather it acted like a wind, blowing corrupt humours and vapours away from the heart.[80] Thirdly the effect of cold drinks on the digestive system was at issue. Those in favour argued that the cold strengthened the stomach and increased appetite whilst the opposition stated that it slowed digestion making it harder for the body to digest food.[81] Some said the cold fluid dried out waste products, leading to blockages, but also accused it of causing cases of 'flux' and dysentery.[82] Finally, even its supporters adopted Galen's caveats, recommending that its use was best confined to a relatively small group of users: those with hot constitutions; those with responsibility for many things, or tied up in many affairs such as governors, kings, and ministers; those who exercise or labour a great deal; those who are very

---

[74] Nicolas Monardes's tract was first translated into Italian in 1574 as *Trattato della neue*. See David, *Harvest*, 6, and de Planhol on this and the broader context, *L'Eau de neige*, 226.

[75] De Planhol finds seven in Latin. This figure excludes discussions contained within more extended medical texts. For a detailed chronology and analysis see his *L'Eau de neige*, 227–8. For a scientific tract see Bartoli, *Del ghiaccio*. For England see Smith, *Clean*, 216–23.

[76] e.g. Persio, *Del bever caldo*, 43. Berti, *Discorso*, 21.

[77] Pisanelli, *Trattato*, 178–80.

[78] Salini, *Trattato del ber fresco*, 9–10.

[79] 'bever con la neve se ben non nuoce di presente, lo fa poi con longhezza di tempo.' Bertaldi, *Regole della sanità*, 65.

[80] Berti, *Discorso*, 23; Peccana, *Del bever*, 31.

[81] Fuscone, *Trattato del bere caldo*, 131; Salini, *Trattato del ber fresco*, 10.

[82] On cold and blockages see Persio, *Del bever caldo*, 42; Mercurio, *De gli errori*, 357. By contrast see Paschetti on heating, blockages, and pestilence, *Del conservare*, 287.

busy; and those engaged in military exercises.[83] The old, the young, and the sick were generally to avoid it and opponents seized gleefully on these restrictions as a sign of how damaging the practice could be.[84]

A lack of clear guidance from ancient texts on the subject contributed greatly to the intensity of the debate. Some tried to overcome this by piling up layer upon layer of quotations from multiple antique sources, presumably hoping that the sheer weight of authority would impress their readers.[85] Monardes suggested that since cold drinking was practised almost 'universally', this legitimized its use in Italy.[86] Another tactic which shows the immediacy of the debate and the extent to which it was grounded in practice, was to cite recent public health events as proof of the benefits or dangers of cold drinking. Pisanelli in his 1583 tract cited as evidence the 'fact' that the annual death rate in the city of Messina had plunged by about one thousand ever since snow had been made widely available to the populace.[87] Although ridiculed by Persio, who pointed out that any number of reasons could explain this improvement in the death rate, the example was recycled several times over the coming decades. Persio then countered the example of Messina with that of Venice, where licences had recently been awarded for the provision and sale of snow in the city. He claimed public health had immediately been compromised, with people suffering from stomach pains and other illnesses, such that the licences had quickly been revoked.[88] Authors also looked for individual proofs, citing either personal experiences of patients or their own bodies or contemporary anecdotes about the health of famous people.[89] However, in different ways most of these assertions represented a profound threat to traditional authority. The appeal to the 'universality' of cold drinking for example was contrary to the underlying ethos of Galenic medicine which was tailored to the individual's constitution; and even to Hippocratic medicine, based on the needs of different peoples rooted in their different locations and climates.[90] This more evidence-based approach meanwhile raised the problem of whether individual and universal experiences actually constituted a proof, and if so, which carried more weight: and crucially, whether experience could really be considered a valid alternative to ancient authorities.

As the debate on drinking gathered pace, it also became more personal and shows us how publishing was used to make and break reputations. Some texts sported lengthy lists of those physicians who supported the same views, noting particularly those with any claims to fame, such as papal physicians.[91] Cassiani

---

[83] These lists vary. This is from [Monardes], *Trattato della neue*, 222.

[84] See Pisanelli, *Trattato*, 178–80.

[85] esp. Bacci and Persio.

[86] [Monardes], *Trattato della neue*, 227.

[87] Pisanelli, *Trattato*, 178.

[88] Persio, *Del bever caldo*, 63.

[89] e.g. Fuscone, on cold drinkers who lived to a great age, *Trattato del bere caldo*, 225; and Persio on some who died suddenly after a cold drink, *Del bever caldo*, 43.

[90] See Fuscone's refutation of universally appropriate remedies or foods, *Trattato del bere caldo*, 57.

[91] Theodoro Meyden lists eight names of those who have written in favour of cold drinking in *Trattato della natura del vino*, 55, 118. Cassiani adds four more physicians from Rome in *Risposta*, 10. To these we can add Gio Battista Berti (1616), Alessandro Peccana (1627), and Gio Battista Vallegio (1664).

ridicules the expertise of his opponents and even more daringly, he questions their integrity, suggesting that they have ceded to pressure—even perhaps bribes—to support a proposition they don't believe in.[92] This comment suggests that the cold drinking debate may have been generated through conflicts between men with vested interests in the snow trade—whether holding local monopolies on snow, or running the snow shops—and kept alive by the reactions of men with medical authority.[93]

The role of 'snow' entrepreneurs in promoting cold drinking emerges in the introduction to Cassiani's anti-cold-drinking tract of 1603, in which he describes how he had spent several days staying in the shop of a snow seller in Bologna. The *bottega*, like most commercial premises, had a sign hanging outside indicating the nature of the business, and he noticed that attached to this sign was a small anonymous pamphlet entitled *Discorso sopra il bever fresco cavato da autori antichissimi e principalissimi dove si mostra l'utilità del bever fresco* (Discourse on Cold Drinking Taken from the Most Ancient and Most Eminent Authors, in Which the Utility of Cold Drinking Is Demonstrated).[94] It was 'just two pages long', merely a compilation of texts by other writers and according to him had been 'rushed' into print following a debate on the topic in one of the city's learned academies which had declared cold drinking to be unhealthy. Dangling as it was from the shop sign, the anonymous tract represents an early manifestation of the uses of print for health advertising and certainly suggests it had been commissioned by someone fearing a loss of trade resulting from the critiques of cold drinking. Outraged at what he perceived to be an irresponsible promotion of cold drinks, and wishing to spread his appreciation for hot drinking (to be discussed later) Cassiani then rushed out his forty-page reply within the year. His publication, too, elicited a response, although a more considered one, which was published three years later in Latin.[95]

Two years later, further up the peninsula in Genoa, the debate on cold and hot drinking was still raging and we are given a glimpse of some of the other channels through which medical ideas and texts circulated.[96] The Roman doctor Paolo Fuscone describes how when visiting a gentleman patient named Sig. Conestaggio, he was shown a printed pamphlet and a handwritten 'piece of advice' which Conestaggio had been handed by Agostino Doria, Duke of Genoa. They were both 'recently composed praises of drinking hot'.[97] These were then passed on to the Prince of Massa, and not long afterwards, to the Marquis of Torriglia. Fuscone claims that all four gentlemen then asked him his opinion on the matter and seeing

---

[92] 'Sforzati non solo di dire ma di operare anche nelle cose della professione loro stessa a gusto di alcuni maggiorenni della Corte, si come non mancano di quegli, che spontaneamente gli lusingano.' Cassiani, *Risposta*, 11.

[93] And thus supports Elizabeth David's speculation that the future Duke of Tuscany, interested in taxing snow, may have commissioned the first translation of Monardes's tract in 1574, *Harvest*, 5–7.

[94] Cassiani, *Risposta*, 7.

[95] G. Castiglioni, *De frigido*.

[96] Fuscone, *Trattato del bere caldo*.

[97] He calls it a 'consiglio che in lode del bere caldo erano stati modernamente composti'; Fuscone, *Trattato del bere caldo*, introd. (unnumbered).

such uncertainty amongst his illustrious clients he decided to compose his own advice tract.

The comments prefacing these two texts reveal not only the intensity and vitality of the drinking debate, but demonstrate that it belonged to a wide 'community of conversation'. It was not just a theoretical debate in Latin restricted to learned academies and scholars, but as Fuscone put it, a subject which was 'familiar, curious and necessary for all kinds of people'.[98] And it seems the advice really was heard and discussed, not only in the palaces and villas of the nobility, but also out in the streets. Although what survives in our libraries is largely evidence of the debate as it was articulated at the top end of the market, Cassiani's account shows that it was fuelled by cheap pamphlets of just a few pages. These were not only more affordable but undoubtedly more readable than the weighty tomes by men such as Fuscone. But even he hoped that by publishing in Italian he would reach a wider audience. It also reveals just how easily and quickly medical authors—or those peddling medical ideas to promote goods—were able to get their ideas into print and circulate them.

In retrospect we can see that the battle in favour of cold drinking had probably been won long before most of the publications in its favour even appeared; and although medical opinion was initially opposed to the practice, by the early seventeenth century there were certainly more writers in favour of it than against.[99] Moreover, in several regimens even though authors start by listing the potential hazards of cold drinking, they often end up by quietly accepting the practice with a few general caveats. Paschetti for example concludes his lengthy analysis rather lamely with 'Cold drinking, as is commonly practised these days . . . by the majority of people . . . remains expedient for the pleasure it gives and for health.'[100]

Indeed, one of the ways in which physicians sought to regain their authority on cold drinking whilst accepting the inevitability of fashion was by shifting the terms of debate away from blanket condemnation or acceptance, to a more subtle focus on specific issues related to usage and formulating rules for safe cold drinking. They explained the different 'degrees' of cold and 'how cold' a cold drink should be; they focused on the dangers and advantages of the many methods used to cool drinks down; and they decried cold drinking at inappropriate times of day, when the body was overheated, as well as excessive cold drinking.[101] Meanwhile physicians also managed to 'rewrite' the ground rules regarding the appropriateness of cold drinking for different social groups—presumably in an attempt to keep it as a mark of social distinction. Although Galenic teaching had deemed it suitable only for those who were fatigued and overheated by their physical labours, in mid-seventeenth-century Spain

[98] 'Come anche per trattarsi di materia familiare, curiosa e necessaria ad ogni sorte di persona.' Fuscone, *Trattato del bere caldo*, introd. (unnumbered).

[99] Only Cosimo Salini and Meyden seem to favour moderate or 'temperate' drinking. Only Persio and Cassiani are definitely in favour of hot drinking.

[100] 'Il bever fresco, come communemente si usa . . . così d'inverno come di estate, sì come osservato viene dalla maggior parte così rimane al gusto e alla sanità . . . molto convenevole.' Paschetti, *Del conservare*, 284. Likewise Petronio, *Del conservar*, 319.

[101] De Planhol, *L'Eau de neige*, 249–54.

physicians now approved of it only for the social and intellectual elites. Custom, they said, underpinned use by the former, and the excessive internal heat generated through the use of the intellect justified it for the latter. Labourers and those engaged in the 'mechanical' arts meanwhile were warned that because they lacked the abundant nourishment enjoyed by the wealthy, the sudden penetration of cold would endanger their stomachs.[102]

The Spada-Veralli correspondence suggests that although cold drinking was standard practice within the family, there was a clear awareness that it could be dangerous, implying that the caution advised by physicians had in fact prevailed. Certainly snow seems to have been a regular feature of daily life, judging from a letter from early April 1678 when Maria Veralli notes that she is not surprised that Cardinal Rocco 'has sent for snow' because the weather has suddenly warmed up.[103] Yet it seems that they drank cool but not cold drinks, and also feared the over-chilling of fruits, since we find Eugenia reassuring her mother that 'she needn't worry' about the ill effects of her drinking too much cold wine since she doesn't put hers 'in snow' and hasn't yet 'seen' any fruit.[104] There are also comments made during the summer months which reveal considerable caution about the dangers of drinking too much cool liquid when the body is overheated. In August 1662 Eugenia writes that it is very hot 'but what is good is that I am not very thirsty'.[105] A few years later in the same vein she notes, 'don't worry that drinking will make me ill because I don't drink too much and the Marquis pays attention to whether I do'; the following year it is his turn to 'feel all hot' which makes him 'drink often', something evidently worthy of a special comment.[106]

NEW DRINKS

One of the most vigorous rejections of cold drinking was written by Persio in 1593. He not only opposed cold drinking but in its place proposed the opposite: that people should take up the newly invented practice of 'hot' drinking which, unlike cold drinking, appears to have been driven initially by its health benefits rather than by fashion.[107] Traditionally, the only occasions when one might have drunk something hot was when taking a medicinal 'decoction' to warm the body. Persio's innovation was to recommend heating water nearly to boiling point and to

---

[102] Our gloss on two texts, one from 1637, the other from 1670 transcribed in de Planhol, *L'Eau de neige*, 250.

[103] 'Non mi meraviglio che il D Card. Rocci habbia mandatao a pigliare la neve.' ASR, FSV, B.618, 2.4.1678.

[104] 'Non abbia paura che mi faccia male il vino fresco perchè non lo faccio mettere in neve e li frutti ancor non se ne scorgono.' ASR, FSV, B.410, 26.6.1656.

[105] 'Fa un gran caldo ma quel che è buono è che non ho una gran sete.' ASR, FSV, B.1115, 27.8.1662.

[106] 'Ma non abbia paura che il bevere mi faccia male perchè non bevo troppo e il Marchese mio bada più se io bevo troppo.' ASR, FSV, B.410, 9.8.1656. 'Ma tanto il sig. Marchese beve spesso perchè lui per tutto sente caldo.' ASR, FSV, B.1115, 1.8.1657.

[107] The two main tracts in defence of hot drinking are by Persio, *Del bever caldo*; and Cassiani, *Risposta*.

add this to one's wine. It was not the wine itself which was heated, since this would have altered its beneficial properties in some way.[108] This differed, according to some, from the ancients, who had heated water, 'not in order to drink it hot, but to drink it cooked', since they subsequently placed the vase of cooked water to be chilled by placing it in snow.[109]

This new trend was very likely a response to recent accounts of practices from overseas, such as Father Gio. Pietro Maffei's account of travelling in the East Indies, China, and Japan.[110] Paschetti also recalls a recent visit to Italy by some princes from the Far East, noting that in China and Japan, despite the availability of grapes for wine, they shun alcohol making a drink called 'chia' from 'healthy herbs', or just drinking 'pure hot water'.[111] Persio conveys the novelty of the new practice by claiming that he devised it as a result of his and a friend's personal experiments.[112]

The medical reasons adduced in favour of 'hot drinking' were many, including propositions such as that the heat of the drinks is restorative of natural heat, helps with colics and stomach pains and with the digestion, and, as we have seen, cooked water being lighter, passes more quickly through the body.[113] Interestingly, although comparatively few voices were raised in particular favour of hot drinking, little could really be said against it presumably because hot drinking had always been recommended for the ill. Furthermore, it seems likely that even if drinking hot wine did not really catch on, the acceptability of a beverage taken at a hot temperature paved the way for the assimilation of two new drinks into the Italian diet: coffee and hot chocolate. As previously unknown foods which had appeared from the New World and the East, physicians struggled to accommodate them within the Galenic framework; however, the fact that both were usually drunk very hot went virtually unremarked by all commentators.[114] Coffee was considered to promote internal heat, stimulate the heart and spirits, dry up damp humours, and dispel vapours—almost a panacea therefore. Chocolate presented far more problems to physicians.[115] Having first appeared officially in Europe in 1585, chocolate was well established amongst wealthy Italians during the second half of the seventeenth century.[116] It was only consumed as a drink with added sugar and spices and was usually drunk hot. Physicians agreed generally that the cocoa bean

[108] Although Persio makes an exception for very weak wines, *Del bever caldo*, 33. See also Fuscone, *Trattato del bere caldo*, 1.

[109] 'Non dico per berla calda, ma per berla cotta.' Peccana, *Del bever*, 14.

[110] Cassiani cites Maffei's book which was first published in Latin in 1588 and Italian in 1589, *Risposta*, 27. See Maffei, *Le istorie*.

[111] 'Acqua pura e calda'; Paschetti, *Del conservare*, 271. Cassiani cites Maffei who has travelled to Japan as his source on their practices, in *Risposta*, 27.

[112] 'Tempratone ciaschedun di noi un bicchiero di vino nel bevemmo con nostro non picciol gusto.' Persio, *Del bever caldo*, 2. Cassiani adds a similar account in *Risposta*, 25.

[113] Persio, *Del bever caldo*, 52–6.

[114] For discussions of New World foods see Gentilcore, *Pomodoro*; and Earle, '"If You Eat Their Food"'. See also Albala, 'The Use and Abuse'.

[115] Surviving tracts on coffee are Rambaldi, *Ambrosia arabica*; and Magri, in *Virtú del caffe*. The first tract in favour of chocolate printed in Italian (from the Spanish) was Colmenero, *Della cioccolata*.

[116] It was already being drunk in Florence and Venice by 1595; Huetz de Lemps, 'Colonial Beverages', 385.

presented contradictory qualities; on the one hand nutritious and restorative and therefore beneficial for health, whilst other properties conspired to make it liable to cause blockages, particularly to the digestion.[117] Both explained the tendency of those who drank large amounts of chocolate to get fat; none suspected the role played by the copious amounts of sugar used to sweeten the drink, since sugar was considered to be a 'perfect' and 'corrective' ingredient.

What then was the impact of these debates about different kinds of drinking on the Spada-Veralli family? From the letters we know that Orazio Spada drank much hot chocolate, and the inventory of Bernardino's goods taken after his death suggests that he did too. He owned a 'flat bottomed beaker [*bicchiere*] made of rhinoceros horn and three little bowls of Indian wood'.[118] These sound identical to the *tazze* or *coppe* made of coconut which were used for drinking hot chocolate in the earlier seventeenth century, in imitation of practices in Mexico, examples of which have been traced in other Roman inventories from the period (see Fig. 7.5).[119] Orazio also owned four 'gilded cups with handles' which may have served the same purpose, since the presence of handles suggests a drink too hot to handle easily.[120]

Elsewhere we learn of Orazio's predilection for chocolate thanks to his wife's worries about its damaging effects on his digestion. In the spring of 1678 she worries that 'by drinking too much chocolate he is making himself ill'.[121] In the autumn of the same year Orazio is, indeed, suffering from a bad stomach and Maria reminds her husband that he has been advised by his doctor not to take chocolate 'especially not as thick as he drinks it', and particularly without due regard for the time of day, or proximity to mealtimes.[122] Early the next year she reprimands him again, begging him not to carry on having 'meals of just chocolate', explaining that this makes the stomach lazy and weakens the complexion, which was particularly serious given that it was Lent, when the other foods he was eating were also difficult to digest.[123] This last comment however seems to indicate that she was not aware that there was serious disagreement amongst theologians as to whether or not chocolate was indeed a 'food' or a 'drink' and the appropriateness of drinking chocolate at all during Lent.[124] As had been conducted only in Latin we can presume that this debate had not yet impinged on Orazio Spada's conscience, although it was to gather pace in Italian publications in the later eighteenth century.[125]

---

[117] See Albala, 'The Use and Abuse'.

[118] ASR, Notai AC, vol. 5933, 'Inventario bonorum Cardinal Bernardino Spada', 23.11.1661, 739ʳ: 'Un bicchiero di noceronte senza piede e tre scudelle di legno all'indiana'.

[119] These are described by Patrizia Piscitello in her account of the evolution of vessels and cups used for making and drinking hot chocolate in 'Serviti da cioccolata'. She also identifies one in the 1663 inventory of Cardinale Giovan Carlo de' Medici, 'Serviti da cioccolata', 20–1.

[120] 'Tazza indorata con le sue maniche.' ASR, Notai AC, vol. 5933, Inv. Spada, 23.11.1661, 743ʳ.

[121] 'Il pigliar troppo spesso la cioccolata non gli sia di pregiuditio.' ASR, FSV, B.618, 26.3.1678.

[122] 'Massime... se la piglia così fitta e senza ordina e regola dal pasto.' ARS, FSV, B.618, 5.10.1678.

[123] 'Fare i pasti con la semplice cioccolata', ASR, FSV, B.618, 9.3.1679.

[124] On chocolate and Lent in the Spanish context, see Forrest and Najjaj, 'Is Sipping Sin', 42.

[125] For Italy see Concina, *Memorie storiche* which summarizes the history of the debate. See also a modern reprint of the important *De chocolatis potu*, by Cardinal Francesco Maria Brancaccio, as *La tazza di cioccolata*. This has a list of all the individual publications on chocolate from 1516 to 1900 at pp. 83–108.

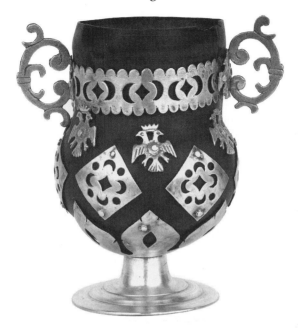

Fig. 7.5. This Tuscan goblet was probably made in the late sixteenth century in Mexico from tropical gourd and then mounted in silver. Imitating the *jicaras* used in Mesoamerica it would have been a fashionable object, used for drinking hot chocolate.

THE MATERIAL CULTURE OF DRINKING

The novelty of first cold, and then hot, drinking created a need for new objects which could deliver very cold or very hot water safely and elegantly to the diner. Lengthy passages in the regimens explained the relative merits and drawbacks of traditional methods of cooling water and wine and in theory fountain water was ideal. But ultimately none of these methods could bring the temperature down low enough to obtain the much-lauded medical benefits, nor satisfy the early modern Italians' desire to serve extremely cold drinks to their guests on a hot summer's night. The answer most definitely was not to add snow to the water; snow melt was 'metallic, foamy, dirty, and unpleasant' wrote Peccana, whilst Mercurio explained that both snow and ice were 'raw' and 'damaging'.[126] Peccana sang the praises of ice which was 'incomparable for its cleanliness and practicality' and ice-harvesting became more popular in some areas in the seventeenth century.[127] But on the whole authors preferred cooling methods which prevented the coolant from coming into contact with the drink.

[126] 'Secchiosa, schiumosa, sporca e spiacevole.' Peccana, *Del bever freddo*, 50. Mercurio, *De gli errori*, 358ᵛ.
[127] 'Alla fine é tollerabile modo, e non ha paragone con nissun de gli altri di politezza e commodità.' Peccana, *Del bever freddo*, 51. See Elizabeth David on the preference for ice and development of ice-pits in Tuscany, *Harvest*, 16–17.

The most healthy solution for keeping large quantities of water cool was also the simplest: taking a large bucket or other container of snow and placing the flasks or carafes of water or wine in them an hour before eating. It should be noted that most authors disapproved of placing the wine flask directly into snow, since it chilled it excessively, so in theory it was only the water which was cooled, though one has the impression from the admonishments in texts that this was not necessarily heeded. For those concerned with appearances, the bucket could be replaced by a beautifully decorated metal container, sometimes standing on low legs, which could be placed on the table, or more usually on the floor, called a *rinfrescatore*. This would be filled with snow or ice and flasks of water could be buried or placed on top (see Fig. 7.6). Cardinal Bernardino Spada owned a fine example of one made of silver with gilded lilies embossed on it as well as a technically more elaborate one made of tin, which was divided into various compartments into which the 'various rounded glass vases' could presumably be inserted.[128] It is quite possible that each flask could contain a different wine or dilution of wine suiting the particular health requirements of each diner. The 1621 inventory of a man who was probably a goldsmith contained a *rinfrescatore* with its 'companion' *fiasco*, suggesting that these objects were generally made as matching pairs or sets.[129] The copper *rinfrescatore* found in the inventory of a cobbler's widow, and those amongst the possessions of several former prostitutes, shows us that such objects were also present in the homes of the lower echelons of society.[130]

There was evidently considerable choice as regarded the vessel which was placed in the water cooler. Paschetti recommended using a jug or flask (*vaso*) of tin-plated copper, or silver, called a *bombola* to plunge into the snow to cool the drinking water.[131] This was perhaps what in Rome was described as a *fiasco da neve*, an object which appears in several inventories and was probably not a luxury object since we find two in the inventory of a hard-up former prostitute.[132] Intriguingly however, the inventory of a glass-maker from 1603 shows that he had a mound of *fiaschi da neve* in his workshop, suggesting they could also be made of glass.[133] An early seventeenth-century painting showing a man seated at a table shows us several vessels which, in the light of this, were presumably connected to cold drinking (Plate 20).

More intriguing than a *rinfrescatore* in terms of design is Monardes's recommendation to use a metal cylinder filled with snow or ice which could be placed inside a large vase or jug of liquid to be cooled.[134] The solutions adopted for keeping one's drink cool when at table are even more ingenious. Scipione Mercurio writes that in Rome he had seen little lids for glasses made of thin metal which

[128] 'Rinfrescatore di argento fatto a foggia di giglio dorato', and 'Un rinfrescatore di latta e diverse boccie e spartimenti'; ASR, Notai AC, vol. 5933, Inv. Spada, 23.11.1661, 742ᵛ–743ʳ.

[129] ASR, TCG, Notai UG, vol. 177, 1618–23, 564ʳ–565ᵛ and 610ʳ⁻ᵛ, Carlo Bomplano, 1.10.1621, 565ʳ.

[130] ASR, TNC, Uff. 2, vol. 218, Maddalena Bartoloccia, 4.08.1660, 258ʳ–259ᵛ and 268ʳ⁻ᵛ. e.g. 'Concolina di rame et rinfrescatore di rame'; ASVR, MCI, Isabella, 13.01.1606, 99ʳ.

[131] Paschetti, *Del conservare*, 307.

[132] ASVR, MCI, Lucia di Antonio del Prato Bolognese, 25.5.1605, 32ʳ–33ʳ.

[133] ASR, TNC, Uff. 4, vol. 71, Concorni, 25.2.1603, 328.

[134] 'Un canone lungo di lama da milano', [Monardes], *Trattato della neue*, 240ᵛ.

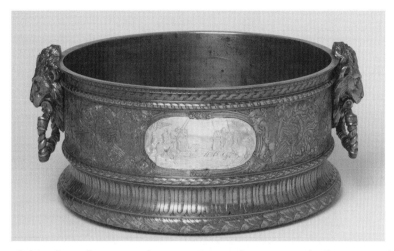

Fig. 7.6. This fine early seventeenth-century Venetian brass wine cooler (h. 19.5 cm, diam. 42.5 cm) would probably have stood on the floor near the table, filled with snow or ice.

had a depression in them which reached halfway down the glass, in which ice or snow was placed to cool the drink as it stood on the table. The advantage to this was that it cooled the drink down slowly rather than too quickly, which harmed the quality of the water.[135] This sounds similar to a vessel, described by Elizabeth David, in Tuscany known as a *cantinplore*, a glass decanter which had an 'ice-pocket' in the side which kept the wine chilled.[136] In the inventories of the wealthy we find other objects evidently designed to chill drinks. In 1604 Jo Baptista Serlupi owned amongst other cooling equipment a 'crystal jar for freezing', which was perhaps similar to the 'thick [?] gilded silver cup for freezing' owned by Cardinal Bernardino.[137] Three decades later eminent lawyer Polidoro Neruzzi Senese also had 'two cork vessels lined with tin for putting wine to cool'.[138]

One of the arguments made in favour of drinking hot was that it was much cheaper and easier to procure hot water than it was to obtain ice or snow. Yet actually heating the water to drink, and particularly keeping it hot on the table throughout the meal, posed as many if not more technical problems as did keeping it chilled. Although water could simply have been heated up in any domestic vessel over the kitchen fire, Persio advocated the use of a kind of small dedicated water heater. It was intended to fulfil the combined requirements of heating sufficient quantities of water without it becoming dirty or being tainted by other flavours, whilst simultaneously being placed on the dining table so as to provide piping hot

[135] Mercurio, *De gli errori*, 358ᵛ.   [136] David, *Harvest*, 20–1, 381–2.

[137] 'giaciatore di cristallo', ASR, TNC, Uff. 4, vol. 77, Jo Baptista Serlupi, 23.02.1605. 'Tazza d'argento spesa indorata per aggiaciare', ASR, Notai AC, vol. 5933, 'Inventario bonorum Cardinal Bernardino Spada', 23.11.1661, 742ᵛ.

[138] 'Due Sugari, da mettere in fresco il vino foderati di latta'; ASR, Notaio AC, vol. 3180, 857ʳ–882ʳ, inventory of Polidoro Neruzzi Senese, 18.11.1641.

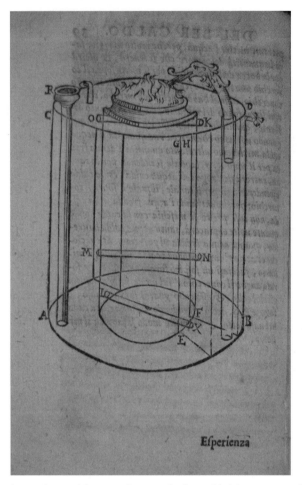

Efperienza

Fig. 7.7. The design for a table water heater which could deliver instant hot water for adding to one's wine was included in Persio's treatise on hot drinking in 1593.

water for guests. Since no such object existed, Persio first describes a rather complicated ancient Roman prototype, then explains that a distinguished friend has designed a simpler modern version and handed the plans to a local master craftsman to make out of brass. This was, perhaps, the earliest documented European kettle. Unfortunately five months later, at the time of going to press, the 'kettle' was still not ready (we will never know whether it was ever finished) but he provided the readers with a diagram and meticulous written instructions so they could make one for themselves (Fig. 7.7).[139]

Persio also reassured his reader that 'when we have had it made, we will communicate the result so that everyone can make one for themselves, or have one

---

[139] Persio, *Del bever caldo*, 34–7, for the ancient prototype, and 40–2 for his design.

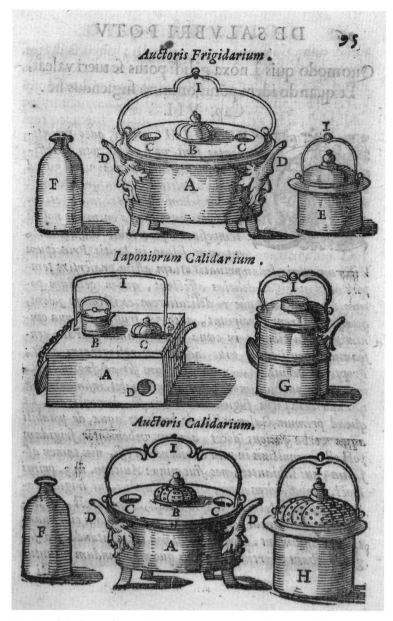

Fig. 7.8. Scacchi's design for a table water heater, and cooler, and a Japanese prototype, from his 1622 treatise in Latin.

made quite easily'. The fact that some thirty years later another doctor saw fit to propose his rather more elegant design for a water heater and cooler shows that Persio was not alone in pondering the technical issues raised by these new drinking trends (Fig. 7.8). In the meantime Persio suggests using small individual flasks, just big enough to hold a glassful of water, with round bellies and long narrow necks which can be placed in a metal cauldron of water which is kept boiling.[140] Being small, the water will heat up quickly, whilst the long neck will prevent the boiling water from entering the vase, and make it possible to pick them out of the cauldron water without burning oneself.

Finally the debate on drinking sheds light on the ways in which the shape of glasses was considered to affect one's health because of the way in which shape determined the speed of the flow of liquids. Any glass which encouraged one to drink too quickly was problematic, partly because it made one gulp too much air, and partly because a rush of fluid would lead to undigested food floating around in the stomach.[141] If the wine was chilled these dangers were exacerbated because the body's natural inner heat could be 'suffocated' by the rush of cold fluid.[142] Avicenna's authority was cited in support of these warnings, and his advice repeated: as a precaution, one should drink chilled drinks—either from 'a narrow mouthed flask' (*vaso*), or a carafe, ampoule, or 'beaked glass' (*bicchiero da becco*).[143] Camaffi added that big glasses with 'wide orifices' also encourage excessive 'licence' when drinking, and in the same vein Mercurio specified that a glass shouldn't be able to contain more than 6 or 7 ounces of wine.[144] However, presumably in thrall to the dictates of fashion, Camaffi then provided his readers with a loophole, by commenting that drinking from a 'flat *tazza* of fine crystal' was pleasant in summer and tasted better. Persio meanwhile condemned the flat, wide-topped *tazze* in his discussion of hot drinking because the liquid made 'certain waves', as it rushed towards the mouth, leading to gorging and slurping. To avoid this he also advocated the use of tall narrow glasses, explaining that the narrow shape ensured that the wine travelled more 'nimbly' to the lips.[145] The fact that these injunctions on shape and size were drawn from Avicenna suggests that they were probably quite well known and raise intriguing possibilities about the purpose of a particular kind of small, rounded bottle with a narrow neck represented in paintings by contemporary artists but also found in large quantities in archaeological excavations in Pisa.[146]

One feature of the material culture of Renaissance drinking for which we have no direct textual explanation is the comparatively large number of lids on glasses to be seen on the shelves of the Victoria and Albert Museum in London.[147] (See Figs. 7.9 and 7.10.) Making a lid for a glass was presumably not a simple proce-

---

[140] He then says that they are similar to earthenware vases used for heating water for the sick in Bologna called *cuogoli*, Persio, *Del bever caldo*, 40.

[141] Mercurio, *De gli errori*, 355.

[142] Camaffi, *Reggimento*, 111. He also adds that it tastes better.

[143] Both Monardes and Camaffi cite the need for a 'vaso di bocca stretta'. Monardes adds the other narrow-necked vessels. [Monardes], *Trattato della neue*, 220; Camaffi, *Reggimento*, 110–11.

[144] 'Tazza di cristallo fino piana.' Camaffi, *Reggimento*, 111. Mercurio, *De gli errori*, 355.

[145] Persio, *Del bever caldo*, 32–3.

[146] Omodeo, *Bottiglie e bicchieri*, 79; Stiaffini, 'I reperti', 78. Stiaffini says those found resemble the small flasks in the Allori painting (Plate 7).

[147] The Victoria and Albert Museum have numerous examples, some dated to the late 15th century.

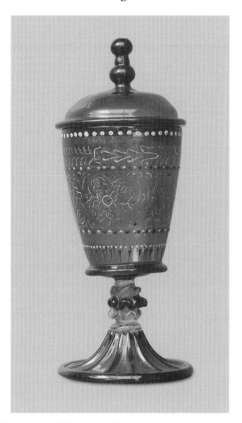

Fig. 7.9. This enamelled and gilded lidded goblet (h. 22 cm, d. 7 cm.) was made in Venice in *c*.1475–1510. The lid may have denoted the importance of the glass in a set, have protected the wine from dust and insects, or preserved it from the air.

dure—given the technicalities of making them fit—nor would they be easy to pre-serve intact, yet their survival suggests they were not uncommon. Our only fairly contemporary reference is a single inventory found by Ago, from 1702, noting the purchase of 'thirty-six little glass lids' and other drinking glassware by the wealthy Santacroce family.[148] Given that wine was nearly always drunk watered down it does not seem very likely that the lids were to conserve the flavour, as suggested by one scholar, and there may have been health-related reasons for them. A lid protected the wine and water from dust and from insects but also could have protected it from penetration by noxious airs. Monardes for example notes that one of the drawbacks of leaving wine to cool in the open air was that the air could be 'imprinted' with bad qualities and corruption.[149] Also basins of water left out to cool overnight were to be

---

[148] Ago, *Il gusto*, 169.
[149] 'Perché l'aere é elemento, che riceve ogni alteratione, e corruttione; e per questo si può imprimere d'ogni mala qualitá facilmente.' [Monardes], *Trattato della neue*, 225.

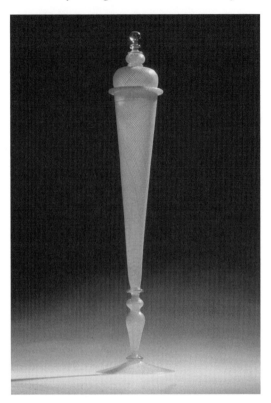

Fig. 7.10. An elegant seventeenth-century Venetian filigree glass with its lid (h. 40.7 cm, w. 10 cm, d. 97 mm.), which looks almost identical to those portrayed in the painting in Plate 21.

covered for the same reason.[150] In paintings from the sixteenth century to the early eighteenth century we also note arrangements in which several glasses and flasks are shown, in which only one large, goblet-like glass has a lid; surrounding glasses do not (see Plate 21). Perhaps the central, covered chalice contained 'neat' wine, because it stood for longer and wine could then be poured out of that into the individual smaller glasses when needed, and mixed with cool water from a jug or flask, according to the specific health requirements of each individual drinker.

CONCLUSIONS

The evidence provided by the Spada-Veralli letters shows a family whose food choices, for the most part, were undoubtedly affected by medical notions of healthy and unhealthy foods, even if different members of the family demonstrated different

---

[150] Mercurio, *De gli errori*, 258; Bacci, *Del teuere*, 147.

degrees of compliance. Maria Veralli dispensed advice to the whole family and we presume she also followed it herself; certainly Eugenia seems to have tried hard to do so. Orazio appears to have been more ambivalent, as his wife frequently remonstrated with him, whilst Cardinal Bernardino Spada was evidently renowned for his flagrant disregard for the advice of his physicians! Whether this gendered pattern of obedient women and defiant men bore any relationship to broader concepts of gendered behaviour is open to question. However, even the women's acceptance of dietary regulation was not unquestioning, and we sense from their comments just how much they struggled to comply with the Lenten rule since it clearly contradicted their understandings of what was and was not healthy.

The debate on cold drinking illuminates a moment in which medical authority was put under pressure on several fronts. Fashionable drinking practices fuelled by commercial interests clashed with traditional medical views; classical authority was undermined by its internal lack of consensus, and by the challenge of new practices from outside Christian Europe. It also reveals the difficult position in which doctors could find themselves, on the one hand seeking to uphold tradition as their main source of authority and on the other keeping apace with contemporary debates, practices, and social as well as political pressure.[151] Yet, the dispute also shows us how 'up to date', how engaged with contemporary culture, controversies, and practices many physicians were, as they seized the opportunity to use the printed word to wade into heated debates. It also brings into focus the extent of the dialogue between medicine and material culture, as physicians engaged with innovative designs, and sought—in some cases literally—to shape the material culture of drinking.

---

[151] There were clear similarities with debates over the origins and treatments of syphilis in the early 16th century; Arrizabalaga, Henderson, and French, *The Great Pox*, esp. 56–87.

8

Excretions as Excrements: The Hygiene of the Body

In the late Renaissance hygiene was conceptualized differently to modern times, as a way of removing the impurities that were constantly deemed to come out of the body, rather than as a cleansing of the dirt deposited on the body surface. As such, personal hygiene was seen to play a key role in enabling the regular purging of the body and therefore in maintaining its health. Indeed the literature on healthy living devotes considerable space to the need to regularly wipe off the impurities the body produces, as these are understood to be residues generated by the third concoction that transforms food into blood, tissues, and other corporeal matters. It was assumed that this waste was expelled from the body through various types of excretions. But, as this chapter will suggest, fear grows considerably during the early modern period that such superfluities may remain trapped inside and in turn generate obstructions that would prevent the elimination of further waste and trigger a range of serious pathologies.[1] Clearly, these fears assign a new role to hygiene.

Rising anxiety about the morbid nature of residual waste lay behind the shift in terminology that seems to occur in health advice literature. From the turn of the sixteenth century, the expression 'excrements' increasingly denotes the various types of superfluities that need to be regularly eased out of the body and, unlike today, these include a range of body matters, fluids, and vapours and not just faeces and urine. These consist, firstly, of the impurities that some authors define as 'excrements of the head' since they are expelled through the mouth, nose, eyes, and ears—seen as conduits for excretions situated in this organ—and, secondly, of the superfluities that are understood to insensibly flow out of the body through the pores of the skin. The first category encompasses the mucus expelled from the chest through the mouth and nose, and the discharge of the eyes and of the ears. These matters are regarded as particularly harmful since they are released during the digestive process and ascend from the stomach to the head at night, endangering the vulnerable brain lodged inside it. Moreover, hair itself is conceptualized as an excrement of the head, that is as one of the natural ways through which this organ purges itself.[2] As for the excrements evacuated through the skin, these are

---

[1] Andrew Wear has valuably documented the fear of processes of internal putrefaction that characterizes early modern narratives of disease. Wear, *Knowledge*, 134–43.

[2] *Di Galeno*, 25; Gropretio, *Un breue*, 374; Lennio, *Della complessione*, 27; and Viviani, *Trattato*, 115 and 124–5.

invisible substances and their expulsion is involuntary. Hence the expression 'insensible perspiration' or 'transpiration' used to describe a process of self-clearing of the body, which unlike other forms of body cleansing occurs unnoticed. Sweating is certainly one of the forms taken by this process; another outcome of insensible transpiration is the grime that encrusts the skin and sticks on the shirt, blackening it. But late Renaissance doctors also firmly believed in the existence of finer and subtler vapours that continuously exude from the porous skin without leaving any odour or sign.[3] Well before the Italian doctor Santorio Santorio in his *De statica medicina* (1614) devised a machine that measured the consistency of these invisible excrements by enabling a comparison between the weight of the food he ingested and that of his solid and liquid excrements, his predecessors were aware of the purging role of insensible transpiration.[4] Indeed by the sixteenth century 'excrements of the head' and those expelled through this invisible means are by far the most widely discussed forms of bodily waste in health-advice literature.

Surprisingly, excrements in the modern sense (faeces and urine), are dealt with only by a few authors who advise about how to keep the body 'lubricated' (*lubrico*) by certain diets and the correct order of food intake (eating cooked plums, apples, or pears at the start of the meal and avoiding fried or roasted foods as a first course) or by ingesting manna in broth or broth and sugar and, in extreme cases, by inducing vomiting or applying enemas.[5] Also artificial evacuations—through emetics or bloodletting—receive little attention, in spite of the prophylactic role that humoral physiology traditionally assigns to them.

In general, the focus of preventive advice shifts away from what are now regarded as violent ways of triggering evacuation and much greater attention is devoted to the performance of daily hygiene. This explains the importance that the morning toilette acquires in health prescription. Early modern regimens provide detailed instructions about the techniques to be used in removing the excrements that accumulate in the passages of the head during the night and in easing the expulsion of superfluities through the pores. Being clean becomes synonymous with being healthy as well as a sign of refinement and respect for other people. Moreover these procedures are now prescribed as regular routines: one should purge the body every day as animals do, following the example of birds which diligently clean their feet and beak, roll and wash in rivers, and terrestrial animals which scratch themselves against walls and trees.[6]

---

[3] On sweat: Stolberg, 'Sweat'. He maintains that sweat and insensible transpiration were understood as the same thing while Italian authors see the former as just one form, and not the most significant, of the latter. For a clear differentiation between forms of insensible perspiration: Fonseca, *Del conservare*, 101.

[4] Medical historians have given Santorio an exaggerated role in the identification of invisible excrements. For example, Shigehisa Kuriyama has stated that 'although the idea of porous elimination was ancient no one has ever suspected such a staggering flood'. Her assertion that before Santorio doctors' concern for evacuations had concentrated on urine and faeces is also contradicted by the Italian sources. Kuriyama, 'The Forgotten Fear', 416. See also Smith, *Clean*, 202.

[5] Salando, *Trattato*, 9–11; Durante, *Il tesoro*, 34; Viviani, *Trattato*, 105–6; and Frediano, *Arca novella*, 192–3 and 196. Elaborate instructions about when vomit is advisable are given in Petronio, *Del vivere*, 216–17, 464.

[6] Frediano, *Arca novella*, 200.

In this chapter we will explore these changing ideas in detail and ask whether they were uniformly shared by medical professionals and laypeople. To what extent did people conform to medical recommendations and alter their hygienic practices and culture of the body? And what was the impact of new concepts of cleanliness on the home and its material culture? Many authors have suggested that the use of baths for hygienic purposes declines in this period. We lack, however, specific studies of the Italian states. Does this trend also apply to Italy? And are the explanations put forward to justify this change confirmed in the Italian case?

THE HYGIENE OF THE HEAD

Basic instructions about cleaning the teeth, the nose, and the mouth were already present in some medieval regimens, but these operations were not classified as ways of purging the head but rather as a means of preserving the function of the organ in question—speech, hearing, sight. Hence removing the superfluities of the ears was advisable since they hinder hearing ('gravano l'udire') and washing the mouth and tongue is encouraged because it would speed up speech.[7] The word 'excrement' is also rarely found in this literature to describe the superfluities gathering in the conduits of the head nor is particular emphasis placed on the damage deriving from failing to remove them. These residues are seen more benevolently as hampering the proper working of the organ; moreover, their removal is advisable for aesthetic reasons, since it improves appearance. Though the need to clear the brain of the superfluities which ascend from the stomach is a familiar concept in medieval texts, this is achieved through fumigations of scented substances that the person is supposed to inhale rather than through hygienic practices.[8] Only combing the hair is already recommended as an operation that contributes to the cleansing of the brain.[9] Indeed the idea that superfluities from the third concoction leave the body through the pores, including those of the scalp, is already found in medieval regimens, though these residues are removed through exercise rather than through hygienic procedures aimed at cleansing the skin.[10]

From the end of the fifteenth century, regimens begin to assign personal hygiene a specific role in the removal of dangerous residues—now obsessively described as degenerating 'excrements'—from the head and the pores. Ficino was the first author to pay detailed attention to daily hygiene. In a text published in vernacular in the 1540s but circulated in Latin since 1489 he recommended allowing half an hour for the purging of 'excrements' from each of the pores on the scalp.[11] Later in the sixteenth century other authors give more precise guidelines about the

---

[7] They were therefore dealt with in the section concerning the health of the various parts of the body, not under the rubric purges (this encompassed instead the applying of enemas, emetics, and the use of baths). Aldobrandino, *Le Régime*, 85–95; Maineri, *Opera utilissima*, ch. 7; Alderotti, *Libello*, 6.

[8] Alderotti, *Libello*, 7; Manente, *Col nome di Dio*, XVIIᵛ. Some early modern authors still recommend fumigations, e.g. Lennio, *Della complessione*, 226; Traffichetti, *L'arte*, 226.

[9] Alderotti, *Libello*, 6.

[10] Maineri, *Opera utilissima*, 33.   [11] Ficino, *De le tre vite*, 12ᵛ–13ʳ.

procedures to follow in the morning toilette, recommending spitting and coughing to purge the chest, blowing one's nose and sneezing to evacuate the brain,
and removing night residues from the eyes.[12] To the catalogue of noxious substances that need to be regularly removed Fonseca adds the 'bilious, greasy and
bitter excrement of the brain that is retained in the depth of ears'.[13] Dental care
(rubbing the gums and the teeth with a coarse cloth, aromatic leaves and woods,
and coral or alum powders) is important to keep them firm and maintain their
whiteness but also to prevent the release of malodorous and morbid vapours
from the rotting teeth that would then ascend through the mouth and the nose
to the brain.[14] Hands and face should also be regularly washed in the morning—the hands because they keep the organs from which the superfluities of
the brain are excreted (ears, eyes, and nose) clean, coming into contact with
the excrements of the head; and the face because of the filth it produces and
since it is particularly exposed to dust and smoke as well as to internal
exhalations.[15]

However, the operation that receives most attention from an early date is the
deep cleansing of the scalp. Ficino already recommends rubbing the head with the
nails and a coarse cloth, then combing the hair with a comb (with at least forty
strokes), and presents it as a key moment of the morning toilette.[16] Later in the
sixteenth century Durante specifies that this comb should be made of ivory. Other
authors provide the rationale for this procedure, explaining that it is intended to
remove the grease and excremental dandruff generated by the head which would
otherwise prevent the evaporation of the morbid vapours generated by the digest-
ing stomach during sleep which rise to the head and seek to escape through the
large pores of the scalp.[17] Combing therefore was understood as a salutary operation rather than being merely a ritual of beautification. This explains the physical
characteristics of combs in this period (see Fig. 8.1). Their fine teeth (at least on
one of the two rows) were employed for scrubbing the head, sometimes with the
aid of bran, sponges, and pieces of rough cloth specific 'for the head'—other paraphernalia for head-care mentioned both in regimens and household inventories.[18]

---

[12] Rangoni, *Consiglio*, 15; Boldo, *Libro*, 218; Durante, *Il tesoro*, 14–15; Viviani, *Trattato*, 123–5;
Frediano, *Arca novella*, 203; and Auda, *Breue Compendio*, 254–5.

[13] 'quell'escremento bilioso, grasso e amaro che nelle caverne delle orecchie si aduna é il purga-
mento del cervello'; Fonseca, *Del conservare*, 102. The coarseness of ears was already mentioned by
Manfredi, *Il perché*, 61. See also Viviani, *Trattato*, 125; Frediano, *Arca novella*, 203; and Auda, *Breue
Compendio*, 254.

[14] Durante, *Il tesoro*, 16; Rosaccio, *Avvertimenti* (unnumbered); Fonseca, *Del conservare*, 143;
Frediano, *Arca novella*, 202; and Auda, *Breue compendio*, 254–5.

[15] Durante, *Il tesoro*, 15; Frediano, *Arca novella*, 206; and Auda, *Breue compendio*, 253–4.

[16] Ficino, *De le tre vite*, 11^v–12^r. While vigorous combing is advocated by others (e.g. Durante, *Il
tesoro*, 14) Petronio disagrees, advising moderation and slow speed, otherwise the head will overheat;
Del vivere, 211.

[17] Durante, *Il tesoro*, 16. 26–8; Viviani, *Trattato*, 124–5; Frediano, *Arca novella*, 202; and Auda,
Breue compendio, 254.

[18] Interestingly regimens do not mention parasites of the head and the fact that fine-toothed combs
might also have been employed in removing lice.

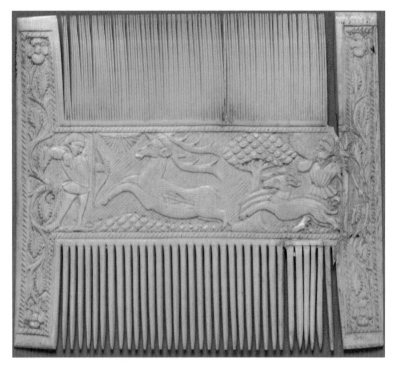

Fig. 8.1. An early and rare example of an intact ivory comb (h. 11.5 cm, w. 16.5 cm, d. 1.2 cm) from fifteenth-century northern Italy. Far from being used just for styling the hair, the close teeth of such combs enabled the user to scrape 'excrements' from the scalp.

As the vivid language employed in regimens indicates, the emphasis on their excremental nature made the superfluities clustering in the upper body passages appear increasingly disgusting. Similarly, the injunction that the comb used for the head should not be the same as the one used for the beard suggests that it was seen as unhygienic to mix the two functions and that the matter gathered from the scalp induced revulsion.[19] Moreover, there are intriguing changes in this period in the material culture of hygiene for the head that confirm this line of thought. For example we observe the disappearance of the display value of objects such as ear-cleaners and toothpicks. In the first decades of the sixteenth century these objects often took on the appearance of jewellery—being made of precious stones and metals—and they figure prominently in a series of male and female portraits of the 1520s and 1530s, hanging from gold chains on the chests of affluent Italians, or depicted in the act of being used (as in the example in Plate 22).

However, no further examples of this genre of portraiture are found in Italy in the following decades.[20] By mid-century objects for the hygiene of the ears and the

---

[19] Durante *Il tesoro*, 14–15 and Rosaccio, *Avvertimenti* (unnumbered).
[20] See the portraits of Lucina Brembati by Lorenzo Lotto, and those by Alessandro Olivieri and Bartolomeo Veneto, all three painted in the 1520s and 1530s.

mouth made of precious metals and with pearls and rubies mounted in them also disappear from the written record, while in the 1520s and 1530s their actual use is attested by their presence in Venetian household inventories.[21] The fashion for exhibiting objects that hinted at hygienic practices seems to have been definitely rejected in Italy by mid-century, when toothpicks worn around the neck are deplored in Della Casa's *Galateo* as a vulgar form of ostentation.[22] This does not mean that the use of such hygienic tools died out, but simply that it was no longer tactful to parade them. As a consequence their status as luxury objects declined and they were more likely to be made of ordinary materials. Indeed instructions for domestically manufactured 'picks for cleaning the teeth' are found across the period in the widely popular recipe books, pointing to a diffusion of practices for the hygiene of the head and of the technology associated with it also among the less prosperous.[23]

Interestingly, in a period in which we would expect their presence to be widespread, combs are notable by their absence from the records. While regimens encourage patients to use ivory combs for their morning toilette, and they feature prominently in the iconography of the naked Venus or Susanna at the bath that became a favourite subject of sixteenth-century painting, combs are apparently uncommon in households, being only found in six of our ninety inventories, and only in the costly ivory version. Two of these listings refer to the possessions of noblemen and, interestingly, three to those of former prostitutes, for whom haircare was particularly important because of the erotic appeal that late Renaissance culture attributes to hair.[24] The extremely rare presence of a household object that we would expect to be ubiquitous has also been noted by Renata Ago in her study of material culture in seventeenth-century Rome and taken to mean that grooming practices were not common.[25] But is this absence from the record evidence of a real absence? It may be that precisely because the use of combs and other devices for hygienic purposes had become widespread these objects assumed a more prosaic and unpretentious appearance and therefore fell into the category of tiny possessions of too little value to be recorded in household listings (which by and large only included saleable items, ones that could find a buyer on the second-hand market).[26] The chances of being recycled might also have been reduced for these objects by the increasingly negative attitude to bodily excretions—think of how

[21] Penny, 'Introduction', 581. In the German lands, however, these kinds of depictions are still found at a later date. An example is represented by the portrait of the Palatinate Count Philippe Ludwig de Neuburg (1547–1614) by Lucas Kilian (Munich, Bayerisches Nationalmuseum).

[22] Penny, 'Introduction', 583. It should also be noted that in the Italian context, all examples of portraits of this kind concern a provincial milieu; even Lorenzo Lotto did not enjoy much fame and mainly worked for clients in the provinces.

[23] e.g. Piemontese, *Dei secreti... Parte terza*, I. 63: 'Stiletti perfetti da nettare i denti'.

[24] ASR, Misc.Fam., B.158, b.1, Duca Francesco Sanesi (1651), 18; ASR, TNC, Uff. 1, vol. 12, Agata Silvestri (1553), 105; and ASVR, MCI, vol. 198 (1605), Caterina Foresti da Viterbo, 82; Margerita Arnisse, 62; Beatrice de Mendoz Hispana, 6. Inventory of the wardrobe of Cardinal Giustiniani (1600–11) in Danesi Squarzina, *La collezione Giustiniani*, vol. i, *Inventari I*, 59.

[25] Ago, *Il gusto*, 176.

[26] The low cost of combs is confirmed by inventories of barbershops, where even those described as ivory ones are often worth just few *baiocchi*; Pediconi, 'The Art', appendix.

combs might have been encrusted with dandruff and grease after protracted use. Indeed, family accounts of the nobility show that combs, in the plural, were frequently bought, and this may suggest they were often disposed of and replaced by new ones.[27] The life of an object so closely connected with disgusting bodily residues might therefore have been a relatively short one.

The flourishing of a material culture of the head is proven in any case by the presence, in the houses of the affluent, of *pettiniere* (comb-boxes) for travelling, including, when the content is described, a mirror, comb, sponge, and other *fornimenti* (equipment), showing that it is the single comb that does not make it to the inventory; when it is part of a set of items for hygienic procedures it acquires value and is therefore more likely to be listed.[28] Moreover, *quadretti di tela da nettar la testa* (squared hemp cloths to clean the head) and *pezze da testa* (cloths for the head) are also found in seventeenth-century inventories;[29] so are *scopette per nettare i capelli* (little brushes to clean the hair) and even a brush for the moustache or brushes for the beard (*scopettino da mostacci, spazzola da barba*).[30] But then *scopette* (little brushes) with no further specification of function are frequently listed and we cannot exclude that as well as being used for clothes some of them may have been destined for the head, the beard, or the moustache. Similarly undifferentiated is household linen; here, too, some of the items may have been used specifically for the rubbing and cleaning of the head, though this is not specified in the listing.

Clearly grooming practices centring on the head were common, as is also shown by the widespread custom of regularly attending the barbershop or, in the case of the affluent, being cared for by a barber in one's home. And barbers in this period did not just trim and dress beards and hair but were responsible for the hygiene and appearance of the whole upper body—cleaning nails, ears, teeth, and pores, as well as washing the head, tasks for which barbers had a set of tools.[31] Members of the upper classes like Bernardino Spada even had a personal barber among their domestic staff, who followed the master on his travels, stays at the spas, and at the villa.[32]

Rather than just being a matter of personal decorum, the regular trimming of hair and beards was also understood as a procedure necessary for maintaining

---

[27] For evidence from family accounts Ago, *Il gusto*, 176.

[28] ASR, TNC, Uff. 4, vol. 77, 150ʳ–157ʳ, Camillo Traversari (1605); Notai AC, vol. 3180, 857ʳ–882ʳ, Polidoro Neruzzi (1641); Misc.Fam., B.158, b.1, c1, Duca Francesco Sanesi (1651); TNC, Uff. 10, vol. 240, 271ᵛ, Maddalena Parentini (1666); Inventory of the wardrobe of Cardinal Giustiniani (1600–11) in Danesi Squarzina, *La collezione Giustiniani*, vol. i, *Inventari I*. 57. The use of *pettiniere* is also mentioned in household management books such as Liberati, *Il perfetto*, 41 and Frigerio, *Arte*, 89.

[29] ASR, Notai UG, vol. 177, 564, Carlo Bomplano (1621); and inventory of Francesco Negrelli (1628), cited in Ago, *Il gusto*, 176.

[30] ASR, TNC, Uff.4, vol. 75, 601ʳ, Margarita Savigiane (1604); Misc.Fam., B.61:6, 793–6, Gió Maria Contelori (1617); Misc.Fam., B.158, b.1, 12ᵛ, Duca Francesco Sanesi (1651); Inventory of Francesco Raspantini (1667), cited in Ago, *Il gusto*, 176. *Scopettoni* or *scopette da testa* and various undefined *scopette* are also found in barbershops' inventories, Pediconi, 'The Art', 172–3, 182, and 185.

[31] See Cavallo, *Artisans*, ch. 2.

[32] Among the many references to this figure in the Spada letters: ASR, FSV, B.491, 22.10.1638; B.619, 27.5.1647; and B.491, 13.6.1655, 1.7.1655, and 7.7.1655.

health. Hair was regarded as one of the excrements of the head; hence from the late sixteenth century people are advised to keep hair and beard short as a form of hygiene. Lennio even encourages shaving head and beard during warm weather, though this would be dangerous in winter.[33] As Viviani explains, 'the longer the hair is, the more resistant it is to expulsions'. This view is reiterated in occupational tracts for barbers: for Tiberio Malfi 'bushiness of hair' does not only produce a proliferation of vermin and filth but the blocking of poisons to be let out of the body, injuring the brain and the sensory faculties.[34]

One wonders whether the fashion for short hair that takes hold in the second half of the sixteenth century and the subsequent reduction of full beards—to goatees on the chin or narrow and pointed ones that characterize the following century—could also be put down to a growing awareness of the unhealthy effects of long hair.[35] In any case, medical ideas at the turn of the seventeenth century were giving their blessing to these new fashions.

Preoccupations concerning the health of the brain prompted anxieties not only about hairstyle but also about washing the head. Whether it was a harmful practice was subject to debate. Medieval authors had described it as a salutary operation to be performed especially in winter and in general twice a month.[36] In the early modern period, however, considerable uncertainty seems to surround the practice. Traffichetti is the only author who praises it unconditionally, since among all the organs of the body the head was the part most in need of being kept clean and fresh, due to the plethora of excrements it attracts—though he concedes that those who are not used to washing the head should continue to avoid doing so as the change in habit would be detrimental. By now, however, as the same author informs us, head-washing (like washing the feet) is seen by many to represent a threat to health: 'nor do I understand the reasons of those who said that one should seldom wash the feet, often the hands, and never the head'.[37] This negative view is upheld, for example, in the popular regimen authored by Rosaccio in 1594 and also in the more learned work by Lennio.[38] The former concedes that one can wash the head some, but not many, times in winter as long as one always makes sure it does not stay wet and is dried immediately afterwards. Durante is more ambivalent: on the one hand he encourages his readers to disregard the old saying that one should wash the hands often, seldom the feet, and never the head, and acknowledges that occasionally washing the head greatly comforts the brain. However he then introduces several elements of caution, listing the specific herbs, soaps, and other substances to be employed in different

---

[33] Durante, *Il tesoro*, 16; Rosaccio, *Avvertimenti* (unnumbered); Camaffi, *Reggimento*, 240; and Lennio, *Della complessione*, 98.

[34] 'quanto piú lunghi sono i capelli, tanto piú resistono all'espulsiva'; Viviani, *Trattato*, 124–5. Also Malfi, *Il barbiere*, 24.

[35] On changing hair and beard styles Levi-Pisetzki, *Storia*, iii. 153 and 331.

[36] Maineri, *Opera utilissima*, 23 and 38 (no less than every 20 days, no more than once a week).

[37] 'né so da che ragione siano mossi coloro che dissero che rade volte si debba lavare i piedi, spesso le mani e mai il capo'; Traffichetti, *L'arte*, 170.

[38] Rosaccio, *Avvertiment* (unnumbered); Lennio, *Della complessione*, 100.

seasons in head-washing. Like Rosaccio, he also stresses the precautions to be taken afterwards: drying the wet head immediately with warm cloths so that no humidity remains that would exacerbate the already wet nature of the brain and abstaining from exposing it to air immediately after washing—so it is better to wash it in the evening, before dining.[39]

It is significant that precisely this favourable view of head-washing was one of the targets of the fierce rebuke of Traffichetti's errors published four years later by Doctor Bruno. Here the physician from Rimini contended that one could well do without all that washing with water and, with much less fatigue and more safety, manage to keep the head dry and clean by frequently combing and rubbing it with cloths and sponges.[40]

Clearly, the experts were divided on the subject and there was an ongoing debate. Did similar reservations about head-washing extend to non-professionals? Both letters and recipe books document that soaps specific for washing the head were in use, thus confirming that this was in fact regarded as a delicate operation that required special cleaning agents.[41] At the same time the differentiation in soaps suggests that head-washing was a common practice and this is also confirmed by the presence, in two particularly detailed inventories, of a 'towel for the head' ('asciugatore da testa') among household linen and of a 'washstand with a basin and a copper bucket to wash the head' ('lavamano con piede e sua conca e secchio di rame per lavar la testa') (see Fig. 8.2).[42]

Overall, epistolary exchanges present an ambivalent attitude to head-washing, perceived both as a necessary hygienic operation, to be performed no less often than every twenty days, and as a challenge for the body, to be avoided when one was unwell. In October 1599, for example, Giulia Benzoni complains in a letter to her husband that she hasn't washed her head for twenty-two days since it was painful to bend and she is now affected by a sore throat as a result of this negligence.[43] Washing the head was indeed not done lightly; it was avoided when one had a cold and was seen as potentially harmful in pregnancy.[44] In 1656, pregnant for the first time, Eugenia sought her mother's advice on whether she could continue to wash her head in her new condition or should dispense with it for three or four months, as her mother-in-law suggested. Maria gave her blessing, maintaining that it would not harm her—though whether she washed bending over or backward was a matter for discussion.[45] The clash of opinions between Maria and her mother-in-law suggests that among laypeople too, the matter was controversial. Considerable anxiety surrounded the practice and when five years later Eugenia suffered a

---

[39] Durante, *Il tesoro*, 16.					[40] Bruno, *Discorsi*, 126–7.

[41] 'Soap balls to wash the head' were dispatched, for example, by Maria Spada to her daughter in Viterbo; ASR, FSV, B.410, 14.6.1656.

[42] ASR, Notai AC, vol. 3180, 857ʳ–882ʳ, Polidoro Neruzzi (1641), and Inventory of Cardinal Benedetto Giustiniani (1621), in Danesi Squarzina, *La collezione Giustiniani*, vol. i, *Inventari I*, 153.

[43] 'V. S. non si maravigli se io so breve, perché non so me basta l'animo de scrivere, perché non me sento tropo bene della gola per non heseme io lavata la testa, perché non me facesi male lo star cina et hogi sono 22 doi [sic] giorni che non me la so lavata.' ASR, FSV, B.449, 10.10.1599.

[44] ASR, FSV, B.410, 3.12.1656.

[45] ASR, FSV, B.410, 19.11.1656 and 26.11.1656.

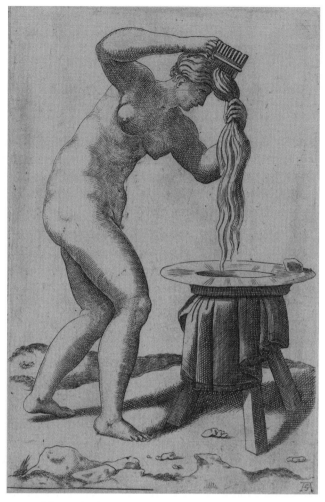

Fig. 8.2. In spite of the medical reservations that surround washing the head, erotic representations of the female body which hint at this practice are frequent in the iconography of the time. This print by Adamo Scultori (1530–85) also illustrates the use of washstands for the hygiene of the upper body that were commonly found in Italian households by 1600.

miscarriage she blamed it on the fact that 'she had decided to wash her head and got considerably tired as a result and two days later she grew even wearier doing something else she can't recollect now'.[46] In spite of the fairly relaxed attitude to head-washing that seems to have been common in the Spada family, the practice was still perceived as a health hazard.

---

[46] 'io ho dato la colpa che mi volsi lavare la testa, e mi strachai assai, e dói giorni doppo mi afatigai a fare non so che.' ASR, FSV, B.1115, 17.4.1661.

THE HYGIENE OF THE PORES

> Among all the evacuations the one that occurs through insensible transpiration from
> all over the body via the pores, through which the air continuously comes in and goes
> out, is particularly worthy as it disperses the subtle excrements that, if retained in the
> skin, cause filthiness and waste... [and] this excrement... should be removed from the
> boundary of the body not only in name of cleanliness but to make [the body] light,
> porous [*traspirabile*] and healthy.[47]

If we are to believe the instructions provided in regimens, the opening and cleansing of the pores so strongly recommended by Frediano was to be achieved through
three main means: by rubbing the body with the hands or with the aid of rough
cloths and odorous balsams, by changing personal linen and bedlinen regularly,
and by the parsimonious use of baths.

On the issue of rubbing, however, regimens remain elusive. Some authors do
not mention it at all, others only briefly and in very general terms. Described as an
alternative to exercise—which, as we have seen in Chapter 5, was also understood
as a means of easing the elimination of superfluities through the pores—frictions
are said to be suitable especially for the elderly.[48] In complete contrast with the
specific instructions concerning the morning toilette, there is a lack of specific
detail about how these frictions (*fregagioni, fricazioni*) were to be performed, and
no references to the gestures and the objects employed in the procedure, to the
extent that one wonders whether they were really practised. It is likely that, as suggested in 1565 by the Dutch doctor and astrologer Lennio, an advocate of this
ancient custom: 'amongst us the habit of rubbing and anointing has become
obsolete'.[49]

Many regimens, in contrast, have a section on baths, but while medieval texts
present them as integral to the expedients aimed at maintaining health, early modern doctors describe bathing as something that may or may not be performed.[50]
Unlike the cleaning of the openings on the head and the scalp, taking baths is not
depicted as a regular procedure but as a practice that, like head-washing, makes the
body prone to health hazards. Many restrictions thus apply: as in medieval regimens, not only are baths discouraged before eating and passing one's stool, but also
one should not eat or drink immediately afterwards. Several caveats and warnings
are also raised about the kinds of bodies or conditions not suited to taking baths:
from those who suffer from constipation or from the opposite condition, to those

---

[47] 'tra tutte le evacuationi si deve stimar molto quella che si fa con l'insensibile traspirazione che
segue per tutto il corpo attraverso i meati per i quali entra e esce continuamente l'aria, esalando da
questi i più sottili escrementi che ritenuti in pelle vi causano le sorditie e l'immondezza... qual essendo
escremento... doversi levare dal confine del corpo non solo per la politezza ma per renderlo leggiero e
traspirabile e sano.' Frediano, *Arca novella*, 200.
[48] For examples of a brief reference to rubbing: Ficino, *De le tre vite*, 56 and 58; Paschetti, *Del
conservare*, 154; Boldo, *Libro*, 219; and Durante, *Il tesoro*, 13. Petronio only devotes few lines in his
400-page regimen to the topic, stressing their limited impact on health; *Del viver*, 294 and 407.
[49] 'presso di noi venuto in desuetudine l'uso di fregare e ungere.' Lennio, *Della complessione*, 56.
[50] On the medieval medical literature on the subject: Lallouette, 'Bains'.

who have a weak stomach, a tendency to vomit, or whose nose easily bleeds.[51] Moreover, in order not to be debilitating, baths should not be protracted and definitely cease when the flesh is swollen; and they should not be too hot but tepid since hot water would prompt the pores to squeeze and lock up. By contrast, the opposite preoccupation, about the harmful effects of cold baths, is only found in medieval regimens and by the mid-sixteenth century is no longer an issue since, as Boldo explains, 'the cold pool is now disused'.[52] Clearly, the fears associated with exposing the body to the cold have heightened in the early modern period and led to the abandonment of the custom. These fears are also echoed in the recommendations not to leave the bath all of a sudden but gradually, giving the body a chance to grow accustomed to the cold external air.[53]

By the last decades of the sixteenth century, therefore, considerable anxiety has grown around the practice of washing by soaking the body, or even sections of the body, in water. We have already noticed that serious concern surrounds head-washing but reservations are also raised in relation to feet-washing. While this practice was encouraged in medieval texts and seen to preserve sight and hearing, later it is treated with greater caution and seen to trigger gout in the elderly. It can be performed only using mild lye, boiled red roses, and salt, and when there is no pain in the body.[54] However it is not water that is seen as the harmful agent in these practices but the humidity resulting from immersion in water, combined with the impact of air on the wet body.

The decline in the habit of washing by immersion signalled by the medical literature is confirmed from the mid-sixteenth century by the disappearance of bath chambers in most palaces. This is a recent development. In the previous decades baths modelled on Roman classical precedents had undergone a sort of revival in residential architecture.[55] So-called baths *all'antica*, inspired by the writings of Vitruvius and other classical authors and by surviving examples of ancient Roman baths, were built between the 1470s and the first decade of the sixteenth century in the residences of the ruling elite such as the Urbino palace, the castle of Ostia, near Rome, and the Vatican palace. These bathing complexes included: heated changing rooms, spaces for massaging and anointing the body and for hot, tepid and cold pools in which to plunge, as well as a sweating room and a room furnished with daybeds for resting afterwards. Defined, according to classical terminology, as *tepidarium, calidarium, sudatorium* or *laconicum*, and *frigidarium*, these structures were equipped with running water, drains, and furnaces to heat both water and rooms, and a complex system of pipes running beneath the floor and embedded in the walls in which the hot air circulated, keeping some of the rooms warm. In the next thirty years the fashion for bath chambers became less exclusive and in Rome it also extended to the residences of professionals, merchants, artists,

---

[51] Petronio, *Del vivere*, 313. See also Paschetti, *Del conservare*, 203–4.
[52] 'il solio freddo oggi é disusato.' Boldo, *Libro*, 257.
[53] Auda, *Breue compendio*, 255.
[54] Durante, *Il tesoro*, 16. For a medieval example: Maineri, *Opera utilissima*, 38.
[55] This paragraph is based on Bruno Contardi and Henrik Lilius, *Quando gli dei*; Frommel, 'Abitare'; and Pediconi, 'The Art'.

and architects. These were modest versions of the bathing complexes found in the palaces of the elites, since they offered the combination of cold and warm pools and sweating closet in one or two rooms that in most distinguished residences spread over several rooms, but shared with their more distinguished counterparts the sophisticated hydraulic and piping system of heating, ventilation, and drainage already described.

As architectural historians have suggested, however, by the late sixteenth century baths were excluded from new palatial building programmes. In early seventeenth-century Rome, the inclusion in the Borghese palace built in 1612–14 of a rather simple bathroom is a unique example, followed three decades later by the bath built in Palazzo Barberini (1640s), which presents a similar plan.[56] However, the technology employed is already much less sophisticated than in the baths *all'antica* in fashion a century earlier. These recent examples simply consist of a room for the bathtub and an adjacent one for the stove in which the water was heated and then manually carried to fill the tub. So the fashion for reviving the experience of classical baths seems to have died out quite quickly in Rome. By the late sixteenth century bathing was scarcely practised by the city aristocracy as, apart from these two examples, none of the Roman palaces studied by Waddy include baths. Around 1625 the practice is also said to have been 'virtually discontinued' by a contemporary anonymous commentator.[57]

The disappearance of baths in the sixteenth century is a leitmotif in the historiography of hygiene.[58] Yet the evidence from Italy is not as consistent as the received view would suggest. It shows hints of regional and micro variation. For example, in his 1602 regimen, Doctor Paschetti addresses his discussion of the benefits of baths to the citizens of Genoa: 'since you use baths a great deal in your city, as there are very few houses which do not have one and do not resort to it often'.[59] Indeed, a recent study has confirmed that baths were still a common feature in Genoa at the turn of the seventeenth century: in this period at least thirteen private palaces and villas contained bathing rooms.[60] Here, too, their presence was no longer inspired by the wish to re-create the bathing culture of the ancients; rather it was a product of Genoa's trading connections with the Ottoman Empire and of the influence of Oriental practices, namely Turkish baths, well known to Genoese merchants.[61] Moreover, the fact that *maestro di casa* handbooks such as Timotei's *Il Cortegiano* (1614) list a *stufarolo* (stover) among the standard members of staff of an aristocratic residence, suggests that in the most distinguished social milieus a culture of bathing and sweating had not disappeared. He, together with the barber, would have been in charge of the hygiene of the master of the house, though it is likely that bathing was done much more gently and in a more simplified manner

---

[56] Waddy, *Seventeenth-Century Roman Palaces*, 48–9.
[57] Waddy, *Seventeenth-Century Roman Palaces*, 48.
[58] Vigarello, *Concepts of Cleanliness*, ch. 1; and Smith, *Clean*, 179–80.
[59] 'essendo pocchissime case, che non l'habbiano, e che non l'essercitino sovente.' Paschetti, *Del conservare*, 202.
[60] Hanke, 'Bathing', 675.   [61] Hanke, 'Bathing', 700.

than in the classical model.[62] Finally, bathing facilities aimed at the lower ranks of the population also survived until later, at least in Rome, where public baths continued to be built at the end of the sixteenth century.[63]

That opinions about the benefits of baths were controversial is also acknowledged, by the mid-seventeenth century, in medical literature. In 1656, Frediano argues polemically that baths cannot be harmful if taken now and then in the evening in a protected place, diluting scented substances in the water, and resting in bed for an hour afterwards.[64] The debate about the advantages of drinking cold water that develops, as we have seen, at the turn of the sixteenth century might have contributed to generate a more positive attitude to bathing. In Camaffi's regimen, for example, praise for the positive effects of fresh water also extends to plunging in rivers (though in summer alone), since 'the use of fresh water both inside and outside [the body] is to be commended'.[65]

This scattered evidence suggests that the disappearance of a bathing culture from the early modern landscape was not as thorough and homogeneous as often assumed. Even in the medieval period, on the other hand, the frequency of bathing and the meanings associated with it seems to have varied significantly in different European countries.[66]

The reasons that triggered the decline in the use of baths as a hygienic practice may also vary in different contexts. There has been a tendency to offer unified, overarching explanations for this shift in attitudes to washing that apply to both Protestant and Catholic countries, urban and rural milieus, and different social conditions. The arguments put forward centre on the one hand on the fear of getting infected with the plague, in a period that saw repeated outbreaks of the epidemic, or with syphilis, a relatively new disease. The infection would have occurred either through the physical contact created—especially in public baths—by bathing with others, or through the penetration of corrupted air, carrying the disease into the body through the pores opened by the steam of the bath.[67] Another common line of explanation attributes the origin of a negative attitude to bathing to the puritanical attitudes of religious reformers (Protestants and Counter-Reformation Catholics). Who increasingly saw it as conducive to lewdness and indulgence in carnal pleasures.[68] From the Italian viewpoint, however, these arguments appear largely speculative and alien to contemporary accounts of this shift. In the Italian states, medical and lay writers certainly acknowledge that a demise of baths has occurred but they do not depict bathing as a morally despicable custom nor do they put its disappearance down to concerns for exposure to physical contagion or

---

[62] Timotei, *Il cortegiano*, 104–5. Similar evidence exists for the court environment of northern Italian states such as the Turin ducal court; Cavallo, *Artisans*, 41, 64, 69.

[63] Pediconi, 'The Art', ch. 3.

[64] Frediano, *Arca novella*, 201.

[65] 'l'uso dell'acqua fresca tanto di dentro, come di fuora è lodato'. Camaffi, *Reggimento*, 11.

[66] Archibald, 'Did Knights'.

[67] On this view see esp. Vigarello, *Le Propre*, ch. 1.

[68] For a summary of the arguments see Smith, *Clean*, 180.

to the infiltration of morbid air into the body.[69] The idea that disease may enter the body through the pores appears particularly alien to early modern medical thinking, as authors do not conceptualize air as a carrier of disease but consider it as dangerous or beneficial to health according to its temperature and level of dryness or humidity. Moreover, they interpret the porosity of the skin positively, preoccupied as they are—we have repeatedly seen this—with keeping the body 'breathing' (*respirabile*) so as to avoid the blockage of impurities within the body. What makes baths risky in their view is exposure to the cold which would narrow the pores and prevent the regular expulsion of internal dirt. Hence only one among our authors talks of the opening of the pores caused by bathing as a health hazard; in his view, however, it is not disease that threatens to penetrate the body but rather the superfluous humidity created by the bath, which then may settle somewhere in the body and generate an illness similar to the French disease.[70]

The success that mineral therapeutic baths continued to enjoy in the late sixteenth century and in the early decades of the following one (amongst the Spada-Verallis, too) throws further doubt upon the classic explanations for the decline of the hygienic bath: surely spas were also an occasion for promiscuity and for infection through the skin pores, yet they were held in high esteem by the medical community.[71] Spas baths were not taken lightly, as with the hygienic bath their debilitating effect and the risks of exposing the body to the cold were recognized and rigid rules prescribed how long one should stay in the water and how long one should rest afterwards.[72] But clearly there was a difference between taking a course of particularly beneficial waters when specific health conditions required it under medical supervision, and using ordinary baths regularly, as a form of cleanliness. The latter was to be avoided.

Rather than being a result of fear, the change in hygienic customs that takes shape in the second half of the sixteenth century is presented by contemporaries as a sign of progress and social distinction and we would like to suggest that this interpretation deserves to be taken seriously. Starting with Mercuriale in 1559, the decline in washing regularly (three or four times a month, or, if one liked to sit down clean to a meal, even once a day) is presented as an acquired freedom, connected with the spread of linen underwear that efficiently collects dirt and residues emerging from the skin and spares the early modern person the burden of washing.[73] (See Figs. 8.3 and 8.4.) This becomes the standard interpretation, then repeated

[69] Sadoleto, author of a 1533 educational tract, is among the non-medical commentators who mention the subject. *Del ben ammaestrare*, 111. For a medical example: Frediano, *Arca novella*, 201.

[70] Panaroli, *Discorso*, 19: 'coloro li quali frequentano queste stufe s'imbattono in due mali: o nella scaranzia, o in un male simile al mal franzese, sebbene non é, perché quelle humiditá superflue per il moto, e per lo strofinar che si fa la carne, e per altre cause, trovando li pori aperti penetrano dentro il corpo, e vagando un tempo si radicano al fine in qualche parte, ancorché quelli poverelli non habbiano mai conosciuto donne di Partito'.

[71] Among the many studies on Italian spas, Palmer, ' "In this" '; Chambers, 'Spas'; Nicoud, 'Les Médecins italiens'; and Boisseuil and Nicoud (eds.), *Séjourner au bain*.

[72] ASR, FSV, B.491, 10.9.1642; and B.619, 5.9.1642.

[73] Mercuriale, *De arte gymnastica*, 103.

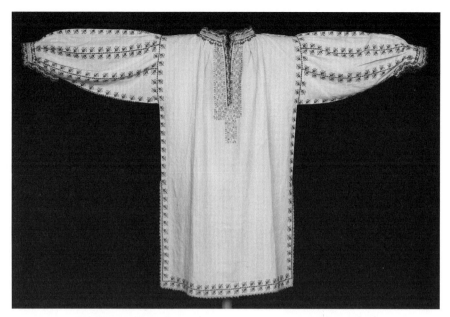

Fig. 8.3. Multiple linen shirts that could be changed and washed frequently became a regular component of the wardrobe across the social scale in the course of the sixteenth century. This finely embroidered example would have belonged to a wealthy gentleman.

with small variations and more direct references to the bath by Petronio in 1592 and Paschetti in 1602:

> [The bath] was the discovery of the ancients for keeping the body fresh and clean, for since they did not have the custom of wearing linen garments, or even if they did these were used by few, they were apt to become covered in dirt of all kinds...but in our own times since all, rich and poor alike, are accustomed to wear shirts and thereby more easily keep the body clean, the bath is neither so widely nor frequently employed as in the times of the ancients.[74]

This view is also reproposed by non-medical authors such as Tassoni (1608); his comments suggest that the bath is now seen as an effeminacy, confined to people who live in unnecessary luxury.[75]

---

[74] Petronio, *Del vivere*, 312; and Paschetti, *Del conservare*, 202: '[il bagno] fu trovato dagli antichi per tenere i corpi netti e mondi perciò che non avendo quelli in uso le vesti di lino o se pur le usavano pochi adoperandole, si riempivano generalmente tutti d'ogni sporchezza...ma a nostri tempi usando tutti universalmente così i poveri come ricchi le camiscie e perciò tenendo più facilmente netti i corpi non è tanto in uso né così frequente come era né tempi antichi'.

[75] Tassoni, *Varietà*, 419: 'I romani erano astretti a tener bagni preparati per tutto (non essendo per altro gente effemminata nè dedita al lusso) soltanto perchè non vestendo su la carne di panni lini nè costumando camicia nè mutande, calzoni, calzette e scarpini erano necessari per conservarsi netti dal sudiciume e dalla polvere di lavarsi ogni giorno.'

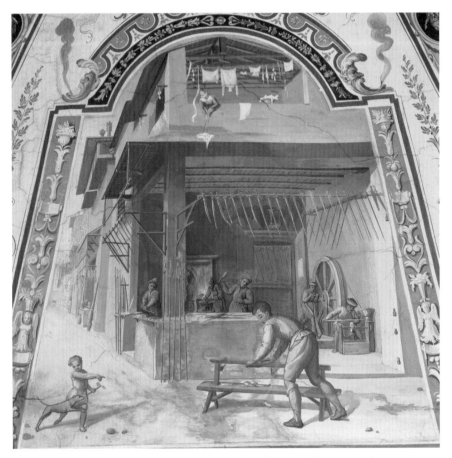

Fig. 8.4. By the late sixteenth century, a wide range of linen undergarments hanging out to dry became a common feature of the urban landscape. Linen vests, collars, underpants, and cloths had become essential accoutrements to keep the body clean.

Changing undergarments and bedlinen regularly is greatly preferred to washing oneself, and both regimens and household management texts give precise prescriptions about it.[76] Washing, in contrast, is increasingly presented as a wearying activity that exposes the body to dangerous changes of temperature and the impact of cold air on the wet skin. Traditionally understood as a form of exercise, the bath follows a similar trajectory. As exercise is increasingly reduced to mild, gentle physical activities, baths are treated with additional caution and replaced by targeted ablutions. The rise of an ideal of comfort and restful life (*vita riposata*) as a model for the true nobleman impelled the elites to abandon the practice, which was

---

[76] Rangoni, *Consiglio*, 11; and Frigerio, *Arte*, 122. Though the replacement of baths with linen underwear as a hygienic tool is standard knowledge in historiography, following Vigarello, the reasons for this shift are normally put down to the fear of water. See n. 66.

regarded as an example of the strenuous physical training commonly performed by the ancients and thus associated with the martial arts, with 'vigorous' (*gagliardi*) movement, scrubbing, and smearing. 'Washing, scrubbing, and anointing provoke great fatigue, besides being superfluous', was the comment of Doctor Fonseca.[77] Therefore an awareness of the delicacy increasingly associated with the gentleman's body is built into the rejection of baths. Bathing however remains a practice suitable for the lower classes, they can be taken once a week by 'those in service' ('corpi alla servitú sottoposta') who are accustomed to immoderate movement, says Fonseca, but were still recommended for the old, who cannot undertake alternative forms of exercise (two or three times a month in the summer, once a month in the winter). For the same reasons, baths were also advised for children under 5 but were discouraged in adult and 'temperate' gentlemen who usually took their exercise walking, out riding, or in carriages. Boldo more specifically associates bathing in cold water with those who live coarse, rough lives ('vivono grossamente') and wear themselves out ('s'affaticano molto');[78] while Fonseca criticizes in particular the use of *stufe* (steam baths), which he disparagingly regards as a German custom that can in no manner be good for health because, among other dangers, the heat can make men effeminate.[79] In the more popular regimens, the practice is even seen as triggering blindness—a malady deemed to be particularly common in the environs of the River Reno, 'where baths and steam baths are much frequented'.[80]

PULITEZZA: CLEANLINESS, APPEARANCE, DECORUM

The decline in the habit of washing by immersion signalled by medical advice and architectural evidence is also confirmed by changes in the material culture of hygiene. In the sixteenth century, bathtubs and other bath accessories disappear from the domestic landscape: they are completely absent from our sample of inventories and likewise from the seventeenth-century palaces studied by Patricia Waddy, while in the previous century they could be found even in artisans' households.[81] By 1600, *lavamani*—washstands consisting of an iron or wooden tripod supporting a copper or maiolica basin (*conca, catino*) and a pitcher to pour water of the same material—have superseded bathtubs, while 'cloths for the face' or 'for the hands' are found in place of bath towels. Normally found in bedrooms or, in palaces, in the small rooms or closets adjacent to the bedroom, these ensembles are

[77] 'Taccino hora gli antichi quelle lor tante lavande fregagioni e unzioni perché oltre all'essere superflue sono ancora di gran fatica'. Fonseca, *Del conservare*, 18.

[78] Boldo, *Libro*, 258–9.

[79] Fonseca, *Del conservare*, 123.

[80] 'Molte cose nuocciono agli occhi, la prima è la stufa overo bagno, offendendo il caldo la loro complessione che naturalmente è fredda...e per questa cagione molti ciechi si ritrovano intorno al fiume Rheno dove comunemente si frequentano i bagni e le stufe'. *Scuola salernitana*, 67.

[81] The evidence comes from our sample of Genoese artisans' inventories. For example, the inventory of a wool worker includes two bath towels (*lenzuola da bagno*), that of a baker a bathtub (*tina da bagno*); ASG, Notai antichi, 544, 30.10.1408 and 25.2.1417. Similar results emerge from a study of 15th-century French houses; Alexandre-Bidon and Piponnier, 'Gestes', 215–16.

increasingly made as a set and testify to the diffusion of daily hygienic practices. Clearly the washstand allows for only limited ablutions that target specific parts of the upper body. Though defined as *lavamani* (hand-washers), it is likely that washstands also served to wash the face and occasionally the head (as indicated by Fig. 8.2) and the parts of the body detailed by Rangoni in 1556 as the ones that require regular cleansing with water. Surprisingly, he also mentions head and feet among the body parts that need washing:

> that the head and feet be washed, the extremities rubbed and superfluities be removed with a linen cloth soaked in wine in which sage has been boiled... the face and eyes be washed with fresh water every day and at least twice a day in summer and be dried with a clean cloth... The neck, neckline, hands and arms be cleaned of superfluities, sweat and grime that nature often deposits in those places.[82]

While washstands are clearly devoted to the morning hygiene of selected parts of the body, the ubiquitous ewer and basin (also made as a set in bronze, copper, or pewter) remain in use for the ritual of hand-washing taking place at the table before and after meals (see Figs. 8.5, 8.6). By the early modern period this had become a well-established ceremony, celebrated in dozens of paintings and taken for granted in conduct books that just prescribe who should offer the *serviette*.[83] In affluent houses, basins, ewers, and hand towels were brought to the table by servants but the presence of the latter (*serviette da mano*) even in households of modest means suggests that the routine was observed across the social scale.

In both regimens and educational tracts, hand-washing before eating is presented as a form of politeness and respect for the other people: in a period in which hands still complement forks in bringing food to the mouth from the serving dish, this is a precaution aimed at 'not fouling the food' and one is encouraged to perform it publicly even when hands are already clean so that those present will be reassured and feel no disgust at sharing the table with one.[84]

The repeated and ostentatious hand-washing ritual also betrays the fact that hands are perceived as the main vehicle of contagion in this period, not so much from the plague (a disease virtually absent from regimens and conduct books) but from disgusting skin diseases such as *rogna* (scabies). Worries about contact with hands that are full of *rogna* are encountered frequently in letters, books for household management, and other primary sources. Though medical historians have paid very little attention to this infection, scabies—a highly contagious skin condition, caused by an infestation of tiny mites that burrow into the skin and can only

---

[82] 'Si lavi il capo, e piedi, si freghi le parti estreme, si netti le superfluità... con una pezza di lino bagnata nel vino, nella quale sia bollita salvia. La faccia e gli occhi ogni giorno la state due volte almeno si lavino con l'acqua fresca e s'asciughino con fazzuol mondo... Il collo, la gola, le mani e le braccia si mondifichino delle superfluità, sudore e sporchezze che la natura spesso spande per quei luoghi'; Rangoni, *Consiglio*, 11–12.

[83] Pascali, *L'aio*, 211.

[84] 'si devono lavar e asciugar le mani altrimenti si fa immondo ciò che si mangi'; Frediano, *Arca novella*, 205; Pascali, *L'aio*, 211–12.

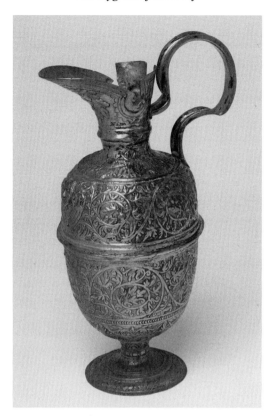

Figs. 8.5–8.6. Bearing the coat of arms of a patrician family and stylistically inspired by Islamic metalwork, this ewer and basin set could have been made for display purposes. However, utilitarian versions of these objects were commonly used for washing hands before meals (M. A.-W.).

be seen with a magnifying glass or microscope—must have been a relatively common disease in the early modern period and one that created much disquiet due to the formation of blisters, pustules, and other visible lesions that created revulsion and panic in the onlooker.[85] Though the condition was conceptualized in medical thought as the result of a humoral imbalance, and more precisely of an excess in phlegm and bile often deriving from improper diet, early modern people seem to have been aware that it could be transmitted through skin-to-skin contact. In March 1678 for example, Maria Spada warned her husband not to handle the things that the farmer had touched since the latter was affected by a bit of *rogna* and this is truly something to avoid.[86] The recommendations recurring in the

---

[85] Apart from informative but antiquarian studies such as Friedman, *The Story of Scabies*, the only recent work on the topic is Nicoud, '"Che manza fichi"'.

[86] 'Mi rallegro che il fattore sia guarito presto, ma V.S. si guardi di non maneggiare le cose che tocca lui, mentre è accompagnato di un po di rogna, essendo mercantia da non c'intrigare.' ASR, FSV, B.618, 26.3.1678.

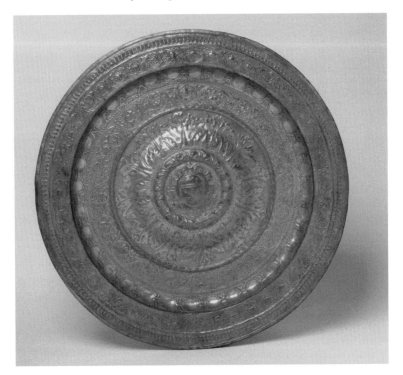

Fig. 8.6.

maestro di casa literature and books of the *scalco* to make sure that the domestic personnel assigned to table service are free from *rogna* also point us in this direction.[87] Though medical theory denied the contagious nature of the disease, in everyday life a parallel was established between scabies and leprosy, thus exacerbating the alarming and threatening nature of the illness in popular perception.[88]

Although baths were abandoned there is little doubt that by the second half of the sixteenth century much more time was spent by men and women alike in grooming and that the distinction between personal hygiene and cosmetics had virtually collapsed. This is betrayed by the polemical remarks of contemporary commentators, who stigmatize the fashion for an excessive culture of the body and try hard to separate what they regard as laudable hygienic practices from the superfluous, effeminizing, and morally despicable polishing of the appearance. 'Combing and washing oneself is healthy cleanliness, but taking great pains over it is more befitting a woman than a man,' states Pascali in 1641.[89] That a very fine line separated necessary and unnecessary grooming is also proven by the increasingly

[87] Evitascandalo, *Dialogo*, 7 and 54; Romoli, *La singolar dottrina*, 3.

[88] For an example of such association see the entry dated October 1615 in Gigli, *Diario*, 45. Scabies is also defined as contagious in the popular regimen by Anguillara, *Vaticinio*, 26.

[89] 'Il pettinarsi e lavarsi é pulitezza salutare ma il far ció con soverchio studio é cosa piú da donna che da uomo.' Pascali, *L'aio*, 207.

ambiguous use of the term *pulitezza* or *politezza* (cleanliness), found to denote both legitimate cleanliness and excessive delicacy. We find a clear example of this ambivalence in Bishop Antoniano's text, where he warns: 'Over-refinement of the body is greatly to be avoided and the immoderate care taken by many in certain fastidious practices [*politezze*] that would plainly ill become women, to say nothing of men'. But a few lines down he feels obliged to clarify: 'now I do not at all dislike cleanliness [*politezza*] in any way, on the contrary I bring it to the attention of our head of household'.[90]

Cutting remarks about artificially changing one's natural appearance—a gift of God and a window into the self—through cosmetics were not new and went back to the classical period.[91] But what marks out the early modern moralizing literature is the full acceptance of the need for regular personal hygiene, now unanimously regarded as an integral component of civilized manners. This, however, makes the task of defining what is to be seen as unnecessary grooming even more difficult. Hence these authors' accounts are sometimes very detailed. In the 1590s, Lombardelli set out to meticulously distinguish the hygienic procedures necessary to health from those that just betray worldly vanity. He concedes that the head is a highly dignified member of the body that requires considerable care 'not only for decorum but for health' ('non solo per la creanza ma per la sanità'), hence the nose should be purged to provoke sneezing, so that the brain, chest, and stomach area are cleared of phlegm; moreover, the hands and face must be washed and the head rubbed.[92] He also admits that it is not good to have discoloured teeth (*rugginosi*), but taking pains to scrape and polish them, and whiten them with instruments or scented waters, with powders or cloths, are 'women's things'.[93] He approves of keeping the hair short and regularly combing it, 'both for refinement and health' ('sia per la delicatezza come per la sanità'), but condemns the great pains taken over having it lightened or curled as women do and in having the beard attended to and carefully groomed. Keeping the nails long and dirty is filthy 'but wasting half a day every time in cutting them, filing them and polishing them is too refined by far'.[94]

The performance of extensive hygienic procedures also prompted the emergence of new spaces and objects devoted to these operations. In palaces these were carried out either in the bedroom or in the recently created adjacent closets, which performed the role of dressing rooms. Likewise in household inventories we witness the development of a material culture of cosmetic and hygienic care made of little vessels and containers for pomades, ointments, and scented waters that the iconography extensively represents lining up on wooden stools, at times covered with a toilette cloth, together with the comb, the soap ball, and the table mirror (see Fig. 8.7).

[90] 'Sia molto da fuggire la troppa delicatezza del corpo e la soverchia cura di molti in certe *politezze* che facilmente disdirebbero alle femmine non agli uomini...ora me non dispice in alcun modo la *politezza*, anzi la ricordo al nostro padre di famiglia' (our emphasis); Antoniano, *Dell'educazione*, 355.

[91] Laughran, 'Oltre la pelle', 49 and 61–3.

[92] Lombardelli, *De gli vfizii*, 150, 157, 210.

[93] Lombardelli, *De gli vfizii*, 159.

[94] Lombardelli, *De gli vfizii*, 164: 'ma il perdervi un mezzo giorno per volta in tagliarle, raschiarle e brunirle ha troppo del delizioso'.

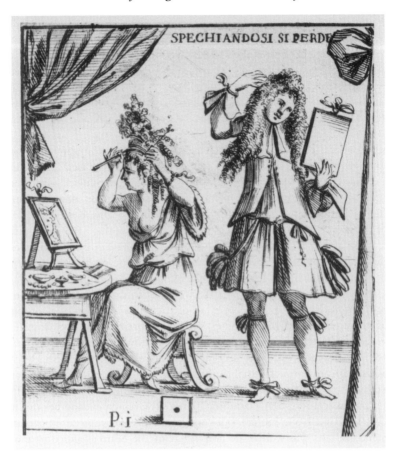

SPECHIANDOSI SI PERDE

P. i

Fig. 8.7. This seventeenth-century engraving satirizes the extended grooming practices which involved men as well as women and illustrates the emergence of specific furnishings for the morning toilette.

While items for hairdressing and skincare were initially placed in niches in the wall or on the *rastello*, a structure with an inbuilt mirror and pegs, the expansion of the equipment for the morning toilette made the use of these rudimentary dressing tables common, while self-standing pieces of furniture made for this purpose made their appearance in Roman noble palaces only at the beginning of the eighteenth century.[95] Moreover, from the mid-sixteenth century onwards in Italy, and more specifically in Venice, which was a hub of trade with the Orient, a great many recipes for beauty and hygienic preparations appeared in books of secrets and in books on the ornamentation of the body. These also attest to the expansion

[95] Thornton traces the evolution of this object, *The Italian*, 239–41. On Rome: Ago, *Il gusto*, 176. Among ruling families, however, examples of purpose-built dressing toilettes were already found in the last quarter of the 16th century; *Le Bain*, 298.

of a culture of body care during this period.[96] Household account books and manuscript recipe collections confirm that many of these products were home-made;
in the Spada palace this was still the case in the 1660s.[97]

The growing attention to the care of one's body also encouraged the appearance of new, specialized domestic staff, in particular the chamber assistant
(*cameriero*), who as well as assisting the master in getting dressed and undressed,
bringing clean linen and dusting clothes, helps him in the various hygienic
operations we have just discussed.[98] Chamber attendants, we learn from the
maestro di casa literature, carried the water for morning ablutions and prepare
the towels, comb-box, and all the other necessary equipment for the lord's
toilette.[99] In the case of the lady, these functions were performed by her maids
and it is in particularly the care of the female body that is frequently represented in the iconography of the period (see Plate 23). These images show
female servants cutting toenails, washing the woman's feet, and dressing her
hair, a skill for which—so we learn from correspondence—female servants were
particularly valued.[100]

Chamber assistants were also responsible for carrying the commode when
needed. Called a *seggetta* (little chair) or *cassetta per far i servizi*, this was a movable
piece of furniture covered in a variety of textiles with a pierced seat which contained a removable pan that could be cleaned after use. Household inventories
reveal that by the late sixteenth century it was preferred to the *destro, agiamento*, or
necessario (a seat set in a niche in the thickness of the wall or in a small closet often
under the staircases) (see Fig. 8.8) by those who could benefit from the service of
domestic staff, probably on account of the foul smells produced by the latrines.

These remained common among the lower ranks of the population but in palaces they were used only by servants and occasional visitors. Attempts had been
made to close them off with doors and cover them with lids to contain the exhalations.[101] Architects also experimented with different ways of ventilating this small
space but clearly the growing availability of servants in the noble house made the
commode a much preferable solution.

It is possible that the expansion of hygienic practices played a significant part in
the fantastic growth in the number of domestic servants employed in noble households that occurs in the second half of the sixteenth century and also in the parallel
masculinization of domestic service. For example, in Venice we find in this period
a ratio of one servant to each member of the family, and sometimes even two;
moreover, there is a decisive increase in the proportion of male to female servants,

---

[96] e.g. [Rosetti], *Notandissimi secreti*; Marinelli, *Gli ornamenti*.

[97] Ago, *Il gusto*, 176.

[98] While the *cameriero* could only be found in court environments in the 15th century, his presence in noble houses spreads in the following century and by mid-17th century he is a regular member
of domestic staff in households such as the Spadas'. Orazio and Bernardino both have one at their
service.

[99] Liberati, *Il perfetto*, 41.

[100] ASR, FSV, B.1115, 24.7.1658 and 2.8.1662.

[101] Pagliara, 'Destri', 65; Waddy, *Seventeenth Century Roman Palaces*, 50–3.

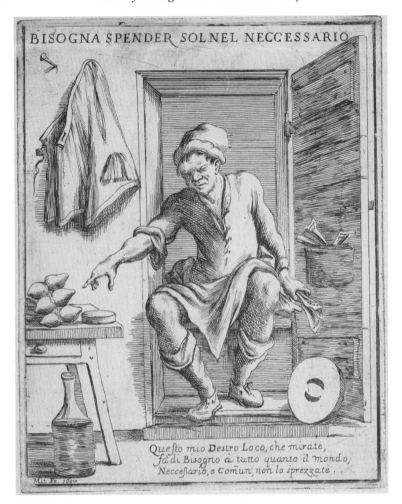

BISOGNA SPENDER SOLNEL NECCESSARIO.

Questo mio Destro Loco, che mirate,
fa di Bisogno à tutto quanto il mondo,
Neccessario, e Comun, non lo sprezzate.

Mit. Fe. 1690

Fig. 8.8. With the advent of the commode, the smelly privy under the staircase, or in a niche of the wall, remained the toilet of the poor, as shown in this seventeenth-century etching.

the former outnumbering the latter in many upper-class households.[102] These transformations have so far been explained in terms of the display role servants (and more precisely male servants) are called to perform. The new self-conscious-ness of the upper classes, argues Romano, 'demanded a larger and more masculine staff'.[103] Male servants wearing the house livery escorted their masters and mis-tresses about the city protecting them from any dangers and offences to their hon-our; they collected their bills and delivered their messages. In Romano's study, and

---

[102] Romano, *Housecraft*, 108–10, 116–17, and 232–4 for comparison with other Italian cities.
[103] Romano, *Housecraft*, 93.

more generally in the literature on service, the role of male domestics in noble households is described as highly public; they are entrusted to represent the status of the family. What is disregarded, however, is the fact that the increased number of male servants is also a consequence of the domestic, private, and intimate roles they are now called to perform in chamber service, in the kitchen, where male cooks replace the female personnel, and in table service.

Interestingly, some contemporary commentators were well aware of these changes. In a household management book published in 1644, the Bolognese Marquis Vincenzo Tanara (b. *c.*1590) recorded the replacement of female with male personnel occurring in the kitchen: 'at the times of our ancestors and still in my first years of life there was in this city a school of women who, to great advantage and convenience, knew how to attend to the kitchen'.[104] But he explained it in ways that differ significantly from what has been suggested by recent historians of domestic service. By then kitchens were populated by men and, according to Tanara, rightly so, for men are far superior to women in trustworthiness, cleanliness, and intelligence, the three attributes required in whoever serves in a kitchen. They are more trustworthy because, unlike women, they have 'honour', thus they cherish their reputation and, if caught stealing from their employer's house, they would never find another job in the city. Secondly, men are cleaner than women because they are less vain and hence they do not constantly adjust their bodies, in particular not touching and rearranging their hair, as women do while cooking; nor do they alternate the cooking with activities such as spinning, that involve spitting on one's fingers to divide the thread.[105] Moreover men are free from 'other things natural to women', a reference to menstruation. Thirdly, men are easier to teach than women who 'are taught something one day and forget it the next', and they enter service at an earlier age than their female counterparts, so that they learn little by little how things are done when they are still boys.[106]

On the one hand Tanara's reasoning sounds familiar; it reiterates the common stereotypes about the scant intellect and fickle temperament of women. However, his representation of women as naturally dirty is intriguing, especially since it is only marginally associated with menstruation, the classic cause of female pollution in the Judaeo-Christian tradition.[107] Rather, he points to the dangers of contact with hair and spit while preparing food. Hair and spit, as we know, were among the many means through which the body was understood to expel the waste that, if locked inside, threatened to poison it. Hair was conceptualized as excrement, as one of the forms through which dangerous phlegm was removed from the body. In this interpretive framework, loose or rebellious female hair may have been seen as

---

[104] 'ai tempi dei nostri antenati e ancor nei miei primi anni era in questa città una scuola di donne quali con molto utile e comodità sapevano servire alla cucina'. Tanara, *L'economia*, 175.

[105] 'la cuciniere posta la pignatta sul fuoco s'acconcia il capo, dapoi nel tempo che le vivande si cuociono con spruzzate dita fila'. Tanara, *L'economia*, 176.

[106] 'altre cose naturali alle donne'; 'oggi le si insegni una cosa e domani non se la ricordano più'; Tanara, *L'economia*, 176.

[107] The idea that women lack cleanliness or have a special need to wash recurs in conduct literature. e.g. Belmonte, *Institutione*, 23–4; Frigerio, *Arte*, 33.

a threat to health, not simply, as often remarked, as an instigation to lust. Indeed, though female hair is not discussed in manuals for healthy living, anxiety about the dangers posed by women's hair is present in conduct literature, especially in advice to the young bride, where emphasis is placed on the need to keep the dressing of the hair decorous and tidy and adopt a sober style.[108] Spitting, on the other hand, is one of the evacuations specifically targeted in books about household service, and precisely in relation to food. The carver (*trinciante*) is admonished to refrain from spitting, sneezing, and coughing when in service—an implicit reference, therefore, to the need to be clean from those excrements of the head now considered so dangerous. And in more elusive terms the cupbearer (*coppiere*) is encouraged to be cleansed of any 'bodily waste' (*immondizie del corpo*) while on duty.[109] Similarly, the butler (*credenziero*) should be healthy and clean in his service 'so that his handling of the food does not make it nauseous'.[110] In these injunctions we find further evidence of the disgust that surrounds bodily emissions.

If we consider Tanara's remarks within the framework of the anxiety about noxious bodily waste that we have seen increasing in the late Renaissance, his explanation of why the most affluent chose male domestic personnel appears less preposterous. The long-haired, unruly female, often unable to adopt restrained, hygienic manners either out of vanity or because of the activities she performs (like spinning and laundering), is a danger to health—also but not exclusively, because of the physiology of her body. These female characteristics seem to justify Tanara's claim that 'as is well known, the dirtiest of men is cleaner than the cleanest of women'.[111] The new gendered division of domestic labour therefore does not appear to be motivated only by the need to employ men in the expanded public roles that servants are expected to perform and are deemed unsuitable for women for reasons of decency. Rather it is arguable that the health significance increasingly attached to cleanliness played a role in the shift from female to male personnel in the most sensitive spheres of service. If we look at which household duties are associated with the requirement of *pulitezza* in the late sixteenth-century literature on service, we find that it is precisely those servants involved in food preparation and table service, and the chamber personnel concerned with the personal hygiene of the master (the chamber attendant and wardrobe attendant), who are expected to be clean in body, hands, dress, and underwear. Moreover, they are responsible for the cleanliness of their utensils and of the spaces in which they operate.[112] As these tasks acquire more importance in the early modern household, it seems sensible to entrust them to a man for the reasons outlined by Tanara: for reasons of temperament and physiology, men are understood to be cleaner.

---

[108] Belmonte, *Institutione*, 24.   [109] Frigerio, *Arte*, 92, 83.
[110] Evitascandalo, *Dialogo*, 54.
[111] Tanara, *L'economia*, 176.
[112] Tanara, *L'economia* , 177; Timotei, *Il cortegiano*, 80, 127–8; Liberati, *Il perfetto*, 33, 40–1.

CONCLUSION

Increasingly in the early modern period, the cleansing of the body was deemed to have an effect on health, rather than just being a matter of personal decorum. It was conducted so as to enable the processing of waste products which lurked within the body and prevent these substances from becoming blocked inside thus provoking pathologies of different kinds. This danger was a crucial concern in early modern medicine and, as medical historians have argued, this preoccupation explains the centrality of practices of evacuation in the therapeutics of the period: patients are purged, bled, made to vomit and sweat.[113] Techniques of bodily hygiene, however, are not normally inscribed under the rubric of evacuation; yet, we have suggested, in the early modern period they must be seen precisely in this light rather than simply in terms of cosmesis and cleanliness of the surface of the body. The greater emphasis on the excremental nature of all sorts of bodily excretions that we see developing during the sixteenth century leads to a redefinition of what constitutes body waste and to the singling-out of the head and the skin as principal channels for the evacuation of noxious residues. The hygiene of the upper body is increasingly described as carrying a salutary value and doctors recommend it is performed daily. Indeed these recommendations seem to have encountered the favour of the population, and the morning toilette becomes a widespread practice, helped by its overlap with the care of the appearance.

The redefinition of the preferred forms of body purging that we have illustrated had a profound impact on the house, its organization, and material culture: it gave meaning to newly created spaces such as dressing rooms, triggered the appearance of specific objects for the hygiene and decoration of the upper body, such as washstands, dressing tables, and table mirrors, and of a plethora of containers for hygienic and beauty products. The diffusion of new hygienic practices transformed the devices that assisted in the removal of 'excrements of the head' from rare and luxurious to everyday objects. It also stimulated the domestic as well as the commercial production of soaps, toothpastes, scented water, and other products for skin and haircare, and led to an extraordinary rise in the popularity of linen underwear, which replaced the hygienic functions previously performed by the bath. Finally, it multiplied the need for body services, boosting the number of domestic servants employed in affluent houses and contributed to shifting the ratio of male to female servants in favour of men.

By the end of the sixteenth century, the hygienic rituals minutely detailed in regimens, as well as in educational tracts, have become so commonly accepted that they are presented as a daily obligation; it is now the excessive care of the body that represents a moral issue. The necessity of being clean in dress, body, and behaviour also extends to those servants whose duties bring them close to the body of the master or his food. A growing disgust surrounds the matters expelled from the body, described as nauseating, and some of them, like the symptoms of the skin infection known as *rogna*, are also understood to be contagious.

---

[113] Pomata, *Contracting*, 129–35. See also n. 1.

The success of daily hygienic routines ties in with various trends we have repeatedly encountered in this book. On the one hand, the fact that personal cleanliness procedures focus on the head and are dominated by preoccupations for the health of the brain confirms the increased importance acquired by this organ in late Renaissance physiology and in popular views. On the other hand, a heightened sense of the delicacy of the gentleman's body plays a key role in making daily cleansing routines appear to be much more appropriate for their refined complexion than traditional purging procedures such as enemas, blood-letting, emetics, or even baths. The former also have the advantage of enhancing the appearance of the body, while the latter—as is now often emphasized—only bring tiredness and hasten ageing. In ancient texts more aggressive forms of bodily cleansing were regarded as central to health maintenance and in late medieval regimens they were seen to perform a preservative role: the *Secretum secretorum*, for example, recommended that vomiting be induced once a month as a form of preventive cleansing.[114] In early modern regimens, however, these means of waste removal are mostly depicted as violent and are exclusively recommended as therapies, to clear entrenched pathogenic obstructions, not as pre-emptive health measures.[115] In lay narratives, too, good health is seen to spring from a limited recourse to these practices: the eulogy written in praise of the late Cardinal Bernardino Spada, for example, celebrates his 'habit of never purging if not for a precise necessity, as it is also customary among the rest of the house'.[116] Even baths survive almost exclusively as a therapeutic measure, practised in the spa resorts. Their decline as a form of hygiene derives from the new emphasis on their debilitating effects rather than from preoccupations about promiscuity and the risk of infection. As for artificial evacuative practices, it is feared that bathing would cause natural heat, or the vital spirits, to leave the body, dramatically cooling and weakening it.[117]

Another form of purging that is increasingly described as debilitating is sexual intercourse. Clearly this is a delicate topic because of the negative view of sexuality propagated by the Church and authors are reluctant to treat it at length. Yet semen was conceptualized as an excrement in medical thinking, hence as a substance from which men need to purge themselves (the physiological effects of sex on women are not considered in regimens), and some guidance needs to be given. Some doctors present sex as necessary to health when practised in moderation, but then introduce a long list of caveats (concerning age, seasons, timing, and physical and mental conditions) that considerably restrict the possibilities of practising it without harm.[118] Other authors praise instead the advantages of abstinence, which prolongs life, preserves from infirmities, and guarantees a healthy

---

[114] Manente, *Col nome di Dio*, XXIᵣ. On ancient authors' views: Smith, *Clean*, 97.

[115] For a dissenting voice Pictorius, *Dialogi*, 63. It does not seem true, as often assumed, that recourse to aggressive purging of the body was ubiquitous, both for prophylaxis and cure. For an example of such assumption Kuriyama, 'The Forgotten Fear', 418.

[116] 'non si purgó mai se non per necessitá precisa come fa il resto della casa'; ASR, FSV, B.463, cap. XXXII.

[117] Lennio, *Della complessione*, 40.   [118] Fonseca, *Del conservare*, 87–8.

old age.[119] As it is to be expected, lay testimonies, too, generally avoid the subject of sexuality but passing references in letters seem to confirm the adherence to a view of sexual intercourse as debilitating and endangering the body. In 1599, Giulia Benzoni comments on the death of a certain Camillo Iano, putting it down to the doctor's decision to bloodlet him twice in a day in spite of the patient warning that 'he had been with women' and was therefore weak as a result of sexual intercourse.[120]

[119] Salando, *Trattato*, 13–15; Camaffi, *Reggimento*, 244–5.
[120] 'era statio con donne.' ASR, FSV, B.449, 7.8.1599.

Conclusions

According to the advice imparted by the health regimens, worrying about the air, fussing about a healthy way to get a good night's sleep, and judiciously regulating one's passions were prerequisites of the day-to-day management of the body for anyone hoping to live a long and healthy life. And by and large, this study finds that such concerns were indeed part and parcel of daily life in late Renaissance Italy. Overall there was a definite receptivity to many of the procedures advocated in vernacular advice books, and our evidence points to a culture of prevention which pervaded daily and domestic life in many ways. Letters and contemporary accounts reproduce the understandings of health hazards found in advice literature, and many aspects of the advice seem to have been taken to heart.

Inevitably, this awareness of preventive health advice would have been more an aspect of life amongst the elites, whose education gave them greater access to such knowledge, and whose wealth provided ample means to implement it; but not exclusively so. The ever-increasing availability of printed books and pamphlets of all sizes and kinds helped disseminate this corpus of medical rules to a far larger public than had ever been conceivable before. Moreover, as we have seen from the dynamics within the microcosm of the Spada-Veralli household, there was a degree to which the inter-class relationships within the palace favoured the circulation of preventive knowledge and the creation of a common language of the body and health, as the literate elite shared the fundamental precepts of health care with their numerous servants. As to having the financial wherewithal to keep healthy, our evidence from inventories suggests that many of the objects needed to protect the body in the home—such as bed-warming pans, portable braziers, and underwear—could be obtained even by the less well-off sectors of society.

Nonetheless, there were also, inevitably, tensions between prescription and social habits, and these are often revealed in the correspondence—sometimes explicitly, and sometimes through omission. For example, the disparaging comments made by Eugenia Spada and her mother about the utility of perfuming and fumigating their letters during the plague suggest a lack of confidence in the precautions advocated by the health authorities. The fear of eating grapes, normally considered one of the healthiest of fruits, is another example. We have also observed that in the Spada family at least there were some blind spots in their adherence to prevailing medical wisdom. As regards diet, Bernardino seems to have ignored much of what he had been told; whilst Orazio was more attentive he obviously struggled to obey the doctor's advice on limiting the amount and density of chocolate that he drank! Maria, so watchful of everybody else's long-term health, is herself reproached for not taking care of her own. Eugenia however is a shining example of someone who seems most eager to implement that which she has been told.

Yet overall, judging by the Spada family, laypeople were well aware of the importance of taking preventive measures and of paying attention to the multiple threats which their environment and lifestyle posed to their health. Their letters suggest that they were particularly sensitive to the dangers of bad foods and overexertion; of bad air, or changing air too swiftly; of over-chilled drinks; and of boredom and melancholy. The letters also sometimes echo some of the confusion and contradiction within the regimens themselves. For example the advice in the regimens on the appropriateness of certain types of exercise for different ages by different classes of people was so confusing that it is not surprising to find that the Spada tended to be quite conservative in their estimation of what was safe. Meanwhile, there are echoes of the most vigorous debate of all—that on hot and cold drinking—as family members sought to avoid excessively cold drinks. Furthermore the extent to which preventive medical advice underpinned lay understandings of health is also revealed in the clash between Lenten prescriptions and the evidently widespread perception amongst the laity—manifest in the Spada letters as late as the 1660s—that the Lenten diet was dangerously unhealthy because it contravened the basic tenets of what they had always been told about healthy eating.

THE MEDICALIZATION OF THE HOME

Andrew Wear has referred to a process by which early modern doctors 'medicalized' ways of living and the evidence from all our sources certainly supports this view.[1] Indeed, we would go even further than this and argue that there was what we might refer to as a 'medicalization of the home', and not just of ways of living. We can see this process starting with the humanist project to recover, translate, and publish texts from antiquity. As well as bringing the Hippocratic *Airs, Waters, Places* to the attention of medics and intellectuals, so too the importance of texts such as the *De architettura* by Vitruvius and the letters of Pliny increased. These ancient authorities concurred in their emphasis on the importance of local climatic influences on the body and also, therefore, on the importance to health of where one lived and particularly of how one's home was designed. The dissemination of such advice could not have been more timely given that it coincided with the rebuilding not only of papal Rome, but also with the urbanization of a recently ennobled patriciate throughout the peninsula. Intense competition between elite families in cities stimulated demand either for newly built palaces and villas, or the rebuilding and modernization of old ones, along with expectations of lavish furnishings. We have seen as an example of this members of the Spada family moving from Brisighella to Bologna and then to Rome, where they bought the former Palazzo Capodiferro. Bernardino then spent most of his life restructuring the palace, as

---

[1] Wear, *Knowledge*, 155.

well as investing in their two suburban villas. This process was however only the beginning. The magnificent homes of this new nobility then needed to be managed efficiently and the well-being of the *famiglia* within attended to. This stimulated the growth in household advice manuals which both assimilated and repackaged the medical advice found in regimens to a different, wider public and contributed to the pervasive presence of this healthy-living culture.

It was not however just the home and its spaces which point to this medicalization of domestic life. It was also the many health routines which took place in and around the home which called upon the use of particular objects. Indeed, shifting definitions of healthy and unhealthy appear to have been a driving force affecting the reshaping of domestic material culture and particular design features of Italian homes in the late Renaissance. A large array of objects which we do not normally associate with health—from leather pillows to bed canopies, from drinking glasses to perfume-burners—was mobilized to assist in the construction of a healthy domestic environment and to enable the pursuit of a healthy lifestyle. In a period which saw a new focus on the home and on domestic life, the attention paid to creating salubrious houses grew considerably. Thus the multiplying worries about the impact of winds and cold damp air upon the body can be linked to the added attention not just on how to locate and design a healthy home but also to new domestic fixtures and furnishings—from the attention to fireplaces and bed curtains to the use of wool and leather wall hangings. The new emphasis in regimens on specific parts of the body, such as the brain and head, or the hands and feet, also had consequences for the style of clothing. There are indications that particular kinds of hats were considered more appropriate for the health of particular kinds of scalps, according to their density and weight. Moreover, according to one writer the popularity of padded clothing is to be attributed to its protective functions, whilst gloves as well as feet-warmers did not just add to one's personal comfort, but were part of the armoury required to prevent one from succumbing to the dangerous consequences of allowing the extremities to chill down.

By recovering the implicit health significance they had for their contemporaries, we have therefore proposed a new way of looking at objects and at the transformations affecting the domestic interior, an aspect that has generally been overlooked. By revealing the forgotten role of medicine in shaping domestic material culture, we suggest that the health perspective should be considered along with the main interpretive paradigms that have framed the narrative of change in the home environment, that is, issues of emulation and display of status, political and religious change, social and gender hierarchies, the logic of economics and the market, the availability of new materials and fashions, and the allegedly growing quest for privacy and comfort.

A DYNAMIC CULTURE OF PREVENTION

By the late seventeenth century, when the publication of regimens started to falter, the genre had already enjoyed a 150-year revival in the Italian peninsula. Whether its decline should be attributed to market saturation or to fading interest in preventive medicine deserves further research. However, we have shown that although broadly following the formula dictated by medical tradition the advice regarding the Non-Naturals had changed significantly both in terms of specific recommendations and the general approach, and that these changes were partly a response to shifting medical ideas, partly driven by social change.

Most obvious, perhaps, were the shifts in how the Non-Naturals were weighted by physicians. Generally speaking, advice on food had lain at the heart of late medieval regimens with the other Non-Naturals forming almost a secondary constellation of concerns around it. Yet by the late sixteenth century, although the food section was often still the longest, it had nonetheless been displaced from its position of pre-eminence in the sense that authors claimed variously that air or sleep or even the quality of water was actually the most important element in a healthy lifestyle. The corresponding sections of the regimens expanded apace and, in the case of air and the debate on hot and cold drinking, even took on a life of their own as separate publications. Although there was little consensus on which was the 'leading' Non-Natural, the overall result was that doctors paid far more comprehensive attention to the whole ensemble of external factors affecting the body.

One of our key observations is the heightened interest in air and that over the sixteenth century the emphasis on the dangers of putrid, miasmatic air diminished. We find instead analyses focused on gauging good and bad air largely by its temperature, density, and humidity levels, such that the primary concerns shifted to the dangers of cold, damp air and winds. This marginalization of miasma during the late sixteenth and seventeenth centuries challenges the widely held perception that putrid air was uninterruptedly regarded as a key health hazard right up to the nineteenth century. Furthermore, our observations also lead us to question the view that physicians were mounting a challenge to the role traditionally ascribed to the air in disease causation in the late sixteenth century.[2] On the contrary, our analysis both of regimens and contemporary letters suggests, if anything, an intensification of concerns about the role played by cold and damp air in illness, coupled with an almost obsessive focus on the importance of seeking out 'good' air for the sake of one's health.

Another aspect of this interest in temperature is the way in which discussions of the influence of the air and winds on the body focus increasingly on their impact on the head, brain, and the pores rather than just the heart. As a cold organ, anything which lowered the temperature of the brain would impair the animal spirits and create a number of serious pathologies; these concerns intensified in our period, becoming particularly relevant in discussions of sleep. Another new set of concerns linked to cold air is fear of the disruption it caused to the excretory processes of the body, since by narrowing the pores it obstructed the exit of noxious excremental matter, with potentially serious results. Included amongst these toxic

---

[2] Cohn, 'Cultures', 200–1.

waste products were the dangerous 'exhalations', 'fumes', and 'vapours' released by poor or incomplete digestion, and from bad oral hygiene. Physicians were particularly worried that if trapped within the body these would damage the brain and animal spirits and block the pores. This observation prompts us to question the universality of the widely accepted scholarly model of the humours as consisting essentially of circulating fluids, since what we find in addition is an emphasis on vapours. This attention to the pores and the release of vapours represents another area of departure for later regimens. Rather than focusing their attention on artificial forms of purging espoused by their predecessors, physicians became far more concerned with the need for daily 'evacuation' of exhalations and other waste products through the skin and scalp and through the orifices on the head. To this end they emphasized the importance of adopting 'gentle' but repetitive hygienic routines thus providing a medical justification for the extended grooming rituals that were becoming common at the time.

Overall, in the later regimens we find that recommendations become longer and more comprehensive, less generic and more specific, less abstract and more practical, than in the medieval and ancient works. This ostensibly superficial change was in fact the result of a fundamental shift in the physicians' approach to humoral theory overall. Rather than giving advice based purely on 'natural' constitutional differences in complexion—such as hot or dry, choleric or melancholic—the vocabularies of differentiation employed by physicians expanded. They increasingly categorized bodies by age, class and occupation, and locality. Body size and physical susceptibilities stemming from individual characteristics that we would now describe as 'metabolism' (for example whether one digested more or less slowly) also became important factors.

It was this tendency to consider additional qualities which added further layers of complexity to the discussion. We can see this in Petronio for example, who in his discussion of exercise and rest offers separate advice for the fat, for those of medium build, and the thin, followed by distinctions according to one's profession, mentioning in particular boatmen, gentlemen, and servants.[3] According to this paradigm each 'body type' reacts slightly differently to the Non-Naturals, and needs more or less sleep or exercise and so on, thus requiring slightly different advice resulting in some extremely unwieldy and impenetrable texts, full of bewildering qualifications and exceptions to the rule.

Class, along with concomitant concepts of gentility and nobility, is a particularly important and common 'category' which emerges, shaping the advice on exercise which was based around a culture of intellectual pursuits and leisure rather than physical effort. Thus sweating, overexertion, displays of vigour, and raw bodily strength were replaced by grace, dexterity, and moderation as the forms of exercise most appropriate to the elites. In Italy the disappearance of bathing, too, seems related to an increased emphasis on its debilitating effects rather than to fears of contagion or promiscuity. Locality is another example of

---

[3] Petronio, *Del viver*, 255.

new forms of differentiation, and we have highlighted the extent to which the influence of place marked discussions of air, sleep, and water quality, even to the extent of the appearance of the city-specific regimen.

SOCIETY CHANGE AND IDEAS OF HEALTHY LIVING

In this study we have suggested that in order to understand the growing interest in healthy living we need to take a broad view, and consider it as the product of a convergence of a number of significant factors—intellectual, social, and religious—which together transformed aspects of Italian society and culture over the period studied. New demands were placed on health regimens which, responding in turn, also changed in certain ways. In one sense this culture of prevention owed its success very largely to the availability of printed books. Printers, editors, and doctors took advantage of the thirst for knowledge about preventive methods: they adapted old texts, reprinted them in new and more appealing formats, and published regimens of diversifying style and length to suit different readerships. As we have stressed, however, it was not purely publications in the medical arena which transmitted this preventive culture, for print facilitated the exchange of precepts and ideals between the different genres of advice literature that flourished in Italy in this period, and medical recommendations were soon included in conduct manuals for stewards, students, and householders. Print however, although clearly the facilitator, by itself cannot entirely answer the question of why there was this surge of interest in preventive medicine and why the regimen was so successful.

Plague has classically been offered as a powerful explanation for the initial surge of interest in preventive medicine and the success of the late medieval regimen. Certainly fear of plague would have been included amongst the many recurring threats to health experienced in sixteenth- and seventeenth-century Italy, but we find that neither the chronology nor the contents of the regimens in this period support the view that the genre as a whole is a response specifically to plague. Moreover their contents betray few, if any, references to the disease itself. Instead, the regimens appear to be responding to a more generalized fear of illness; a broad concern with staying healthy, and fending off the myriad and largely nameless pains, swellings, fevers, and chronic disorders which, as our letters reveal, constantly assailed the early modern body. Interestingly plague is also mentioned only incidentally in the Spada-Veralli correspondence and not as an illness causing them particular concern, other than to despair at the inconvenience caused by the quarantine imposed in 1656. On the other hand we have found that hypochondriac melancholy and scabies are just two examples of conditions which caused as much, if not more, concern at the time, yet have received relatively little attention from historians.

Another way of understanding the role of the preventive discourse, and accounting for its success, is to contextualize it in a society in which understandings of the human body and its place in the world were being not only extended, but also challenged and undermined. The recovery of antique texts by the humanists may have answered some questions, but they raised others, not least regarding the inconsistencies and contradictions between the time-honoured Arab translations of ancient texts and the new 'purer' versions of Hippocrates and Galen. Moreover, these uncertainties were compounded by the reports from travellers who ventured to the new world, and found profoundly different peoples eating different foods and living different lifestyles. Indeed, we can see that the wider dissemination of Hippocratic notions of climate and locality was very timely, providing tools for explaining and justifying differences between peoples based on ancient authority.

In this context we can see how the regimens, by both reaffirming old principles and admitting modifications which showed the author's grasp of contemporary debates, provided reassurance and offered certainties and a sense of control over an increasingly uncertain world. Indeed, it was an era in which, as Wear has argued, there was 'a more active and manipulative view of nature and the body' and a belief that 'nature itself could be mastered'.[4] This desire to 'know' and gain control over nature and, by extension, over their own bodies and health, has recently come to the attention of scholars who have shown that people from all walks of life were dabbling in the search to uncover the so-called 'secrets' of nature.[5] The vernacular regimen can be seen as another expression of this fascination with the arcane knowledge of the body which had long been the province purely of physicians and scholars.

One of the crucial social changes affecting Italian society at this time was the consolidation of a new urban noble class engaged in the painstaking construction of a group identity which would distinguish them not only from the lower classes but also from their less fortunate peers. 'Virtue' was the key word in these discussions, and in the absence of a noble ancestry, it was all important. Virtue was to be constructed—as Castiglione explained in his *Courtier*—by a seamless weaving together of physical and moral attributes, with particular attention paid to the body of the noble; every aspect of his gesture, posture, demeanour, and attitude needed to signify virtue. It was not just managing appearances which mattered, however, and we suggest that care for one's health played an increasingly significant part in the construction of the gentleman over the sixteenth and seventeenth centuries. This is exemplified for us seventy or so years after Castiglione, in 1603, in Paschetti's regimen in which he notes that paying attention to one's health was a sign of one's virtue and nobility. This assertion is made in the introduction, framed as a discussion between several eminent members of the Genoese nobility. This is presumably in response to contemporary critiques that gentlemen and courtiers were overly cautious and concerned with their health, since the speakers seek to defend their 'excessive' concern for their health against external criticism. One speaker asserts defiantly that 'in this house we pay the greatest attention to our lives and to those other things which can offend our bodies'.[6] Another confirms that 'it

---

[4] Wear, 'The History', 1290.
[5] See Eamon, *Science*; also Leong and Rankin, 'Introduction', 1–20.
[6] 'In questa nostra dimora teniamo particolar cura nel vivere, e nelle altre cose parimente, che offender possono i corpi nostri', Paschetti, *Del conservare*, 4.

shows great prudence and great virtue…not cowardliness and fearfulness, to set store by one's health'.[7] It is also portrayed as a public virtue, as he adds, 'how can we fulfil public duties as administrators of the Republic if we are ill in bed?'[8] By the mid-seventeenth century in his guide to domestic economy, Tanara asserts that the 'greatest economy' which a diligent head of household can make is to ensure both his own good health and that of his household and servants.[9] The nexus between paying attention to one's health and one's social, spiritual, and moral worth was also an element in more religiously inspired discourses, as authors of Counter-Reformation conduct manuals emphasized.

The relationship between social practice and medical advice was dynamic and at times the wording in the regimens does lead us to surmise that the stimulus for change in them often came in response to social trends. For example it seems clear that in the advice on exercise, hedged about with increasing detail regarding the activities deemed suitable for gentlemen or noblewomen, we are seeing doctors accommodating the gentler forms of exercise that are already popular amongst the elite. Likewise, although day sleep was excoriated in the late fifteenth century as an extremely damaging practice, the regimens show a gradual relaxation of the advice on sleeping after lunch, increasingly on the grounds of custom and habit. By the start of the seventeenth century, this shifts to a grudging acceptance on the grounds that it is an indulgence commonly granted to young people, and by 1626 there is complete toleration of the practice as being an entirely healthy one. The way in which practice could drive the advice literature is made even starker in the publications on hot and cold drinking. Here doctors acknowledge that over a single generation more and more people have been cooling their drinks with snow, even amongst the lower classes, and they use this as their starting point for either disapproving of or accepting the practice. Moreover discussions of hot drinking refer to previous experiments which prove the healthiness of the practice, one of which had been under way for some twenty years. In cases like this it is clearly practices which are seen to legitimize the appearance of changes and novelties in the advice literature.

This does not mean that the relationship between social habit and medical recommendations was entirely straightforward and sometimes the debates within the genre itself bring into focus areas of conflict. Frediano for example, far from being prepared to accommodate the often immoderate lifestyle choices of his patients and noble readers, was deeply critical of their gentle exercise habits, accusing them in no uncertain terms of laziness. On other occasions we find different authors clashing over what constituted the correct advice, as in the dispute over hair washing, which Traffichetti regarded as safe, and Bruno deemed to be perilous. More blatantly, there was the long-running cold drinking debate, in which some authors

---

[7] 'Prudenza e virtù grande…e egli, e non viltà o timoro lo stimar la propria sanità', Paschetti, *Del conservare*, 5.

[8] 'E come si empiegherà egli ne i magistrati, nelle dignità pubbliche?' Paschetti, *Del conservare*, 6.

[9] Tanara, *L'economia*, 6.

thundered against the habits of cold drinkers, whilst others applauded the fashion as perfectly healthy.

EMPOWERING PATIENTS OR EMPOWERING DOCTORS?

Earlier we noted that through their increasingly detailed guidelines early modern physicians endeavoured to regulate a growing number of the activities performed in domestic life—from how to take one's afternoon sleep to using combs correctly. This was accompanied by increased expectations that people would actually follow these daily guidelines—hence the detail and the references to objects specific to accomplishing them so as to facilitate the practical and material implementation of the advice.

For those who did follow them, all these precautions belonged to a web of strategies which gave people the tools to confront the constant threat of illness in their quest to live 'a long and healthy life'. And undoubtedly there must have been a certain sense of empowerment and reassurance in believing that you knew how to choose a healthy site for your home, or that by drawing the curtains before going to bed you were protecting the brain from cold damp air. Indeed, by expanding the domain of what could be considered preventive and hence affected by human action, the authors of these texts were providing patients with a degree of control over their bodies and their environments.

The dedication to Viviani's 1626 regimen exemplifies this view of the regimen as a personal tool offering its reader 'mastery' over his own body. It was addressed to his wealthy patron the Cardinal Orsini who had asked Viviani to pick out a suitable regimen from those already on the market for him to read. In Viviani's words, this was so that the cardinal could satisfy 'your desire to have some instructions, which, once you have mastered them, will enable you to look after the procedures which maintain health by yourself without jeopardizing your health'.[10] Orsini is also a good example of how lay readers, anxious about the persistent threat of illness, and wishing to feel less vulnerable to disease and more proactive about the maintenance of their health, stimulated the production of health advice.

On the other hand, doctors could only benefit from this process. One might have expected doctors to be perhaps wary of engaging in a genre which, advertised as offering comprehensive instructions on health management, potentially threatened their source of income, supplanting the need for their services. Yet we find no confirmation of this caution. Indeed, after an initial hesitation, it was the physicians themselves who enthusiastically appropriated the genre. Indeed, perhaps ironically, although the early modern regimen empowered the reader to some extent in its immense detail on medical matters, at the same time the increased complexity of recommendations, coupled with the huge number of new

---

[10] 'Il desiderio, che ella haveva d'una instruzione, con l'ammaestramento della quale sapesse da sè stessa regger l'operationi appartenenti al vivere, senza pregiudizio della Sanità.' Viviani, *Trattato*, 2.

qualifications and distinctions between bodies and habits to which we referred earlier, meant that only an expert could ultimately unravel what it was one was supposed to do. Thus in actual fact, far from dispensing with the doctor's expertise, dependence on the physician was, in some cases, increased.

Through vernacular print, doctors were able to acquire authority, articulating their knowledge, arbitrating in disputes, and, rather than falling behind the times, embracing and even shaping new practices through their intervention and emphasis on the health implications. The debate on hot and cold drinking is a good example of this. It was one area in which medical knowledge was clearly in disarray and the educated public were floundering in the interstices between contradictory voices of authority. Although it is an extreme case, it nonetheless illuminates the relationship between physicians, the regimen, and the reading public. The debate on drinking points to a new role which doctors had assumed by the last decades of the sixteenth century—as arbiters over some increasingly contentious issues regarding health and how to preserve it. In the accounts of the hastily produced regimen advertising the health benefits of snow which dangled from a shop sign, and of the drawing room of the Genoan elite, where pamphlets, handwritten advice, and books jostled for attention, there is a sense of real urgency, as people tried to settle one way or another whether indeed it was their drinking habits which was making them ill. Meanwhile in Fuscone's self-aggrandizing account of being asked by his illustrious clients to explain the contours of the debate, and then print his own views on the matter, we get a sense of the importance attached to the printed word and the recognition it conferred upon a doctor.

Finally, Petronio's discussion of melancholy offers another example of the ways in which doctors had gradually extended the domain of their authority, from the body to the soul. Along with several of his colleagues, he evidently felt himself qualified to stray beyond simply managing melancholy through the Non-Naturals, crossing over instead into the territory of the soul. In his case, he ventured further than most, recommending a more confessional or 'psychological' approach whereby the doctor seeks to elicit and 'reveal' those 'deeply rooted' hidden fears or thoughts which are so troubling the patient.

The vestiges of antique culture, promoted with such perseverance by the humanists, discourses of class, gentility, and religious decorum, as well as fashionable practices such as drinking cold, sleeping late, and riding in carriages, all contributed to the dialogue between late Renaissance culture and ancient medicine. All these factors elicited a response from physicians who managed on the one hand to protect and transmit the basic principles of preventive medicine, and on the other to shape their advice in the light of contemporary concerns and habits and it is surely this responsiveness which also helps to explain the regimens' success. The result was a dynamic culture of prevention which is not only reflected in the regimen genre itself, but has left far wider traces, in the letters, objects, images, and buildings of late Renaissance Italy.

Bibliography

MANUSCRIPT SOURCES

Biblioteca universitaria di Bologna

Beluda, Giocondo, 'Trattato del modo di volteggiare e saltare il cavallo di legno di Giocondo Beluda da Pesaro e di Oloizo Annibale Marescalchi Bolognese 22 November 1659', MS2133.

PRINTED SOURCES

Alberti, *Art of Building*

Alderotti, *Libello per conservar la sanità del corpo fatto per maestro Taddeo da Firenze* (Imola: Galeati, 1852).

Aldobrandino da Siena, *Le Régime du corps de Maître Aldebrandin de Sienne: Texte français du XIIIe siècle: Publié pour la première foi...par les docteurs Louis Landouzy et Roger Pépin* (Paris: H. Champion, 1911).

Amico, Giovanni Biagio, *L'architetto prattico in cui con facilità si danno le regole per apprendere l'architettura civile* (Palermo: Gio. Battista Aiccardo, 1726).

Anguillara, Lampridio, *Vaticinio et avertimenti per conservare la sanità et prolongar la vita humana* (Ferrara: Vittorio Baldini, 1589).

Antoniano, Silvio, *Dell'educazione christiana e politica de' figlioli libri tre* (1584; Turin: Paravia, 1926).

Aristotle, *Aristotle on the Parts & Progressive Motion of Animals, The Problems, On Indivisible Lines...* trans. Thomas Taylor (Sturminster Newton: The Prometheus Trust, 2004).

Arnaldi de Villanova, *Opera medica omnia*, X.1, *Regimen sanitatis ad regem aragonum*, ed. L. García Ballester, and M. R. McVaugh (Barcelona: Universitat de Barcelona, 1996).

Auda, Domenico, *Breue compendio di marauigliosi secreti rationali...Con vn trattato...per conseruarsi in sanità* (Roma: Ignatio de' Lazari, 1652).

Avicenna, *A Treatise on the Canon of Medicine of Avicenna Incorporating a Translation of the First Book by O. Cameron Gruner* (London: Luzat, 1930).

Bacci, Andrea, *Del Teuere...libri tre, ne' quali si tratta della natura, & bontà dell'acque...* (Venice: Aldo Manuzio, 1576).

Bartoli, Daniello, *Del ghiaccio e della coagulatione: Trattati del padre della compagnia di Giesú* (Bologna: Gio' Recaldini, 1682).

Belmonte, Pietro, *Institutione della sposa...fatta principalmente per madonna Laudomia* (Rome: eredi Gigliotto, 1587).

Benzi, Ugo, *Tractato utilissimo circa lo regimento et conservatione de la sanitade...* (Milan: Petromartire, 1508).

Bertaldi, Giovanni Lodovico, *Regole della sanità et della natura de cibi di Ugo Benzo medico e filosofo Senese con le annotazioni di Giò Ludovico Bertaudo* (Turin: Tarino, 1618).

Berti, Gio Battista, *Discorso sopra il bere fresco* (Rome: Giacomo Mascardi, 1616).

Bini, Pietro di Lorenzo, *Memorie del calcio fiorentino* (Florence: Stamperia di SAS alla Condotta, 1688).

Boldo, Bartolomeo, *Libro della natura et virtú delle cose, che nutriscono, et delle cose non naturali, con alcune osseruationi per conseruar la sanità...prima per M. Michele Savonarola medico padoano poi di nuovo con miglior ordine ordinato, accresciuto e emendato e quasi fatto un altro per Bartolomeo Boldo medico bressano* (Venice: Domenico & Gio. Battista Guerra fratelli, 1575).

Borromeo, Carlo, *Sermoni familiari…fatti alle monache dette angeliche dell'insigne monastero di S Paolo raccolti fedelmente dalla viva voce del santo per Agata Sfondrata, e pubblicati ora la prima volta da' codici manuscritti per opera di D Gaetano Volpi* (Padua: G. Comino, 1720).

Brancaccio, Francesco Maria, *La tazza di cioccolata*, ed. Luigi Sada, trans. P. P. A. Chetry and G. Pagliaruolo (Bari: Edipuglia, 1979).

Bruno, Matteo, *Discorsi…sopra gli errori fatti dall'eccell.te M. Bartolomeo Traffichetti da Bertinoro: Nell'arte sua di conseruar la sanità tutt'intiera…* (Venice: Andrea Arriuabene, 1569).

Burton, Robert, *Anatomy of Melancholy* (Oxford: Lichfield and Short, 1621).

Caggio, Paolo, *Iconomica…* (Venice: Andrea Arrivabene, 1552).

Camaffi, Luc'Antonio, *Reggimento per viver sano nei tempi caldi…* (Perugia: Stamparia Augusta, 1610).

Capra, Antonio, *Nuova architettura civile* (Cremona: Giuseppe Forbici, 1717).

Carroli, Bernardino, *Instrutione del giovane ben creato* (Ravenna: G. Corelli, 1581).

Cartegeni, Giovan Battista, *Trattato de' centi in quanto si appartiene al medico e del sito della città di Pisa* (Pisa: Lionardo Zeffi, 1628).

Cassiani, Piero, *Risposta di Piero Cassiani al discorso sopra il bever fresco* (Bologna: Vittorio Benacci, 1603).

Castiglione, Baldassare, *The Book of the Courtier*, trans. and ed. George Bull (Penguin: London, 1976).

Castiglioni, Giuseppe, *De frigido et calido potu apologeticus* (Rome: Guglielmo Facciotto, 1607).

Ciccolini, Barnaba, *L'oro della sanità ritrovato nel clima romano…* (Rome: Gioseppe Vannacci, 1697).

Cobarubias, Pietro di, *Rimedio de' givocatori* (Venice: Valgrisi, 1566).

Colle, Francesco, *Refugio over ammonitorio del gentiluomo* (s.l.: s.n., 1532).

Colmenero, Antonio, *Della cioccolata discorso diviso in quattro parti, medico e chirurgo della città d'Ecija nell'Andaluzia* (Rome: Alessandro Vitrioli, 1667).

Commentarii di M. Arnaldo da Villanova Cattellano, in *Scuola salernitana del modo di conseruarsi in sanità* (Perugia: Petrucci, 1587).

Concina, Daniele, *Memorie storiche sopra l'uso della cioccolata in tempo di digiuno: Esposte in una lettera a monsig. Illustriss. Reverendiss. Arcivescovo in Venice* (Venice: Simone Occhi, 1748).

Cornaro, Luigi, *Trattato de la vita sobria…* (Padua: Perchacino, 1558).

Corti, Matteo, *De prandii ac caenae modo libellus* (Rome: Paolo Manuzio, 1562).

Croce, Giulio Cesare, *Comiato dato dai Beccari ai pescatori nel fine di Quadragesima…* (Bologna: Eredi di Gio' Rossi, 1604).

Del Riccio, Agostino, 'Del giardino di un rè', in Detlef Heikamp (ed.), *Il giardino storico italiano: Problemi di indagine: Fonti letterarie e storiche* (Florence: Olschki, 1981), 59–124.

Di Galeno, Delli mezzi, che si possono tenere per conseruarci la sanità: Recato in questa lingua nostra da m. Giouanni Tarcagnota (Venice: Tramezzino, 1549).

Du Laurens, André, *Discours de conservation del la veue; des maladies melancholiques; des catarrhes et de la viellesse* (Paris: Mettayer, 1597).

—— *A discourse of the preservation of the sight: of melancholike diseases; of rheumes, and of old age*, trans. Richard Surphlet, introd. Sanford V. Larkey (London, 1599), published for the Shakespeare association by H. Milford (Oxford: Oxford University, 1938).

Du Laurens, André *Discorsi della conseruatione della vista, delle malattie melanconiche, delli catarri, e della vecchiaia... tradotti in lingua italiana e commentati da Fr. Gio. Germano* (Naples: L. Scorigio, 1626).

—— 'Discorso della malinconia', in Giacomo Ferrari, *Democrito et Eraclito: Dialoghi del riso, delle lagrime e della malinconia...* (Mantua: Aurelio & Lodovico Osanna fratelli, 1627).

—— *Il tesoro della vecchiezza...* (Venice: Il Ginammi, 1637).

Durante, Castore, *Herbario novo... con figure che rappresentano le vive piante, che nascono in tutta Europa, & nell'Indie Orientali, & Occidentali...* (Rome: Iacomo Bericchia & Iacomo Tornierij, 1585).

—— *Il tesoro della sanità* (Venice: Andrea Muschio, 1586).

Evitascandalo, Cesare, *Dialogo del maestro di casa* (Rome: Martinelli, 1598).

Ferrari, Giacomo, *Democrito et Eraclito: Dialoghi del riso, delle lagrime e della malinconia* (Mantua: A. et L. Osanna fratelli, 1627).

Ficino, Marsilio, *De le tre vite, cioè, a qual guisa si possono le persone letterate mantenere in sanità...* (Venice: Tramezzino, 1548).

—— *Three Books on Life: A Critical Edition and Translation*, trans. Carol V. Kaske and John R. Clark (Binghamton, NY: Medieval and Renaissance Texts and Studies, 1989).

Filarete, Antonio Averlino, *Trattato di architettura*, ed. Anna Maria Finoli and Liliana Grassi (Milan: Edizioni il Polifilo, 1972).

Firmano, Annibale, *Convito del Primo dì d'Agosto, ove piacevolmente si ragiona in che modo si possano conosere e emendare gli affetti e vitij dell'animo* (Rome: Valerio Dorico, 1563).

Fonseca, Rodrigo, *Del conservare la sanitá* (Florence: Semartelli, 1603).

Franco, Cirillo, *Una lettera... scritta al cavaliero U. Gualtierazi nella quale si lamenta molto che la musica moderna non produca quegli affetti che produceva l'antica* (s.l., 1650?).

Frediano, Elici, *Arca novella di sanità trattato fisico morale con alcune regole per conservarsi sano...* (Lucca: Iacinto Paci, 1656).

Frigerio, Bartolomeo, *Arte d'acquistar e conservar la robba e la reputazione d'una famiglia e d'una corte...* (Rome: Grignani, 1650).

Fuscone, Pietro Paolo, *Trattato del bere caldo e freddo* (Genoa: G. Pavoni, 1605).

Galen, *De sanitate tuenda: A Translation of Galen's Hygiene*, ed. and trans. Robert Montraville Green (Springfield, Ill.: Thomas, 1951).

—— *On the Passions and Errors of the Soul*, ed. Walther Riese (Columbus: Ohio State University Press, 1963).

—— *Galen On the Elements According to Hippocrates*, ed. Phillip De Lacy (Berlin: Akademie Verlag, 1996).

Gallina, Francesco, *Tratto della natura de' cibi et del bere, del sig. Baldassare Pisanelli... Ridotto in vn'assai bell'ordine, et aggiontoui di molte dotte, et belle annotationi sopr'ogni capo dal sig. Franc. Gallina* (Carmagnola: Marc' Antonio Bellone, 1589).

Gallo, Agostino, *Le dieci giornate della vera agricoltura, e piaceri della villa* (Venice: Giovanni Bariletto, 1566).

Giacinto Gigli, *Diario di Roma*, ed. Manlio Barberito (Rome: Colombo, 1994).

Giamboni, Giovanni, *Capitolo... In lode della villa* (Florence: Francesco Tosi, 1575).

Giuliani, Gio Francesco, *Dialogo di un medico con un secretario et un palaferniere di un principe romano: Del modo, & utilità di far la quadregesima, acquistar la sanità, e conseruarla insino al fine della vita* (Rome: Gio' Pietro Colligni, 1655).

Giustiniani, Vincenzo, 'Discorso sopra il giuoco del pallamaglio' (1626), in Claudio Bascetta (ed.), *Sport e giochi, trattati e scritti dal XV al XVIII secolo* (Milan: Il Polifilo, 1978), 326–32.

Grassi, Latino de, *Opera nuova... universale e salutifera... La quale impara a perlongare la vita, e conservarsi sano* (Venice: s.n., c.1550).

Gropretio, Roberto, *Un breue et notabile trattato del reggimento della Sanità,* annexed to Domenico Romoli, *La singolare dottrina...* (Venice: Tramezzino, 1560).

Guazzo, Stefano, *La civil conversazione,* ed. Amedeo Quondam (Rome: Bulzoni, 2010).

Gufferi, G. Francesco, *Il biasimo dello tabacco overo l'uso pernicioso di esso* (Palermo: s.n., 1645).

Hippocrates, *Airs, Waters, Places,* trans. W. H. S. Jones (London: William Heinemann; New York: G. P. Putnam's Sons, 1923).

Laguna, Andrés, *De victus et exercitii ratione* (Rome: A. Blado, 1547).

Lanteri, Giacomo, *Della economica... nel quale si dimostrano le qualità che all'uomo e alla donna convengono nel governo della casa* (Venice: Valgrisi, 1560).

Lennio, Levino, *De gli occulti miracoli, e varii ammaestramenti delle cose della natura* (Venice: Nicolino 1563).

—— *Della complessione del corpo humano libri tre* (Venice: Domenico Nicolino, 1564).

Liberati, Francesco, *Il perfetto maestro di casa* (1658; Rome: Franzini, 1668).

Libro di Arnaldo di Villa Nuova, medico et filosofo acutissimo del modo di conservar la gioventù e ritardar la vecchiezza, annexed to Pictorius, *Dialogi...* (Venice: Bottega d'Erasmo di Vincenzo Valgrisi, 1550).

Lollio, Alberto, *Lettera... in laude de la villa, scritta a messer Hercole Perinato* (Venice: Sigismondo Bordogna, 1544).

Lombardelli, Orazio, *Della tranquillità dell'animo: Sopr'il dialogo di Florenzio Voluseno... divisa in quattro libri* (Siena: Luca Bonetti, 1574).

—— *De gli vfizii, e costvmi de' giovani libri IIII* (Florence: Gio' Marescotti, 1584).

—— *Il giovane studente* (Venice: Francesco Uscio, 1594).

Longiano, Sebastiano Fausto, *De lo istituire un figlio d'un principe da li. X. infino à gl'anni de la discretione* (Venice: Bindoni e Pasini, 1542).

Lutii, P., *Opera bellissima nella quale si contengono molte partite e passeggi di gagliarda* (Perugia: Orlando, 1589).

Maffei, Giovanni Pietro, *Le istorie delle Indie Orientali, con una scelta di lettere scritte dell'Indie* (Venice: Damoan Zenaro, 1589).

Magagni, Giovanni, *Compendio de la sanità corporale et spirituale* (Milan: Gotardo da Ponte, 1527).

Magri, Domenico, *Virtú del caffe bevanda la piu salutifera e la men connosciuta, introduotta nuovamente nell'Italia* (Venice: Michele Hercole, 1716).

[Maineri, Maino de], *Opera utilissima di Arnaldo da Villanova di conservare la sanità* (Venice: Tramezzino, 1549).

Malfi, Tiberio, *Il barbiere... Ne' quali si ragiona dell'eccellenza dell'arte...* (Naples: Beltrano, 1626).

Manente, Giovanni, *Col nome de Dio: Il segreto de segreti...* (Venice: Zuan Tacuino da Trino, 1538).

Manfredi, Girolamo, *Libro intitolato Il perché... Con mostrar le cagioni d'infinite cose appartenenti alla sanità...* (Venice: Lucio Spineda, 1622).

Manilli, Giacomo, *Villa Borghese fuori di Porta Pinciana* (Rome: Lodovico Grignani, 1650).

Marinelli, Giovanni, *Gli ornamenti delle donne tratti dalle scritture d'una reina greca* (Venice: De Francesci, 1562).

—— *Le medicine partenenti alle infermità delle donne: Scritte per M. Giouanni Marinello, nuouamente da lui ampliate, & ricorrete* (Venice: Giovanni Valgriso, 1574).

Martini, Francesco di Giorgio, *Trattati di architettura, ingegneria e arte militare,* ed. Corrado Maltese, 2 vols. (Milan: Il Polifilo, 1967).

—— *Trattato di architettura di Francesco di Giorgio Martini: Il codice Ashburnham 361 della Biblioteca Medicea Laurenziana*, ed. Pietro Marani (Florence: Giunti Barbera, 1979).

Meduna, Bartolomeo, *Lo scolare...Nel quale si forma a pieno vn perfetto scolare* (Venice: Pietro Fachinetti, 1588).

Mercuriale, Girolamo, *De arte gymnastica*, trans. Vivian Nutton (Florence: Olschki, 2008).

Mercurio, Scipione, *La comare o ricoglitrice...divisa in tre libri* (Venice: G. B. Cioti, 1596).

—— *De gli errori popolari d'Italia* (Padua: Francesco Bolzetta, 1645).

Meyden, Theodoro, *Trattato della natura del vino e del ber caldo, e freddo* (Rome: Giacomo Mascardi, 1608).

[Monardes, Nicholas], *Trattato della neue e del bere fresco, raccolto per M. Giouan Batista Scarampo, dal trattato del Monardo medico di Siuiglia, & ridotto in lingua toscana* (Florence: Bartolomeo Sermatelli 1574).

Montaigne, Michel de, *Viaggio in Italia* (Bari: Laterza, 1991).

Montanari, Massimo, *Convivio: storia e cultura dei piaceri della tavola dall'antichità al medioevo* (Laterza: Bari, 1989).

Oldradi, Angelo degli, *Capitolo del palamaglio...* (Rome, 1552).

Opera nuova intitolata Dificio di ricette (Venice?: s.n., 1525).

Paleario, Aonio, *Dell'economia, overo del governo della casa*, ed. S. Caponetto (Florence: Olschki, 1983).

Palladio, Andrea, *Quattro libri di architettura* (Venice: Dominico de' Franceschi, 1570).

Panaroli, Domenico, *Abuso nel governo dei putti* (Rome: Marciani, 1642).

—— *Aerologia cioè discorso dell'aria, trattato utile per la sanità...* (Rome: Domenico Marciani, 1642).

—— *Discorso delle stufe da bagni di Roma e suoi nocumenti* (Rome: Robletti, 1646).

Pascali, Lelio, *L'aio del capitano Lelio Pascalli dd. all'ecc.mo sig.or duca Iacomo Salviati* (1641; Rome: Heredi Corbelletti, 1648).

Paschetti, Bartolomeo, *Del conservar la sanità* (Genoa: Giuseppe Pavoni, 1602).

Peccana, Alessandro, *Del bever freddo* (Verona: Angelo Tamo, 1627).

Persio, Antonio, *Del bever caldo costumato dagli antichi Romani* (Venice: Gió Battista Ciotto, 1593).

Petronio, Alessandro Trajano, *Del viver delli Romani, et di conservar la sanità...libri cinque* (Rome: Domenico Bassa, 1592).

Piccolomini, Alessandro, *De la institutione di tutta la vita dell'homo nato nobile* (Venice: Geronimo Scoto, 1542).

—— *Della institutione de la felice vita de l'homo nato nobile...* (Venice: Giovanmaria Bonelli, 1552).

Pictorius, Georg, *Dialogi...del modo del conseruare la sanità: Nuouamente dalla lingua latina nella uolgar italiana tradotto...* (Venice: Bottega d'Erasmo di Vincenzo Valgrisi, 1550).

Piemontese, Alessio, *Secreti...* (Rome: Antonio Blado, 1555).

—— *Dei secreti di diversi eccellentissimi huomini...Parte terza* (Milan: Giovann'Antonio de gli Antonij, 1559).

Pietragrassa, Bartolomeo, *Politica medica per il governo conservativo del corpo humano* (Pavia: Gio. Andrea Magri, 1649).

Pino, Paolo, 'Dialogo di pittura', in Paola Barrocchi (ed.), *Trattati d'arte del Cinquecento: fra manierismo e controriforma*, i (Bari: Laterza, 1960).

Pisanelli, Baldassarre, *Trattato della natura de' cibi* (Bergamo: Comino Ventura & C., 1587).

Platina, Bartolomeo, *On Right Pleasure and Good Health: A Critical Edition and Translation of De Honesta Voluptate et Valetudine*, ed. Mary Ella Milham (Tempe, Ariz.: Medieval and Renaissance Texts and Studies, 1998).

Pontormo, Iacopo da, *Diario fatto nel tempo che dipingevo il coro di San Lorenzo 1554–1556* (Rome: Gremese, 1998).

Rambaldi, Angelo, *Ambrosia arabica overo della salutare bevanda café* (Bologna: Longhi, 1691).

Rangoni, Tommaso, *Thomaso philologo da Rauenna: Come l'huomo può viuere piu de CXX anni* (Venice: Matheum Paganum a Fide, 1556).

—— *Consiglio del magnifico cavaliere eccellent. fisico M. Tomaso Filologo da Ravenna: come i venetiani possano vivere sempre sani… tradotto novamente da Jacomo Pratello Montefiore, medico* (Venice: F. de' Patriani, 1565).

Regesti di bandi, editti, notificazioni e provvedimenti diversi relativi alla città di Roma ed allo Stato pontificio, 5 vols. (Rome: Cuggiani, 1920–58).

Romoli, Domenico, *La singolare dottrina…* (Venice: Tramezzino, 1560).

Rosaccio, Giuseppe, *Avvertimenti a tutti quelli che desiderano regolatamente vivere…* (Florence: G. Caneo, 1594).

[Rosetti, Giovanventura], *Notandissimi secreti de l'arte profumatoria: A fare ogli, acque, paste, balle, moscardini uccelletti, paternostri e tutta l'arte intiera* (Venice: Francesco Rampazetto, 1560).

Rusconi, Giovanni Antonio, *Della architettura di Giovanni Antonio Rusconi*, ed. Anna Bedon (Vicenza: Centro Internazionale di Studi di architettura Andrea Palladio, 1996).

Sadoleto, Jacopo, *Del ben ammaestrare i figlioli* (1533; Venice: Giovanni Tavernini, 1755).

Salando, Ferdinando, *Trattato sopra la regola del vivere nelle sei cose chiamate non naturali* (Venice: Angelo Tamo, 1607).

Salini, Cosimo, *Trattato del ber fresco* (Rome: Guglielmo Facciotti, 1609).

Sansovino, Francesco, *Venetia città nobilissima* (Venice: I. Sansovino, 1581).

Savonarola, Michele, *Libreto… de tutte le cose che se manzano comunamente… e de sei cose non natural: & le regule per conseruare la sanità de li corpi humani* (Venice: Bernardino Benalio, 1515).

Scaino, Antonio, *Trattato del gioco della palla diviso in tre parti* (Venice: Gabriel Giolito dei Ferrari e Fratelli, 1555).

Scamozzi, Vincenzo, *L'idea dell'architettura universale* (1615; Bologna: Forni, 1982).

—— *Intorno alle ville: Lodi e comodità delle 'fabriche suburbane' e 'rurali'* (1615), ed. Lionello Puppi and Lucia Collavo (Turin: Umberto Allemandi, 2003).

Scuola salernitana del modo di conseruarsi in sanità, trans. Serafino Razzi (Perugia: Petrucci, 1587).

Serlio, *Architettura civile: Libri sesto, settimo e ottavo nei manoscritti di Monaco e Vienna*, ed. Francesco Paolo Fiore (Milan: Edizioni Il Polifilo, 1994).

Stella, Benedetto, *Il tabacco medico, morale curiosa* (Rome: Mancini, 1669).

Svegliarino alli signori veneziani per poter con sicurezza viver di continuo in sanità sino agli anni cento e dieci (Venice: Leonardo Pittoni, 1691).

Taegio, Bartolomeo, *La Villa: Dialogo di M Bartolomeo Taegio* (Milan: Moscheni, 1559).

Tanara, Vincenzo, *L'economia del cittadino in villa* (1644; Venice: Bertani, 1661).

Tartaglini, Leone, *Opera nuoua nella quale se contiene la natura dil sonno cioé come l'huomo debbe dormire per mantenersi sano…* (Venice: Tartaglini, 1551).

Tassoni, Alessandro, *Varietà di Pensieri* (Modona: eredi di G. M. Verdi, 1612).

—— *Pensieri e scritti preparatori*, ed. Pietro Puliatti (1612; Modena: Edizioni Panini, 1986).

Timotei, Michele, *Il cortegiano christiano* (Rome: Mascardi, 1614).

Traffichetti, Bartolomeo, *L'arte di conservar la salute tutta intiera trattata in sei libri…* (Pesaro: Girolamo Concordia, 1565).

Traffichetti, Bartolomeo, *Idea dell'arte di conseruare la sanità... et hora per il medesmo diffesa dalle false oppositioni di M. Matteo Bruni il medico da Rimino* (Venice: Bindoni & fratelli, 1572).

Ugoni da Brescia, *Dialogo della vigilia, et del sonno...* (Venice: Pietro da Fine, 1562).

Vitruvius, *Ten books on Architecture*, ed. Ingrid D. Rowland, Thomas Noble Howe, and Michael J. Dewar (Cambridge: Cambridge University Press, 1999).

Viviani, Viviano, *Trattato del custodire la sanità* (Venice: Girolamo Piuti, 1626).

Zacchia, Paolo, *Del vitto quaresimale: Ove insegnasi, come senza offender la sanità si possa viver nella Quaresima* (Rome: Pietro Antonio Facciotti, 1637).

—— *De mali hipochondriaci: Libri due* (Rome: Pietro Antonio Facciotti, 1639).

Zanini, Giuseppe Viola, *Della architettura... Libri II* (1627; Padua: F. Bolzetta, 1629).

SECONDARY SOURCES

Accademia della Crusca, *Vocabolario degli Accademici della Crusca*, 5th impression, vols. 1–11 (Florence, 1863–1923).

Aga-Oglu, Mehmet, 'About a Type of Islamic Incense Burner', *Art Bulletin*, 27 (March 1945), 28–45.

Ago, Renata, 'Gerarchia delle merci e meccanismi dello scambio nella Roma del primo seicento', *Quaderni storici*, 96 (1997), 663–83.

—— *Economia barocca: Mercato e istituzioni nella Roma del seicento* (Rome, 1998).

—— *Carriere e clientele nella Roma barocca* (Bari, 1999), 68–71.

—— *Il gusto delle cose: Una storia degli oggetti nella Roma del Seicento* (Rome, 2006).

Ajmar-Wollheim, Marta, and Dennis, Flora (eds.), *At Home in Renaissance Italy* (London, 2006).

——, ——, and Matchette, Ann (eds.), 'Approaching the Italian Domestic Interior: Sources, Methodologies, Debates', *Renaissance Studies*, 20/5 (2006), 623–8.

Albala, Ken, *Eating Right in the Renaissance* (Berkeley, Los Angeles, and London, 2002).

—— 'The Use and Abuse of Chocolate in 17th Century Medical Theory', *Food and Foodways*, 15 (2007), 53–74.

—— 'The Ideology of Fasting in the Reformation Era', in Ken Albala and Trudy Eden (eds.), *Food and Faith in Christian Culture* (New York, 2011), 41–58.

Alexandre-Bidon, Daniele, and Piponnier, Françoise, 'Gestes et objets de la toilette aux XIVème et XVème siècles', in Denis Menjot (ed.), *Les Soins de beauté* (Nice, 1987), 211–44.

Andretta, Elisa, 'Les Régimes de santé des papes dans la deuxième moitié du XVIe siècle', in Catherine Lanoe, Mathieu da Vinha, and Bruno Laurioux (eds.), *Cultures de cour, cultures du corps XIV–XVIII siècles* (Paris, 2011), 69–84.

—— *Roma medica: Anatomie d'un système médical au XVIe siècle* (Rome, 2011).

—— and Nicoud, Marylin (eds.), *Être médecin à la cour: Italie, France et Espagne, XIII–XVIII siècles* (Micrologus Library 52; Florence, 2013).

Arcangeli, Alessandro, 'I gesuiti e la danza', *Quadrivium*, NS 1/2 (1990), 21–37.

—— 'La disciplina del corpo e la danza', in Paolo Prodi (ed.), *Disciplina dell'anima, disciplina del corpo e disciplina della società tra medioevo ed età moderna* (Bologna, 1994), 417–36.

—— 'Dance and Health: The Renaissance Physicians' View', *Dance Research*, 18/1 (2000), 3–20.

—— *Recreation in the Renaissance: Attitudes towards Leisure and Pastimes in European Culture, c. 1425–1675* (Basingstoke, 2003).

—— 'Una controversia veronese su ginnastica e medicina', in Alessandro Pastore and E. Peruzzi (eds.), *Girolamo Fracastoro: Fra medicina, filosofia e scienze della natura* (Florence, 2006), 163–71.

Archibald, Elizabeth, 'Did Knights Have Baths?', in Corinne J. Saunders (ed.), *Cultural Encounters in the Romance of Medieval England* (Cambridge, 2005), 101–16.

Arikha, Noga, *Passions and Tempers: A History of the Humours* (New York, 2008).

Arrizabalaga, Jon, Henderson, John, and French, Roger, *The Great Pox: The French Disease in Renaissance Europe* (New Haven and London, 1997).

Attardi, Luisa, *Il camino veneto del cinquecento* (Vicenza, 2002).

Austern, Linda Phillis, 'Musical Treatments for Lovesickness: The Early Modern Heritage', in Peregrine Horden (ed.), *Music as Medicine: The History of Music Therapy Since Antiquity* (Aldershot, 2000), 213–45.

Aynsley, Jeremy, and Grant, Charlotte, 'Introduction', to Jeremy Aynsley and Charlotte Grant with assistance from Harriet McKay (eds.), *Imagined Interiors: Representing the Domestic Interior Since the Renaissance* (London, 2006), 10–20.

Baernstein, Renée, 'Reprobates and Courtiers: Lay Masculinities in the Colonna Family 1520–1584', in David S. Peterson and Daniel E. Bornstein (eds.), *Florence and Beyond: Culture, Society and Politics in Renaissance Italy* (Toronto, 2008), 291–303.

Bareggi di Filippo, Claudia, *Il mestiere di scrivere: Lavoro intellettuale e mercato librario a Venezia nel cinquecento* (Rome, 1988).

Barisi, Isabella, Fabiolo, Marcello, and Madonna, Maria Luisa (eds.), *Villa d'Este* (Rome, 2003).

Bascetta, Claudio, *Sport e giochi, trattati e scritti dal XV al XVIII secolo* (Milan, 1978).

Behr, Charlotte, Usborne, Cornelie, and Wieber, Sabine, 'Introduction: The Challenge of the Image', *Cultural and Social History*, 7/4 (2010), 425–34.

Behringer, Wolfgang, *A Cultural History of Climate*, trans. Patrick Camiller (Cambridge, 2010).

Beier, Lucinda M., 'In Sickness and in Health: A Seventeenth-Century Family Experience', in Roy Porter (ed.), *Patients and Practitioners: Lay Perceptions of Medicine and Pre-industrial Society* (Cambridge, 1985), 108–28.

Bell, Rudolph, *How to Do It: Guides to Good Living for Renaissance Italians* (Chicago and London, 1999).

Bergdolt, Klaus, *Wellbeing: A Cultural History of Healthy Living* (Cambridge, 2008), 87–93.

Boisseuil, Didier, and Nicoud, Marilyn (eds.), *Séjourner au bain: Le Thermalisme entre médecine et société, XIVe–XVIe siècle* (*Collection d'histoire et d'archéologie médiévales*, vol. 23; Lyons, 2010).

Boiteux, Martine, 'Jeux equestres à la cour de Rome', in Franca Varallo (ed.), *La Ronde: Giostre, esercizi cavallereschi e loisir in Francia e Piemonte fra Medioevo e Ottocento* (Florence, 2011).

Bonfield, Christopher A., 'The *Regimen sanitatis* and Its Dissemination in England c.1348–1355' (University of East Anglia, PhD thesis, 2006).

Bonhomme, Guy, 'Le Cheval comme instrument du mouvement humain à la Renaissance', in Jean Céard, Marie-Madeleine Fontaine, and Jean Claude Margolin (eds.), *Le Corps à la Renaissance: Actes du XXX colloque de Tours 1987* (Paris, 1990).

Bos, J., 'The Rise and Decline of Character: Humoral Psychology in Ancient and Early Modern Medical Theory', *History of the Human Sciences*, 22 (2009), 29–50.

Bottari, G., *Raccolta di lettere sulla pittura, scultura e architettura scritte da' piu celebri personaggi dei secoli 15, 16, e 17* (Milan, 1980).

Bound Alberti, Fay, 'Emotions in the Early Modern Medical Tradition', in Fay Bound Alberti (ed.), *Medicine, Emotion and Disease, 1700–1950* (Basingstoke, 2006), 1–21.

Boutier, Jean, 'Le nobiltà del Gran Ducato', in Jean Boutier, Sandro Landi, and Olivier Rouchon (eds.), *Firenze e la Toscana: Genesi e trasformazioni di uno stato (14.–19. secolo)* (Florence, 2010).

Britton, Piers, '"Mio malinchonico, o vero…mio pazzo": Michelangelo, Vasari, and the Problem of Artists' Melancholy in Sixteenth-Century Italy', *Sixteenth Century Journal*, 34/3 (2003), 653–75.

Brizzi, Gianpaolo, *La formazione della classe dirigente nel sei–settecento: I seminaria nobilium nell'Italia centro-settentrionale* (Bologna, 1976).

Brockliss, Laurence, and Jones, Colin, *The Medical World of Early Modern France* (Oxford, 1997).

Brunelli, Giampiero, *Soldati del papa: Politica militare e nobiltà nello stato della chiesa, 1560–1644* (Rome, 2003).

—— 'Identità dei militari pontifici in età moderna', in Claudio Donati and B. R. Kroener (eds.), *Militari e società civile nell'Europa dell'età moderna secoli XVI–XVIII* (Bologna, 2007), 313–50.

Burke, Peter, 'The Invention of Leisure in Early Modern Europe', *Past and Present*, 1337 (1995), 136–50.

—— *Eyewitnessing* (London, 2001).

—— 'Interrogating the Eyewitness', *Cultural and Social History*, 7/4 (2010), 435–44.

Burnett, Charles, '"Spiritual Medicine": Music and Healing in Islam and Its Influence in Western Medicine', in Penelope Gouk (ed.), *Musical Healing in Cultural Contexts* (Aldershot, 2000), 85–91.

Burns, Howard, 'Letti visibili e invisibili nei progetti architettonici del Rinascimento', in Aurora Scotti-Tosini (ed.), *Aspetti dell'abitare in Italia tra XV e XVI secolo: Distribuzione, funzioni, impianti* (Milan, 2001), 133–40.

Cabantous, Alain, *Histoire de la nuit: XVIIe–XVIIIe siècle* (Paris, 2009).

Cabré, *Montserrat*, 'Women or Healers? Household Practices and the Categories of Health Care in Late Medieval Iberia', *Bulletin of the History of Medicine*, 82/1 (2008), 18–51.

Carlino, Andrea, 'Introduction', in Andrea Carlino and Michel Jeanneret (eds.), *Vulgariser la médecine: Du style médical en France et en Italie (XVIe et XVIIe siècles)* (Geneva, 2009), 9–13.

Carpané, Lorenzo, 'Libri, librai tipografi nella Verona del '500', in A. Contò (ed.), *Studi in memoria di Mario Carrara*, Bollettino della Biblioteca Civica di Verona, 1 (1995), 203–34.

Carré, Antònia, and Cifuentes, Lluís, 'Girolamo Manfredi's *Il perché*: I. The *Problemata* and its Medieval Tradition', *Medicina e storia*, 19–20 (2010), 13–38.

——, ——, 'Girolamo Manfredi's *Il perché*: II. The *Secretum secretorum* and the Book's Publishing Success', *Medicina e storia*, 19–20 (2010), 39–58.

Carrera, Elena, 'Madness and Melancholy in Sixteenth- and Seventeenth-Century Spain: New Evidence, New Approaches', *Bulletin of Spanish Studies*, 87/8 (2010), 1–15.

—— 'Understanding Mental Disturbance in Sixteenth- and Seventeenth-Century Spain', *Bulletin of Spanish Studies*, 87/8 (2010), 105–36.

Casali, Elide, '"Economica" e "creanza" cristiana', *Quaderni storici*, 41 (1979), 555–75.

Casanova, Cesarina, 'Le donne come "risorsa": Le politiche matrimoniali della famiglia Spada', in *Memoria: Rivista di storia delle donne*, 21 (1987), 56–78.

Castelli, Patrizia, *L'estetica del rinascimento* (Bologna, 2005).

Cavallo, Sandra, 'The Artisan's *Casa*', in Marta Ajmar-Wollheim and Flora Dennis (eds.), *At Home in Renaissance Italy* (London, 2006), 352–55.

—— *Artisans of the Body in Early Modern Italy: Identities, Families, Masculinities* (Manchester, 2007).

—— 'Secrets to Healthy Living: The Revival of the Preventive Paradigm in Late Renaissance Italy', in Elaine Leong and Alisha Rankin (eds.), *Secrets and Knowledge in Medicine* (Aldershot, 2011), 191–212.

Chambers, David S., 'Spas in the Italian Renaissance', in David S. Chambers, *Individuals and Institutions in Renaissance Italy* (Aldershot, 1998).

Chartier, Roger (ed.), *A History of Private Life*, iii. *Passions of the Renaissance* (Cambridge, Mass., 1989).

Chittolini, G., 'Il "militare" tra tardo medioevo e prima età moderna', in Claudio Donati and B. R. Kroener (eds.), *Militari e società civile nell'Europa dell'età moderna secoli XVI–XVIII* (Bologna, 2007), 53–102.

Ciappelli, Giovanni, *Carnevale e Quaresima: Comportamenti sociali e cultura a Firenze nel Rinascimento* (Rome, 1997).

Clericuzio, Antonio, 'Chemical medicine and Paracelsianism in Italy 1550–1650', in Margaret Pelling and Scott Mandelbrote (eds.), *The Practice of Reform in Health, Medicine and Science 1500–2000* (Aldershot, 2005), 59–79.

Coffin, David, *The Villa d'Este at Tivoli* (Princeton, 1960).

—— *The Villa in the Life of Renaissance Rome* (Princeton, 1979).

—— *Gardens and Gardening in Papal Rome* (Princeton, 1991).

—— *Magnificent Buildings, Splendid Gardens*, ed. Vanessa Bezemer Sellers (Princeton, 2008).

—— 'Pope Innocent VIII and the Villa Belvedere', in David Coffin, *Magnificent Buildings, Splendid Gardens*, 58–71.

Cohn (Jr), Samuel K., *Cultures of Plague: Medical Thinking at the End of the Renaissance* (Oxford, 2010).

Conrad, Peter, *The Medicalization of Society: On the Transformation of Human Conditions into Treatable Disorders* (Baltimore, 2007).

Contadini, Anna, 'Middle Eastern Objects', in Marta Ajmar-Wollheim and Flora Dennis (eds.), *At Home in Renaissance Italy* (London, 2006).

Contardi, Bruno, and Lilius, Hendrik, *Quando gli dei si spogliano: Il bagno di Clemente VII a Castel Sant'Angelo e le altre stufe romane* (Rome, 1984).

Cook, Harold J., 'Physical Methods', in William F. Bynum and Roy Porter (eds.), *Companion Encyclopedia of the History of Medicine* (London, 1993), ii. 936–60.

—— 'Good Advice and Little Medicine: The Professional Authority of Early Modern English Physicians', *Journal of British Studies*, 33 (1994), 1–31.

Couchman, Jane, and Crabb, Ann (eds.), *Women's Letters Across Europe, 1400–1700: Form and Persuasion* (Aldershot, 2005).

Courtright, Nicola, *The Papacy and the Art of Reform in 16th Century Rome: Gregory XIII's Tower of the Winds in the Vatican* (Cambridge, 2003).

Cowen Orlin, L., 'Fiction of the Early Modern Probate Inventory', in H. S.Turner (ed.), *The Culture of Capital: Property, Cities and Knowledge in Early Modern England* (London, 2002).

Cozzo, P., ' "Aliquando necessarium": Gioco e dimensione ludica nella cultura ecclesiastica di età moderna', in Franca Varallo (ed.), *La ronde giostre, esercizi cavallereschi e loisir in Francia e Piemonte fra Medioevo e Ottocento* (Florence, 2011), 83–95.

Crisciani, Chiara, 'Histories, Stories, *Exempla*, and Anecdotes: Michele Savonarola from Latin to Vernacular', in Gianna Pomata and Nancy Siriaisi (eds.), *Historia: Empiricism and Erudition in Early Modern Europe* (Cambridge, Mass., 2005), 297–324.

D'Amelia, Marina, 'Una lettera a settimana: Geronima Veralli Malatesta al signor fratello 1572–1622', *Quaderni storici*, 28 (1993), 381–413.

—— 'La presenza delle madri nell'Italia medievale e moderna', in Marina D'Amelia (ed.), *Storia della maternità* (Bari, 1997), 3–52.

—— 'Lo scambio epistolare tra cinque e seicento: Scene di vita quotidiana e aspirazioni segrete', in Gabriella Zarri (ed.), *Per lettera: La scrittura epistolare femminile tra archivio e tipografia secoli XV–XVII* (Rome, 1999), 79–110.

D'Onofrio, Cesare, *La Villa Aldobrandini di Frascati* (Rome, 1963).

Dallasta, Federica, *Eredità di carta: Biblioteche private e circolazione libraria nella Parma farnesiana (1545–1731)* (Milan, 2010).

Danesi Squarzina, Silvia, *La collezione Giustiniani*, 3 vols. (Turin, 2003).

Daniels, Rhiannon, *Boccaccio and the Book: Production and Reading in Italy 1340–1520* (Oxford, 2009).

Dannenfeldt, Karl H., 'Sleep: Theory and Practice in the Late Renaissance', *Journal of the History of Medicine and Allied Sciences*, 41/4 (1986), 415–41.

David, Elizabeth, *Harvest of the Cold Months* (London, 1994).

Davis, Robert C., 'Venetian Shipbuilders and the Fountain of Wine', *Past and Present*, 156/1 (1997), 55–86.

Daybell, James (ed.), *Early Modern Women's Letter Writing, 1450–1700* (Basingstoke, 2001).

—— *Women Letter-Writers in Tudor England* (Oxford, 2006).

De Boer, Wietse, *The Conquest of the Soul: Confession, Discipline and Public Order in Counter-Reformation Milan* (Leiden, 2001).

De Bondt, Cees, *Royal Tennis in Renaissance Italy* (Turnhout, 2006).

De la Ruffinière du Prey, Pierre, *The Villas of Pliny from Antiquity to Posterity* (Chicago, 1994).

de Planhol, Xavier, *L'Eau de neige: Le Tiède et le frais: Histoire et géographie des boissons fraîches* (Paris, 1995).

De Renzi, Silvia, 'Medical Competence, Anatomy and the Polity in Seventeenth-Century Rome', *Renaissance Studies*, 21/4 (2007), 79–95.

—— 'Medical Competence, Anatomy and the Polity in Seventeenth-Century Rome', in Sandra Cavallo and David Gentilcore (eds.), *Spaces, Objects and Identities in Early Modern Italian Medicine* (Oxford, 2008), 79–95.

—— 'A Career in Manuscripts: Genres and Purposes of a Physician's Writing in Rome, 1600–1630', *Italian Studies*, 66/2 (2011), 234–48.

—— 'Tales from Cardinals' Deathbeds: Medical Hierarchy, Courtly Etiquette and Authority in the Counter Reformation', in Elisa Andretta and Marylin Nicoud (eds.), *Être médecin à la cour: Italie, France et Espagne, XIII–XVIII siècles* (Micrologus Library, 52; Florence, 2013).

Del Panta, Lorenzo, *Le epidemie nella storia demografica italiana (secoli XIV–XIX)* (Turin, 1980), 117–78.

Delumeau, Jean, *Vie économique et sociale de Rome dans la seconde moitié du XVIe siècle*, 2 vols. (Paris, 1957).

Dennis, Flora, 'Developing a Domestic Culture, 1400–1750', in Jeremy Aynsley and Charlotte Grant, with assistance from Harriet McKay (eds.), *Imagined Interiors: Representing the Domestic Interior Since the Renaissance* (London, 2006), 22–45.

—— 'Music', in Marta Ajmar-Wollheim and Flora Dennis (eds.), *At Home in Renaissance Italy* (London, 2006), 228–43.

—— 'Representing the Domestic Interior in Fifteenth- and Sixteenth-Century Italy: From the Birth of the Virgin to Palaces of Cheese', in Jeremy Aynsley and Charlotte Grant (eds.), *Imagined Interiors: Representing the Domestic Interior Since the Renaissance* (London, 2006), 22–45.

Dixon, Thomas, *From Passions to Emotions: The Creation of a Secular Psychological Category* (Cambridge, 2003).

Domenichelli, Mario, *Cavaliere e gentiluomo: Saggio sulla cultura aristocratica in Europa (1513–1915)* (Rome, 2002).

Donati, Claudio, *L'idea di nobiltà in Italia, secosli 14–18* (Rome, 1988).

Donato, Maria Pia, *Morti improvvise: Medicina e religione nel settecento* (Rome, 2010).

—— and Kraye, Jill (eds.), *Conflicting Duties: Science, Medicine and Religion in Rome 1550–1750* (London, 2003).

Duden, Barbara, *The Woman Beneath the Skin: A Doctor's Patients in Eighteenth-Century Germany* (Cambridge, Mass., 1991).

Duranti, Tommaso, *Mai sotto Saturno: Girolamo Manfredi medico e astrologo* (Bologna, 2008).

Eamon, William, *Science and the Secrets of Nature: Books of Secrets in Medieval and Early Modern Culture* (Princeton, 1994).

—— 'The Scientific Renaissance', in Guido Ruggiero (ed.), *A Companion to the Worlds of the Renaissance* (Oxford, 2002), 403–24.

—— 'Markets, Piazzas and Villages', in Lorraine Daston and Katharine Park (eds.), *Cambridge History of Science*, iii. *Early Modern Science* (Cambridge, 2006), 206–23.

Earle, Rebecca, ' "If You Eat Their Food . . .": Diets and Bodies in Early Colonial Spanish America', *American Historical Review*, 115/3 (2010), 688–713.

Ehrlich, Tracy L., *Landscape and Identity in Early Modern Rome: Villa Culture at Frascati in the Borghese Era* (Cambridge, 2002).

English, Eleanor B., 'Physical Education Principles of Selected Italian Humanists of the Quattrocento and Cinquecento: Exposition and Comparison with Modern Principles' (State University of New York at Buffalo, PhD thesis, 1978).

Faccioli, Emilio, 'La cucina dal Platina allo Scappi', in Ezio Riondato (ed.), *Trattati scientifici nel Veneto fra il XV e XVI secolo* (Vicenza, 1985), 135–46.

Fantoni, Marcello, Matthew, Louisa C., and Matthews Grieco, Sara F. (eds.), *The Art Market in Italy, 15th–17th Centuries* (Modena, 2003).

Findlen, Paula, 'Natural History', in Katherine Park and Lorraine Daston (eds.), *The Cambridge History of Science*, iii. *Early Modern Science* (Cambridge, 2006), 435–68.

Fissell, Mary, 'Readers, Texts and Contexts: Vernacular Medical Works in Early Modern England', in Roy Porter (ed.), *The Popularization of Medicine 1650–1850* (London, New York, 1992), 72–96.

—— 'The Marketplace of Print', in Mark S. R. Jenner and Patrick Wallis (eds.), *Medicine and the Market in England and Its Colonies, c.1450–c.1850* (Basingstoke, 2007), 108–32.

—— 'Introduction: Women, Health and Healing in Early Modern Europe', *Bulletin of the History of Medicine*, 82/1 (2008), 1–17.

—— 'Popular Medical Writing', in Joad Raymond (ed.), *Cheap Print in Britain and Ireland* (Oxford, 2011), 417–30.

Flandrin, Jean-Louis, 'Introduction: The Early Modern Period', in Jean-Louis Flandrin and Massimo Montanari (eds.), *Food: A Culinary History from Antiquity to the Present* (New York, 1999), 349–73.

Flandrin, Jean-Louis, 'From Dietetics to Gastronomy: The Liberation of the Gourmet', in Jean-Louis Flandrin and Massimo Montanari (eds.), *Food: A Culinary History from Antiquity to the Present* (New York, 1999), 418–32.

Forrest, Beth Marie, and Najjaj, April L., 'Is Sipping Sin Breaking Fast? The Catholic Chocolate Controversy and the Changing World of Early Modern Spain', *Food and Foodways*, 15 (2007), 31–52.

Fortini-Brown, Patricia, 'The Venetian *Casa*', in Marta Ajmar-Wollheim and Flora Dennis (eds.), *At Home in Renaissance Italy* (London, 2006), 50–65.

Fragnito, Gigliola, 'La trattatistica cinque e seicentesca sulla corte cardinalizia', *Annali dell'Istituto storico italo-germanico in Trento*, 18 (1991), 135–85.

Friedman, Reuben, *The Story of Scabies* (New York, 1947).

Frigo, Daniela, *Il padre di famiglia: Governo della casa e governo civile nella tradizione della 'economica' tra cinque e seicento* (Rome, 1985).

Frommel, Christopher L., 'Abitare nei palazzetti romani del primo cinquecento', in Aurora Scotti Tosini (ed.), *Aspetti dell'abitare in Italia tra XV e XVI secolo: Distribuzione, funzioni, impianti* (Milan, 2001), 23–38.

—— 'Galleria e loggia: Radici e interpretazione italiana della gallerie francese', in Christina Strunck and Elisabeth Kieven (eds.), *Europaische Galeriebauten: Galleries in a Comparative European Perspective 1400–1800, Römische Studien der Bibliotheca Hertziana 29* (Munich, 2011), 89–103.

Fumerton, Patricia, and Hunt, Simon (eds.), *Renaissance Culture and the Everyday* (Philadelphia, 1999).

Gage, Frances, 'Exercise for Mind and Body: Giulio Mancini, Collecting and the Beholding of Landscape Painting in the Seventeenth Century', *Renaissance Quarterly*, 61 (2008), 1167–1207.

Gallo, Marzia, 'Le livree', in *Farsi portare in carega: Portantine e livree per la nobiltà genovese* (Genoa, 1995), 75–85.

García Ballester, L., 'On the Origins of the "Six Non-Natural Things" in Galen', in García Ballester, *Galen and Galenism* (Aldershot, 2002), 105–15.

Gentilcore, David, *Healers and Healing in Early Modern Italy* (Manchester, 1998).

—— *Medical Charlatanism in Early Modern Italy* (Oxford, 2006).

—— *Pomodoro: A History of the Tomato in Italy* (New York: Columbia University Press, 2010).

—— 'The *Levitico*, or How to Feed a Hundred Jesuits', *Food and History*, 8/1 (2010), 87–120.

Gil-Sotres, Pedro, 'The Regimens of Health', in Mirko D. Grmek (ed.), *Western Medical Thought from Antiquity to the Middle Ages* (Cambridge, Mass., 1998), 291–396.

Girard, Alain, 'Du manuscrit à l'imprimé: Le Livre de cuisine en Europe aux 15e et 16e siècles', in Jean Claude Margolin and Robert Sauzet (eds.), *Pratiques et discours alimentaires à la Renaissance: Actes du colloque de Tours 1979* (Paris, 1982), 107–17.

Gnoli, Domenico, 'Gli orti letterari nella Roma di Leon X', in Gnoli, *La Roma di Leon X: Quadri e studi originali* (Milan, 1938), 13–163.

Goldthwaite, Richard A., *Wealth and the Demand for Art in Italy, 1300–1600* (Baltimore, 1993).

Gouk, Penelope, 'Music, Melancholy, and Medical Spirits in Early Modern Thought', in Peregrine Horden (ed.), *Music as Medicine: The History of Music Therapy Since Antiquity* (Aldershot, 2000), 175–94.

—— 'Raising Spirits and Restoring Souls: Early Modern Medical Explanations for Music's Effects', in Veit Erlman (ed.), *Hearing Cultures: Essays on Sound, Listening and Modernity* (Aldershot, 2005), 87–105.

Gowland, Angus, *The Worlds of Renaissance Melancholy: Robert Burton in Context* (Cambridge and New York, 2006).

Gozzadini, Giovanni, *Dell'origine e dell'uso dei cocchi e di due veronesi* (Bologna, 1864).

Grendler, Paul, *Schooling in Renaissance Italy: Literacy and Learning 1300–1600* (Baltimore, 1989).

—— 'Form and Function in Italian Renaissance Popular Books', *Renaissance Quarterly*, 46 (1993), 451–85.

—— 'Fencing, Playing Ball, and Dancing in Italian Renaissance Universities', in John McClelland and Brian Merrilees (eds.), *Sport and Culture in Early Modern Europe / Le Sport et la civilisation de l'Europe pré-moderne* (Toronto, 2010), 295–319.

Grieco, Allen J., 'The Social Politics of Pre-Linnean Botanical Classification', *I Tatti Studies: Essays in the Renaissance*, 4 (1991), 131–49.

—— 'La gastronomia del XVI secolo: Tra scienza e cultura', in Allen J. Grieco and Gianpiero Nigro (eds.), *Et coquatur ponendo: Cultura della cucina e della tavola in europa tra medioevo ed età moderna* (Prato, 1996), 143–67.

—— 'Food and Social Classes in Late Medieval and Renaissance Italy', in Jean-Louis Flandrin and Massimo Montanari (eds.), *Food: A Culinary History from Antiquity to the Present* (New York, 1999), 302–12.

—— 'From Roosters to Cocks: Italian Renaissance Fowl and Sexuality', in Sara F. Matthews-Grieco (ed.), *Erotic Cultures of Renaissance Italy* (Farnham, 2010), 89–140.

Groebner, Valentin, '*Complexio*/Complexion: Categorizing Individual Natures, 1250–1600', in Lorraine Daston and Fernando Vidal (eds.), *The Moral Authority of Nature* (Chicago, 2004).

Guidi, Giuseppe, *Ragguaglio delle monete, dei pesi, e delle misure attualmente in uso negli stati italiani e nelle principali piazze commerciali d'Europa* (Florence, 1855).

Hamling, Tara, and Richardson, Catherine (eds.), *Everyday Objects: Medieval and Early Modern Material Culture and Its Meanings* (Farnham and Burlington, Vt., 2010).

Hanke, Stephanie, 'Bathing *all'antica*: Bathrooms in Genoese Villas and Palaces in the Sixteenth Century', *Renaissance Studies*, 20/3 (2006), 674–700.

Hardingham, Glenn J., 'The *Regimen* in Late Medieval England' (University of Cambridge, PhD thesis, 2005).

Harkness, Deborah E., 'A View from the Streets: Women and Medical Work in Elizabethan London', *Bulletin of the History of Medicine*, 82/1 (2008), 52–85.

Harris, Neil, 'The History of the Book in Italy', in Michael F. Suarez, SJ and Henry R. Woodhuysen (eds.), *The Oxford Companion to the Book*, 2 vols. (Oxford, 2010), i. 257–69.

Harvey, Karen, *History and Material Culture* (London and New York, 2009).

Hill Cotton, J., 'Benedetto Reguardati: Author of Ugo Benzi's *Tractato de la conservatione de la sanitade*', *Medical History*, 12 (1968), 175–89.

Hohti, Paula, 'Conspicuous Consumption and Popular Consumers: Material Culture and Social Status in Sixteenth-Century Siena', *Renaissance Studies*, 24/5 (2010), 654–70.

Horden, Peregrine, 'Commentary on Part I', in Pergrine Horden (ed.), *Music as Medicine: The History of Music Therapy since Antiquity* (Aldershot, 2000), 44–5.

—— 'Commentary on Part II', in Peregrine Horden (ed.), *Music as Medicine: The History of Music Therapy since Antiquity* (Aldershot, 2000), 103–7.

Horrocks, Thomas A., 'Rules, Remedies and Regimens: Health Advice in Early American Almanacs', in Charles E. Rosemberg (ed.), *Right Living: An Anglo American Tradition of Self-Help Medicine* (Baltimore, 2003), 112–46.

Huetz de Lemps, Alain, 'Colonial Beverages and the Consumption of Sugar', in Jean-Louis Flandrin and Massimo Montanari (eds.), *Food: A Culinary History from Antiquity to the Present* (New York, 1999), 383–93.

Israel, Uwe, and Ortalli, Gherardo (eds.), *Il duello fra Medioevo ed età moderna: Prospettive storico-culturali* (Rome, 2009).

Jackson, Mark (ed.), *Health and the Modern Home* (London, 2007).

Jacquart, Danielle, 'Cœur ou cerveau? Les Hésitations médiévales sur l'origine de la sensation et le choix de Turisanus', *Micrologus*, 11 (2003), 73–96.

—— and Micheau, Françoise (eds.), *La Médecine arabe et l'Occident médiéval* (Paris, 1990).

Janelle, Pierre, *The Catholic Reformation* (Milwaukee, 1948).

Jardine, Lisa, *Worldly Goods: A New History of the Renaissance* (Basingstoke, 1996).

Jeanneret, Michel, 'Ma salade et ma muse', in Tomothy J. Tomasik and Julian M. Vitullo (eds.), *At the Table: Metaphorical and Material Cultures of Food in Medieval and Early Modern Europe* (Turnhout, 2007), 211–20.

Jenner, Mark and Wallis, Patrick, 'Introduction', in Mark S. R. Jenner and Patrick Wallis (eds.), *Medicine and the Market in England and Its Colonies, c.1450–c.1850* (New York and Basingstoke, 2007), 1–23.

Jewson, Nicholas D., 'Medical Knowledge and the Patronage System in 18th-Century England', *Sociology*, 8 (1974), 369–85.

Kamen, Henry, 'Climate and Crisis in the Mediterranean', in Wolfgang Behringer, Hartmut Lehmann, and Christian Pfister (eds.), *Cultural Consequences of The 'Little Ice Age'* (Göttingen, 2005), 369–76.

Koslofsky, Craig, *Evening's Empire: A History of the Night in Early Modern Europe* (Cambridge, 2011).

Krautheimer, Richard, 'Roma verde nel Seicento', in *Studi in onore di Giulio Carlo Argan II* (Rome, 1984), 71–82.

Kraye, Jill, 'Moral Philosophy', in C. B. Schmitt (gen. ed.), Q. Skinner and E. Kessler (eds.), and J. Kraye (assoc. ed.), *The Cambridge History of Renaissance Philosophy* (Cambridge, 1988), 303–86.

—— 'Philologists and Philosophers', in Jill Kraye (ed.), *The Cambridge Companion to Renaissance Humanism* (Cambridge, 1996), 142–60.

—— 'The Revival of Hellenistic Philosophies', in J. Hankins (ed.), *The Cambridge Companion to Renaissance Philosophy* (Cambridge, 2007), 97–112.

Kruft, Hanno-Walter, *A History of Architectural Theory from Vitruvius to the Present*, trans. Ronald Taylor, Elsie Callander, and Antony Wood (London and New York, 1994).

Kunzle, David, *The Early Comic Strip: Narrative Strips and Picture Stories in the European Broadsheet from c1450 to 1825* (Berkeley, 1973).

Kuriyama, Shigehisa, 'The Forgotten Fear of Excrements', *Journal of Medieval and Early Modern Studies*, 38/3 (2008), 413–42.

Lallouette, Anne-Laure, 'Bains et soins du corps dans les textes médicaux (XII–XIV siècles)', in Sophie Albert (ed.), *Laver, monder, blanchir: Discours et usages de la toilette dans l'Occident medieval* (Paris, 2005), 33–49.

Lane, Joan, ' "The doctor scolds me": The Diaries and Correspondence of Patients in Eighteenth-Century England', in Roy Porter (ed.), *Patients and Practitioners: Lay Perceptions of Medicine and Pre-industrial Society* (Cambridge, 1985), 205–48.

Laughran, Michelle, 'Oltre la pelle: I cosmetici e il loro uso', in Manlio Belfanti and Fabio Giusberti (eds.), *La moda* (*Storia d'Italia annali 9*; Turin, 2003), 43–82.

—— and Vianello, Andrea, '*Grandissima gratia*: The Power of Italian Renaissance Shoes as Intimate Wear', in Bella Mirabella (ed.), *Ornamentalism: Accessories in the Renaissance* (Ann Arbor, 2011), 253–89.

Laurioux, Bruno, *Gastronomie, humanisme et société à Rome au milieu du XVe siècle: Autour du* De honesta voluptate *de Platina* (Florence, 2006).

Lazzaro, Claudia, *The Italian Renaissance Garden* (New Haven and London, 1998).

Le Bain et le miroir: Soins du corps et cosmétiques de l'Antiquité à la Renaissance (Paris, 2009).

Leong, Elaine, 'Making Medicines in the Early Modern Household', *Bulletin of the History of Medicine*, 82/1 (2008), 145–68.

—— and Pennell, Sara, 'Recipe Collection and the Currency of Medical Knowledge in the Early Modern Medical Marketplace', in Mark S. R. Jenner and Patrick Wallis (eds.), *Medicine and the Market in England and Its Colonies, c.1450–c.1850* (New York and Basingstoke, 2007), 133–52.

—— and Rankin, Alisha, 'Introduction: Secrets and Knowledge', in Leong and Rankin (eds.), *Secrets and Knowledge in Medicine and Science, 1500–1800* (Farnham, 2011), 1–20.

Levi-Pisetzki, Rosita, *Storia del costume in Italia*, 5 vols. (Milan, 1964), vol. iii.

Lillie, Amanda, *Florentine Villas in the Fifteenth Century: An Architectural and Social History* (New York, 2005).

—— *The Florentine Villa* (Cambridge, 2005).

Lindow, James, *The Renaissance Palace in Florence: Magnificence and Splendour in Fifteenth-Century Italy* (Aldershot, 2007).

Lockwood, Dean P., *Ugo Benzi, Medieval Philosopher and Physician 1376–1439* (Chicago, 1951).

Lotz, Wolfang, 'Gli 883 cocchi della Roma del 1594', *Archivio romano della Società reale di storia patria*, 23 (1973), 247–66.

Loughman, John, 'Between Reality and Artful Fiction: The Representation of the Domestic Interior in Seventeenth-Century Dutch Art', in Jeremy Aynsley and Charlotte Grant with assistance from Harriet McKay (eds.), *Imagined Interiors: Representing the Domestic Interior Since the Renaissance* (London, 2006), 72–97.

Ludke Finney, Gretchen, 'Music, Mirth, and Galenic Tradition in England', in J. A. Mazzeo (ed.), *Reason and the Imagination: Studies in the History of Ideas 1600–1800* (New York and London, 1962), 143–54.

MacDougall, Elizabeth (ed.), *Fons sapientiae: Renaissance Garden Fountains* (Washington DC, 1978).

—— 'L'ingegnoso artifizio', in Elizabeth MacDougall (ed.), *Fons sapientiae: Renaissance Garden Fountains* (Washington DC, 1978), 85–114.

McGeary, Thomas, 'Harpischord Decoration: A Reflection of Renaissance Ideas about Music', *Explorations in Renaissance Culture*, 6 (1980), 1–27.

McIver, Katherine, *Women, Art, and Architecture in Northern Italy, 1520–1580: Negotiating Power* (Aldershot, 2006).

Maclean, Ian, 'Girolamo Cardano: The Last Years of a Polymath', *Renaissance Studies*, 21/5 (2007), 587–607.

—— 'The Diffusion of Learned Medicine in the Sixteenth Century Through the Printed Book' in Ian Maclean, *Learning and the Market Place: Essays in the History of the Early Modern Book* (Leiden and Boston, 2009), 59–86.

McNeil, P., and Riello, G., 'The Art and Science of Walking: Gender, Space, and the Fashionable Body in the Long Eighteenth Century', *Fashion Theory*, 9/2 (2005), 175–204.

McVaugh, Michael R., *Medicine Before the Plague: Practitioners and Their Patients in the Crown of Aragon, 1285–1345* (Cambridge, 1993).

Madignier, Mirabelle, 'Sociabilité informelle et pratiques sociales en Italie: Les Salons romains et florentins au XVIIIème siècle' (European University Institute, PhD thesis, 1999).

Malacarne, Giancarlo, *Sulla mensa del principe: Alimentazione e banchetti alla corte dei Gonzaga* (Modena, 2000).

Mantese, Giovanni, *I mille libri che si vendevano e leggevano a Vicenza alla fine del secolo sedicesimo* (Vicenza, 1968).

Marangoni, Barbara, 'Un medico portoghese nello studio di Pisa–Rodrigo Fonseca', in *Toscana e Portogallo: Miscellanea storica nel 650° anniversario dello Studio generale di Pisa* (Pisa, 1994), 209–15.

Massimo, Vittorio, *Notizie istoriche della Villa Massimo* (Rome, 1836).

Matthews Grieco, Sara F., 'Pedagogical Prints: Moralizing Broadsheets and Wayward Women in Counter Reformation Italy', in Geraldine A. Johnson and Sara F. Matthews Grieco (eds.), *Picturing Women in Renaissance and Baroque Italy* (Cambridge, 1997): 61–88.

Melli, Piera (ed.), *La città ritrovata: Archeologia urbana a Genova 1984–1994* (Genoa, 1996).

Mikkeli, Heikki, *Hygiene in the Early Modern Medical Tradition* (Helsinki, 1999).

Milani, Marisa, 'La fortuna della *Vita sobria* nel mondo anglosassone', *Cultura neolatina*, 40 (1980), 333–56.

—— (ed.), *Scritti sulla vita sobria: Elogio e lettere* (Venice, 1983).

—— 'La tradizione italiana del *secretum secretorum*', *La parola e il testo*, 5 (2001), 209–53.

Miller, Daniel, *Materiality* (Durham, NC and London, 2005).

Morris, Edwin T., *A History of Aromatics* (New York, 1984).

Musacchio, Jacqueline, *Art, Marriage, and Family in the Florentine Renaissance Palace* (New Haven and London, 2008).

Nada-Patrone, Anna Maria, 'I giochi di palla nel Piemonte nel tardo medioevo', in Andrea Merlotti (ed.), *Giochi di palla nel Piemonte medievale e moderno* (Rocca de'Baldi: Museo storico-etnografico A. Doro, 2001), 43–76.

Napoleone, Caterina (ed.), *Villa Madama, Raphael's Dream* (Turin, London, Venice, and New York, 2007).

Neppi, Lionello, *Palazzo Spada* (Rome, 1975).

Niccoli, Ottavia, 'Creanza e disciplina: Buone maniere per i fanciulli nell'Italia della Controriforma', in Paolo Prodi (ed.), *Disciplina dell'anima, disciplina del corpo e disciplina della società tra medioevo ed età moderna* (Bologna, 1994), 929–63.

—— *Il seme della violenza: Putti, fanciulli e mammoli in Italia tra cinque e seicento* (Roma, 1995).

Nicoud, Marilyn, ' "Che manza fichi semina rogna": Problèmes d'identification d'une dermatose au Moyen Âge', *Médiévales*, 26 (1994), 85–101.

—— 'L'Expérience de la maladie et l'échange épistolaire: Les Derniers Moments de Bianca Maria Visconti', *Mélanges de l'École française de Rome*, 116/2 (2000), 85–101.

—— 'Les Pratiques diététiques à la cour de Francesco Sforza', in Bruno Laurioux and Laurence Moulinier-Brogi (eds.), *Scrivere il medioevo: Lo spazio, la santità, il cibo: Un libro dedicato a Odile Redon* (Rome, 2001), 393–404.

—— 'Les Médecins Italiens et le bain thermal', *Médiévales*, 43 (2002), 13–40.

—— *Les Régimes de santé au Moyen Âge: Naissance et diffusion d'une écriture médicale (XIIIe–XVe siècle)* (Rome, 2007).

—— 'Il *Regimen sanitatis salernitanum*: Premessa ad un'edizione critica', in Danielle Jacquart and Agostino Paravicini-Bagliani (eds.), *La scuola medica salernitana, gli autori e i testi* (Florence, 2007), 365–84.

—— 'Formes et enjeux d'une médicalisation médiévale: Réflexions sur les cités italiennes (XIIIe–XVe siècles', *Genèses*, 82 (2011), 7–30.

—— 'Les Savoirs diététiques, entre contraintes médicales et plaisirs aristocratiques', *Micrologus*, 16. *I saperi nelle corti/Knowledge at the Courts* (2008), 233–55.

Nordera, Marina, 'La donna in ballo: Danza e genere nella prima età moderna' (European University Institute, PhD thesis, 2001).

Norris, Rebecca, 'Women on the Edge: The Saletta delle Dame of the Palazzo Salvadego in Brescia', in Deborah Howard and Laura Moretti (eds.), *The Music Room in Early Modern France and Italy: Sound, Space, and Object* (Oxford, 2012), 115–34.

Nuovo, Angela, *Il commercio librario nell'Italia del Rinascimento* (2nd edn., Milan, 2003).

—— ' "Et amicorum": Costruzione e circolazione del sapere nelle biblioteche private del Cinquecento', in Rosa M. Borraccini and Roberto Rusconi (eds.), *Libri, biblioteche e cultura degli ordini regolari nell'Italia moderna attraverso la documentazione della congregazione dell'Indice* (Vatican City, 2006), 106–11.

—— and Sandal, Ennio, *Il libro nell'Italia del Rinascimento* (Brescia, 1998).

Nutton, Vivian, 'Hippocrates in the Renaissance', *Sudhoffs Arch Z Wissenschaftsgesch Beih.*, 27 (1989), 420–39.

—— 'Les Exercices et la santé: Hieronymus Mercurialis et la gymnastique médicale', in Jean Céard, Marie-Madeleine Fontaine, and Jean Claude Margolin (eds.), *Le Corps à la Renaissance: Actes du XXX colloque de Tours 1987* (Paris, 1990), 295–308.

O'Hara May, J., 'Food or Medicine? A Study of the Relationship Between Foodstuffs and *materia medica* from the Sixteenth to the Nineteenth Century', *Transactions of the British Society for the History of Pharmacy*, 1 (1971), 61–97.

O'Malley, Michelle, and Welch, Evelyn, *The Material Renaissance* (Manchester and New York, 2005).

Omodeo, Anna, *Bottiglie e bicchieri nel costume italiano* (Milan, 1970).

Pacifici, Vincenzo, *Ippolito II d'Este, cardinale di Ferrara* (Tivoli, 1920).

Pagliara, Pier Nicola, 'Destri e cucine nell'abitazione del XV e XVI secolo, in specie a Roma', in A. Scotti Tosini (ed.), *Aspetti dell'abitare in Italia tra XV e XVI secolo: Distribuzione, funzioni, impianti* (Milan, 2001), 39–91.

Palmer, Richard, 'Pharmacy in the Republic of Venice in the Sixteenth Century', in Andrew Wear, Richard K. French, and Iain M. Lonie (eds.), *The Medical Renaissance of the Sixteenth Century* (Cambridge, 1985), 100–18.

—— ' "In this our lightye and learned tyme": Italian Baths in the Era of the Renaissance', *Medical History*, 34/S10 (1990), 14–22.

—— 'Medicine at the Papal Court in the Sixteenth Century', in Vivian Nutton (ed.), *Medicine at the Courts of Europe, 1500–1837* (London, 1990), 49–78.

—— 'Health, Hygiene and Longevity in Medieval and Renaissance Europe', *History of Hygiene: Proceedings of the 12th International Symposium on the Comparative History of Medicine* (Tokyo, 1991), 75–98.

—— 'Girolamo Mercuriale and the Plague in Venice', in Alessandro Arcangeli and Vivian Nutton (eds.), *Girolamo Mercuriale: Medicina e cultura nell'Europa del cinquecento* (Florence, 2008), 51–65.

Paniagua, J. A., '*El regimen sanitatis ad regem Aragonorum* y otres presuntos regimens arnaldiana', in *Studia Arnaldiana: Trabajos en torno a la obra medica de Arnau de Vilanova s.1240—1311* (Barcelona, 1995), 335–84.

Park, Katherine, 'The Organic Soul', in C. B. Schmitt (gen. ed.), Q. Skinner and E. Kessler (eds.), and J. Kraye (assoc. ed.), *The Cambridge History of Renaissance Philosophy* (Cambridge, 1988), 464–84.

Pediconi, Angelica, 'The Art and Culture of Bathing in Renaissance Rome' (MA dissertation, Royal College of Art, 2002–3).

Pennell, Sara, 'Mundane Materiality, or, Should Small Things Still be Forgotten?: Material Culture, Micro-Histories and the Problem of Scale', in Karen Harvey (ed.), *History and Material Culture* (London and New York, 2009), 173–91.

Pennuto, Concetta, 'La natura dei contagi in Fracastoro', in Alessandro Pastore and E. Peruzzi (eds.), *Girolamo Fracastoro: Fra medicina, filosofia e scienze della natura* (Florence, 2006), 57–71.

Penny, Nicholas, 'Introduction: Toothpicks and Green Hangings', *Renaissance Studies*, 19/5 (2005), 581–90.

Perini, Leandro, 'Libri e lettori nella toscana del cinquecento', in *Firenze e la Toscana dei Medici nell'Europa del '500*, i. *Strumenti e veicoli della cultura* (Florence, 1983), 577–92.

Petrucci, Armando, 'Alle origini del libro moderno: Libri da banco, libri da bisaccia, libri da mano', *Italia medievale e umanistica*, 12 (1969), 295–313.

Pfister, Christian, 'Weeping in the Snow: The Second Period of Little Ice Age-Type Impacts, 1570–1630', in Wolfgang Behringer, Hartmut Lehmann, and Christian Pfister (eds.), *Kulturelle Konsequenzen der 'Kleinen Eiszeit'/Cultural Consequences of the 'Little Ice Age'* (Göttingen, 2005), 31–86.

Piscitello, Patrizia, 'Serviti da cioccolata: L'Evoluzione della tazza dalla jicara alla termbluse', in Luisa Ambrosio (ed.), *Cio'bi: Quando cioccolato e birra diventano arte: Catalogue of an exhibition held at Museo Duca di Martina, Naples* (Naples, 2011), 20–81.

Pollock, Linda, *With Faith and Physic: The Life of a Tudor Gentlewoman, Lady Grace Mildmay, 1552–1620* (New York, 1993).

Pomata, Gianna, *Contracting a Cure: Patients, Healers and the Law in Early Modern Bologna* (Baltimore, 1998).

—— 'Editor's Introduction', in Oliva Sabuco de Nantes Barrera, *The True Medicine*, ed. and trans. G. Pomata (Toronto, 2010), 1–84.

Porter, Roy, 'The Patient's View: Doing Medical History from Below', *Theory and Society*, 14 (1985), 175–98.

Porzio, Francesco, 'Aspetti e problemi della scena di genere in Italia', in Francesco Porzio (ed.), *Da Caravaggio a Ceruti: La Scena di genere e l'immagine dei pitocchi nella pittura Italiana* (Milan, 1998), 17–41.

Pretty, Jules N., et al., 'Health Values from Ecosystems', in *The UK National Ecosystem Assessment Technical Report: UK National Ecosystem Assessment* (Cambridge: UNEP–WCMC, 2011), 1154–81, <http://uknea.unep-wcmc.org> (accessed 10 October 2012).

Preyer, Brenda, 'The Florentine *casa*', in Marta Ajmar-Wollheim and Flora Dennis (eds.), *At Home in Renaissance Italy* (London, 2006), 34–48.

Price Zimmermann, T.C., 'Renaissance Symposia', in Sergio Bertelli and Gloria Ramakus (eds.), *Essays Presented to Myron P Gilmore*, 2 vols. (Florence, 1978), i. 363–74.

Prinz, Wolfram, *Galleria: Storia e tipologia di uno spazio architettonico* (Modena, 1988).

Quiviger, Francois, *Seeing and Looking in the Renaissance* (Valencia, 2004).

Quondam, Amedeo, 'L'accademia', in Giulio Einaudi (ed.), *Letteratura italiana*, i. *Il letterato e le istituzioni*, ed. Alberto Asor Rosa (Turin, 1982), 842–58.

—— 'Elogio del gentiluomo', in Amedeo Quondam and Giorgio Patrizi (eds.), *Educare il corpo, educare la parola nella trattatistica del Rinascimento* (Rome, 1998), 11–21.

—— and Patrizi, Giorgio (eds.), *Educare il corpo, educare la parola nella trattatistica del Rinascimento* (Rome, 1998).

Rankin, Alisha, 'Becoming an Expert Practitioner: Court Experimentalism and the Medical Skills of Anna of Saxony (1532–1585)', *Isis: Journal of the History of Science Society*, 98 (2007), 23–53.

Ranum, Orest, 'The Refuges of Intimacy', in Philippe Ariès and George Duby (eds.), *A History of Private Life*, iii. *Passions of the Renaissance*, ed. Roger Chartier, trans. Arthur Goldhammer (Cambridge, Mass., 1989), 210–29.

Rather, L. J., 'The "Six Things Non-Natural": A Note on the Origins and Fate of a Doctrine and a Phrase', *Clio Medica*, 3 (1968), 337–47.

Rawcliffe, Carole, ' "Delectable Sightes and Fragrant Smelles": Gardens and Health in Late Medieval and Early Modern England', *Garden History*, 36/1 (2008), 1–21.

—— 'The Concept of Health in Late Medieval Society', in *Le interazioni fra economia e ambiente biologico nell'Europa preindustriale secc. XIII–XVIII* (Florence, 2010), 321–38.

Redon, Odile, and Laurioux, Bruno, 'Histoire de l'alimentation entre Moyen Âge et temps modernes', in Odile Redon et al. (eds.), *Le Désir et le goût* (Paris, 2003), 53–98.

Retford, Kate, 'Thomas Bardwell's The Broke and Bowes Families (1740)', *Cultural and Social History*, 7/4 (2010), 493–509.

Rhodes, Dennis A., *La vita e le opere di Castore Durante e della sua famiglia* (Viterbo, 1968).

Richards, Jennifer, 'Useful Books: Reading Vernacular Regimens in Early Modern England', *Journal of the History of Ideas*, 73/2 (2012), 247–71.

Richardson, Brian, *Printing, Writers and Readers in Renaissance Italy* (Cambridge, 1999).

Riebesell, Christina, 'Sulla genesi delle gallerie di antichità nell'Italia del Cinquecento', in Christina Strunck and Elisabeth Kieven (eds.), *Europaische Galeriebauten: Galleries in a Comparative European Perspective 1400–1800* (Römische Studien der Bibliotheca Hertziana 29; Munich, 2011), 197–217.

Riello, Giorgio, *A Foot in the Past: Consumers, Producers and Footwear in the Long Eighteenth Century* (Oxford, 2006).

Rocca, Julius, *Galen on the Brain: Anatomical Knowledge and Physiological Speculation in the Second Century AD* (Leiden, Boston, 2003).

Roche, Daniel, *A History of Everyday Things: The Birth of Consumption in France 1600–1800* (Cambridge, 2000).

Roggero, Marina, 'L'Alphabétisation en Italie: Une conquête féminine', *Annales histoire, sciences sociales*, 55 (2001), 903–26.

Romano, Dennis, *Housecraft and Statecraft: Domestic Service in Renaissance Venice 1400–1600* (Baltimore, 1996).

Roodenburg, Herman, *The Eloquence of the Body: Perspectives on Gesture in the Dutch Republic* (Zwolle, 2004).

Rosenfeld, M. N., *Sebastiano Serlio on Domestic Architecture: The Sixteenth-Century Manuscript of Book VI in the Avery Library of Columbia University* (Cambridge, Mass. and London, 1978).

Rosignoli, Guia, *Cuoi d'oro, corami da tappezzeria, paliotti e cuscini del Museo Stefano Bardini* (Florence, 2009).

Rowland, Ingrid, *The Culture of the High Renaissance: Ancients and Moderns in Sixteenth-Century Rome* (Cambridge, 1998).

Rozzo, Ugo (ed.), *Biblioteche italiane del cinquecento tra riforma e Contro Riforma* (Udine, 1994).

Ruberg, Willemijn, 'The Letter as Medicine: Health and Illness in Dutch Daily Correspondence 1770–1850', *Social History of Medicine*, 23/3 (2010), 492–508.

Russell, Susan, 'Girolamo Mercuriale's *De arte gymnastica* and papal health at the Villa Pamphilij, Rome', in Alessandro Arcangeli and Vivian Nutton (eds.), *Girolamo Mercuriale: Medicina e cultura nell'Europa del cinquecento* (Florence, 2008), 175–89.

Sarti, Raffaella, *Vita di casa: Abitare, mangiare, vestire nell'Europa moderna* (Rome and Bari, 2000).

—— *Europe at Home: Family and Material Culture 1500–1800* (New Haven, 2002).

Schmidt, Jeremy, *Melancholy and Care of the Soul: Religion, Moral Philosophy and Madness in Early Modern England* (Farnham, 2007).

Schmidt, Sandra, 'Trois dialogues de l'exercise de sauter, et voltiger en l'air: Strategies of Ennoblement of a Bodily Practice in the Sixteenth Century', in John McClelland and Brian Merrilees (eds.), *Sport and Culture in Early Modern Europe* (Toronto, 2010), 377–89.

Scotoni, Lando, 'Raccolta e commercio della neve nel Circondario delle 60 miglia (Lazio)', *Rivista geografica italiana*, 79 (1972), 60–70.

Sears, Elizabeth, *The Ages of Man: Medieval Interpretations of the Life Cycle* (Princeton, 1986).

Semmelhack, Elizabeth, *On a Pedestal: From Renaissance Chopines to Baroque Heels* (Toronto, 2009).

Sherman, William, *Used Books: Marking Readers in Renaissance England* (Philadelphia, 2008).

Sinclair, Sir John, Bart., *The Code of Health and Longevity*, 4 vols. (Edinburgh, 1807).

Siraisi, Nancy, 'The Changing Fortunes of a Traditional Text: Goals and Strategies in Sixteenth-Century Latin Editions of the *Canon* of Avicenna', in Andrew Wear, Robert K. French, and I. M. Lonie (eds.), *The Medical Renaissance of the Sixteenth Century* (Cambridge, 1985), 16–41.

—— *Avicenna in Renaissance Italy: The Canon and Medical Teaching in Italian Universities after 1500* (Princeton, 1987).

—— *The Clock and the Mirror: Girolamo Cardano and Renaissance Medicine* (Princeton, 1997).

—— '*Historiae*, Natural History, Roman Antiquity, and Some Roman Physicians', in Gianna Pomata and Nancy Siriaisi (eds.), *Historia: Empiricism and Erudition in Early Modern Europe* (Cambridge, Mass., 2005), 325–54.

—— *History, Medicine and the Traditions of Renaissance Learning* (Ann Arbor, 2007).

Slack, Paul, 'Mirrors of Health and Treasures of Poor Men: The Uses of the Vernacular Medical Literature of Tudor England', in Charles Webster (ed.), *Health, Medicine and Mortality in the Sixteenth Century* (Cambridge, 1979), 237–73.

Smith, Virginia, *Clean: A History of Personal Hygiene and Purity* (Oxford, 2007).

Soler, Sebastià, *Arnau de Villanova en la imprenta renaixentista, segle XVI* (Manresa, 2002).

Spagnuolo, Vita Vera, 'Gli atti notarili dell'Archivio di Stato di Roma saggio di spoglio sistematico: L'anno 1590', in B. Antolini, A. Morelli, and V. Spagnuolo (eds.), *La musica a Roma attraverso le fonti d'archivio* (Lucca, 1994), 19–65.

Stiaffini, Daniela, 'I reperti della lavorazione del vetro', in Francesco Redi (ed.), *L'arte vetraia a Pisa: Dallo scavo di una vetreria rinascimentale* (Pisa, 1984), 69–95.

Stolberg, Michael, 'Sweat, Learned Concepts and Popular Perceptions, 1500–1800', in Manfred Horstmansoff, Helen King, and Claus Zittel (eds.), *Blood, Sweat and Tears: The Changing Concepts of Physiology from Antiquity into Early Modern Europe* (Leiden, 2012), 503–21.

—— *Experiencing Illness and The Sick Body In Early Modern Europe* (Palgrave Macmillan, 2011).

Storey, Tessa, *Carnal Commerce in Counter-Reformation Rome* (Cambridge, 2008).

—— 'Face, Waters, Oils, Love Magic and Poison: Making and Selling Secrets in Early Modern Rome', in Elaine Leong and Alisha Rankin (eds.), *Secrets and Knowledge in Medicine* (Aldershot, 2011), 143–63.

—— 'Italian Books of Secrets Database: Study Documentation', <https://lra.le.ac.uk/handle/2381/4335> (accessed 10 October 2012).

Swan, Claudia, 'From Blowfish to Flower Still-life Paintings: Classification and Its Images Circa 1600', in Pamela Smith and Paula Findlen (eds.), *Merchants and Marvels: Commerce, Science and Art in Early Modern Europe* (New York, 2002), 109–36.

Tabarrini, Marisa, *Borromini e gli Spada: Un palazzo e la committenza di una grande famiglia nella Roma barocca* (Rome, 2008).

Thomas, Keith, *The Ends of Life: Roads to Fulfilment in Early Modern England* (Oxford, 2009).

Thornton, Peter, *The Italian Renaissance Interior 1400–1600* (London, 1991).

Tlusty, Ann, *The Martial Ethic in Early Modern Germany: Civic Duty and the Right of Arms* (Basingstoke, 2011).

Toscani, Xenio, 'Catechesi e catechismi come fattore di alfabetizzazione', *Annali di storia dell'educazione*, 1 (1994), 17–36.

Tozzi, Simonetta, and Margiotta, Anita, 'Falda, Giovanni Battista', in *Dizionario biografico degli italiani*, xliv (1994); online at: <http://www.treccani.it/enciclopedia/ricerca/Falda,-G-B/Dizionario_Biografico/> (accessed 10 October 2012).

Ulmann, Jacques, *De la gymnastique aux sports modernes: Histoire des doctrines de l'éducation physique* (Paris, 1965).

Vanasse, Claudie, 'Le Jeûne dans le débats confessionnels au XVIe siècle', in Marie Viallon-Schoneveld (ed.), *Le Boire et le manger au XVIe siècle* (Saint-Étienne, 2004), 237–52.

Verrier, Frédérique, *Les Armes de Minerve: L'Humanisme militaire dans l'Italie du XVIe siècle* (Paris, 1997).

Vicini, Maria Lucrezia, *Il collezionismo del cardinale Fabrizio Spada in Palazzo Spada* (Rome, 2008).

Vigarello, Georges, *Le Propre et le sale: L'Hygiène du corps depuis le Moyen Âge* (Paris, 1985).

—— *Concepts of Cleanliness: Changing Attitudes in France Since the Middle Ages* (Cambridge, 1988).

—— 'S'exercer, jouer', in Alain Corbin et al. (eds.), *Histoire du corps*, i. *De la Renaissance aux Lumières* (Paris, 2005), 235–302.

Visceglia, Maria Antonietta, and Fosi, Irene, 'Marriage and Politics at the Papal Court in the Sixteenth and Seventeenth Centuries', in Trevor Dean and Kate J. P. Lowe (eds.), *Marriage in Italy 1300–1650* (Cambridge, 2002), 197–224.

Vogel, Klaus A., 'Cosmography', in Lorraine Daston and Katharine Park (eds.), *Cambridge History of Science*, iii. *Early Modern Science* (Cambridge, 2006), 469–85.

Volpi Rosselli, Giuliana, 'I portoghesi nell'Ateneo Pisano in epoca medicea (1543–1737)', in *Toscana e Portogallo: Miscellanea storica nel 650° anniversario dello Studio Generale di Pisa* (Pisa, 1994), 117–32.

von Tippelskirch, Xenia, *Letture femminili in Italia nella prima età moderna* (Rome, 2011).

Waddy, Patricia, *Seventeenth-Century Roman Palaces: Use and the Art of the Plan* (Cambridge, Mass. and London, 1990).

Wear, Andrew, 'The History of Personal Hygiene', in William F. Bynum and Roy Porter (eds.), *Companion Encyclopedia of the History of Medicine*, 2 vols. (London, 1993), ii. 1283–308.

—— *Knowledge and Practice in English Medicine, 1550–1680* (Cambridge, 2000).

—— 'Place, Health, and Disease: The Airs, Waters, Places Tradition in Early Modern England and North America', *Journal of Medieval and Early Modern Studies*, 38 (2008), 443–65.

Wear, Andrew, Kathleen, and d'Amico, John F. (eds.), *The Renaissance Cardinal's Ideal Palace: A Chapter from Cortesi's* De Cardinalatu (Rome, 1980).

Welch, Evelyn, *Shopping in the Renaissance: Consumer Cultures in Italy, 1400–1600* (New Haven and London, 2005).

—— 'Perfumed Buttons and Scented Gloves: Smelling Things in Renaissance Italy,' in Bella Mirabella (ed.), *Ornamentalism: Accessories in the Renaissance* (Ann Arbor, 2011), 13–39.

Wentworth Rinne, Katherine, *The Waters of Rome: Aqueducts, Fountains, and the Birth of the Baroque City* (New Haven and London, 2010).

Witte, Arnold A., *The Artful Hermitage: The Palazzetto Farnese as a Counter-Reformation Diaeta* (Rome, 2008).

Zarri, Gabriella (ed.), *Per lettera*: *La scrittura epistolare femminile tra archivio e tipografia secoli XV–XVII* (Rome, 1999).

Zarzoso, Alfonso, 'Mediating Medicine Through Private Letters: The Eighteenth-Century Catalan Medical World', in Willhem DeBlecourt and Cornelie Usborne (eds.), *Cultural Approaches to the History of Medicine* (Basingstoke, 2004), 108–26.

Zirpolo, Lilian H., 'Climbing the Social, Political, and Financial Ladders: The Rise of the Sacchetti in Seventeenth-Century Rome', *Seventeenth Century*, 12/2 (1997), 151–71.

Picture Acknowledgements

We thank the following copyright holders for permission to use the following illustrations:

Archivio di Stato di Roma (Figs., 3.4, 3.15, 6.4); Arti Doria Pamphilj s.r.l. (Plate 11; Fig. 3.6a-b); Biblioteca Alessandrina, Rome (Fig. 7.8); Biblioteca Comunale dell'Archiginnasio Bologna (Figs. 3.9, 7.1, 8.7, 8.8); Biblioteca Nazionale Universitaria di Torino (Figs. 1.5, 1.6); Biblioteca Universitaria Bologna (Figs. 1.1, 5.2, 5.3); Cambridge University Library (Figs 1.3, 1.4, 1.7, 1.8, 6.3); Civica Raccolta delle Stampe Achille Bertarelli, Milan (Figs. 3.5, 8.2); Civiche Raccolte d'Arte Applicata, Milan (Plate 8); Devonshire Collection, Chatsworth (Fig. 4.2); Fondazione Querini-Stampalia, Venice (Plate 14); Foto Studio Rapuzzi, Brescia (Plate 19); Galleria Colonna, Rome (Plate 20); Kunst und Gewerbe, Hamburg (Fig. 3.1); Ministero per i Beni e le Attività Culturali (Fig. 3.8); Matthiesen Gallery, London (Plate 23); Museo Bagatti Valsecchi, Milan (Fig. 3.7, 3.14); Musei Civici Fiorentini, Florence (Plates 9, 10, 12); Museo del Tessuto, Prato (Fig. 8.3); Museo di Roma, Rome (Plate 16; Fig. 5.7); Museo Stibbert, Florence (Fig. 5.1); Museum Thyssen-Bornemisza, Madrid (Plate 22); Rare Book & Manuscript Library of the University of Illinois at Urbana-Champaign (Fig. 5.4); Soprintendenza per i Beni Architettonici, Paesaggistici, Storici, Artistici ed Etnoantropologici di Arezzo (Plate 7); Soprintendenza Speciale per il Patrimonio Storico, Artistico ed Etnoantropologico e per il Polo Museale della Città di Firenze (Figs. 3.12, 4.4 7.5, 8.4); Soprintendenza Speciale per il Patrimonio Storico, Artistico ed Etnoantropologico e per il Polo Museale della Città di Roma (Plate 1, 2, 3, 4, 5, 6, 17, 21; Fig. 2.2); Stadlisches Kunstinstitut, Frankfurt (Plate 15); Tagliaferri, collezione privata (Fig. 7.2, 7.3, 7.7); Victoria and Albert Museum, London (Plate 18; Figs. 3.10, 3.11, 3.13, 4.1, 4.3, 5.5, 5.6, 5.8, 6.5, 7.6, 7.9, 7.10, 8.1, 8.5, 8.6); Warburg Institute, London (Figs. 3.2, 3.3); Wellcome Library, London (Figs. 6.1, 6.2, 7.4; Plate 13); <www.openlibrary.org/> (Fig. 1.2).

Index